AIDS and Malignancies

Πάσα επιστήμη χωριζομὲνη της δικαιοσὺνης και της άλλης αρετής, πανουργὶα, ου σοφὶα φαίνεται.

Πλάτων 4ος αιώνας π.χ.

Every field of knowledge that is divorced from justice and the other virtues is evil rather than wisdom.

Plato, 4th century BC

AIDS and Malignancies

Current Concepts and Perspectives

Edited by

Basil C. Golematis

Athens Medical School, Hippokration Hospital, Athens, Greece and

Vincent T. DeVita Jr

Yale Cancer Center, Yale University School of Medicine, New Haven, USA

Associate Editors

Konstantinos N. Syrigos

Royal Postgraduate Medical School, Hammersmith Hospital, London, UK

Manousos M. Konstantoulakis

Hippokration Hospital, Athens, Greece

JOHN WILEY & SONS

Chichester · New York · Brisbane · Toronto · Singapore

Baffins Lane, Chichester,
West Sussex PO19 1UD, England

National 01243 779777
International (+44) 1243 779777
e-mail (for orders and customer service enquiries): cs-book@wiley.co.uk
Visit our Home Page on http://www.wiley.co.uk
or http://www.wiley.com

Other Wiley Editorial Offices

John Wiley & Sons, Inc., 605 Third Avenue,
New York, NY 10158-0012, USA

Jacaranda Wiley Ltd, 33 Park Road, Milton,
Queensland 4064, Australia

John Wiley & Sons (Canada) Ltd, 22 Worcester Road,
Rexdale, Ontario M9W 1L1, Canada

John Wiley & Sons (Asia) Pte Ltd, 2 Clementi Loop #02-01,
Jin Xing Distripark, Singapore 129809

Library of Congress Cataloging-in-Publication Data

AIDS and malignancies : current concepts and perspectives / edited by
Basil C. Golematis and Vincent T. DeVita Jr. ; associate editors,
Konstantinos N. Syrigos and Manousos M. Konstantoulakis
p. cm.
Includes bibliographical references and index.
ISBN 0-471-96714-9 (hbk. : alk. paper)
1. Cancer—Etiology. 2. AIDS (Disease—Complications.
I. Golematis, Basil C. II. DeVita, Vincent T.
[DNLM : 1. Acquired Immunodeficiency Syndrome—complications.
2. Neoplasms—etiology. WC 503.5 A287 1996]
RC268.48.A33 1996
616. 99'4071—dc20
DNLM/DLC
for Library of Congress 96–2979
CIP

British Library Cataloguing in Publication Data

A catalogue record for this book is available from the British Library

ISBN 0-471-96714–9

Typeset in 10/12 Palatino by Vision Typesetting, Manchester
Printed and bound in Great Britain by Biddles Ltd, Guildford and King's Lynn
This book is printed on acid-free paper responsibly manufactured from sustainable forestation, for which at least two trees are planted for each one used for paper production.

Contents

Contributors

Clay J. Cockerell MD Dermatology Laboratories, University of Texas Southwestern Medical Center, Dallas, Texas, USA

Sandra Colombini MD Laboratory of Tumor Cell Biology, National Cancer Institute, National Institutes of Health, Bethesda, Maryland, USA

Vincent T. DeVita Jr MD Professor of Medicine, Epidemiology and Public Health, Director, Yale Cancer Center, Yale University School of Medicine, New Haven, Connecticut, USA

Agamemmon A. Epenetos PhD, FRCP(Lond), FRCP(Glasg) Consultant in Medical Oncology, Professor in Developmental Cancer Therapeutics and Director of Research and Development, Department of Clinical Oncology, Royal Postgraduate Medical School, Hammersmith Hospital, London, UK

Alvin E. Friedman-Kien MD Professor of Dermatology and Microbiology, New York University Medical Center, New York, USA

Robert C. Gallo MD Institute of Human Virology, Medical Biotechnology Center, University of Maryland Biotechnology Institute, University of Maryland at Baltimore, Baltimore, Maryland, USA

Basil C. Golematis FACS Professor and Chairman, 1st Department of Propaedeutic Surgery, Athens Medical School, Hippokration Hospital, Athens, Greece

Jaap Goudsmit MD Professor of Medical Microbiology, Human Retrovirus Laboratory, Academic Medical Centre, University of Amsterdam, Amsterdam, The Netherlands

Kevin J. Harrington FRCS Clinical Research Fellow, Department of Clinical Oncology, Royal Postgraduate Medical School, Hammersmith Hospital, London, UK

Barton F. Haynes MD Frederic M. Hanes Professor of Medicine, Director, Duke University Arthritis Center, Durham, North Carolina, USA

Phyllis J. Kanki DVM, SD Associate Professor of Pathobiology, Harvard AIDS Institute, Harvard School of Public Health, Boston, Massachusetts, USA

Efi Kokkotou MD Research Fellow, Harvard AIDS Institute, Harvard School of Public Health, Boston, Massachusetts, USA

Manousos M. Konstantoulakis MD 1st Department of Propaedeutic Surgery, Athens Medical School, Hippokration Hospital, Athens, Greece

Mathios Konstantoulakis MD, PhD Associate Professor, Athens Medical Centre, Athens, Greece

Jill Lacy MD Associate Professor, Yale University School of Medicine, New Haven, Connecticut, USA

Christine A. Lee MA, MD, FRCP, FRCPath Professor and Director, The Haemophilia Centre, Royal Free Hospital, London, UK

John M. Luce MD Professor of Medicine, Director of the Intensive Care Unit, University of California, San Francisco General Hospital, San Francisco, California, USA

Kenneth H. Mayer MD Chief, Division of Infectious Diseases, Memorial Hospital of Rhode Island, Professor of Medicine and Community Health, Brown University School of Medicine, and Director, Brown University AIDS Program, Brown, Rhode Island, USA

David Mitchell MA, MD, FRCP Consultant in Respiratory Medicine, St Mary's Hospital, London, UK

Theodoros D. Mountokalakis MD Professor of Medicine, Director, 3rd Department of Medicine, Athens Medical School, Sotiria Hospital, Athens, Greece

George N. Pavlakis MD, PhD Head, Human Retrovirus Section, ABL–Basic Research Program, National Cancer Institute–FCRDC, Frederick, Maryland, USA

Panayiotis P. Peveretos MD Professor of Surgery, Athens Medical School, Hippokration Hospital, Athens, Greece

Konstantinos N. Syrigos MD Department of Clinical Oncology, Royal Postgraduate Medical School, Hammersmith Hospital, London, UK

Marc Allan Tack DO Division of Infectious Diseases, Brown University School of Medicine, Brown, Rhode Island, USA

Robert M. Wachter MD Assistant Professor of Medicine and Epidemiology, Director of Housestaff Education, Director of the Intensive Care Unit, San Francisco General Hospital, San Francisco, California, USA

Preface

Over a decade has now elapsed since the acquired immunodeficiency syndrome (AIDS) was first recognized as a separate disease and it is understood that more than 40% of all patients with AIDS will develop a malignant disease at some time during the course of their human immunodeficiency virus (HIV) infection. Furthermore, with the improved survival of patients with AIDS, owing to the better prevention and treatment of infectious complications, there may be an increase in AIDS-related malignancies. Therefore oncologists, surgeons and specialists involved in the treatment of patients with AIDS are expected in the near future to converge more often in this significant, though neglected field.

In the present volume we cover extensively the area of HIV-associated malignancies based on the experience of well-established scientists, emphasizing new developments in clinical and basic research. The authorship consists primarily of those who have made major contributions in the area they have been asked to discuss. Efforts have been made to cover important advances in the field with emphasis on the clinical applications. The authors have attempted to combine their clinical experience with the newest advances in the relevant sciences and to highlight the therapeutic aspects of each topic. The rationale for this policy is the perception that physicians who are acquainted with basis sciences and can use them in the evaluation and treatment of a patient are in a better position to analyse clinical problems and to help their patient. Therefore a portion of this volume is dedicated to the biology and pathogenesis of HIV, presented in an easy-to-understand way. In addition, a few chapters of this book deal with problems that are indirectly related to AIDS-associated neoplasms and we include them in order to offer to the reader a more complete and comprehensive framework of the problems raised in an HIV-infected patient when he or she develops a malignancy. Finally, as HIV infection provides an interesting model for the study of malignancies developed on the ground of immunosuppression, this issue is also discussed in this volume.

In conclusion, the objective of the preparation of this volume was to provide a single, comprehensive source of information on the discipline of

AIDS-related malignancies and to furnish a platform for further investigation towards a better understanding of these two diseases.

The editors are indebted to the authors for their expert contributions. They are also grateful to the publishers John Wiley & Sons Ltd for the commitment and especially to Mr Michael Osuch, Medical Editorial Assistant, and Dr Lewis N. Derrick, Senior Production Editor, for their untiring efforts in assembling this volume. Finally, they extend their gratitude to their patients, students and colleagues for providing them with ongoing education, stimulus and purpose.

Konstantinos Nikolaou Syrigos MD

1
Introduction

Vincent T. DeVita Jr
Yale University School of Medicine, New Haven, Connecticut, USA

Acquired immunodeficiency syndrome (AIDS) is the syphilis of our generation. It seems to mimic all diseases and there are links between AIDS and most illnesses. This book is about cancer and AIDS, and there is indeed a strong link between them. As we approach a book that examines this link it provides us the opportunity to reflect a bit about the impact and significance of this epidemic and all it has wrought, and its enduring relationship to cancer and cancer research.

The major message of the AIDS epidemic is that there are agents out there in the world that, given the proper circumstances, have the potential to wreak havoc with humans. They can 'slip their leash', so to speak, and catch the world by surprise. The AIDS epidemic has reminded us of the need to be ready for these possibilities. Were we ready for this epidemic? In fact, despite frequent protestations to the contrary, we were more ready than most people realize. Even though there is plenty of gloom surrounding the epidemic today, it is important to note that there is no other example in the history of medicine where a disease like AIDS has been described, its natural history defined, its etiology discovered, and the etiological agent characterized in so short a time.

There are some valuable perspectives to be gleaned from the first efforts to understand and control AIDS that can appropriately serve as a prelude to this text. Cancer, of course, was irrevocably linked to the AIDS epidemic from the start when the first cases were identified with Kaposi's sarcoma in Los Angeles, California, USA, in 1981. Discovery of other cancers associated with AIDS followed, most notably lymphocytic lymphomas, and these joined other complications of AIDS as the 'AIDS-defining illnesses'. Then it also became apparent that even when cancer is not a defining illness, cancer that develops in the context of AIDS often is unusual and difficult to manage.

AIDS and Malignancies: Current Concepts and Perspectives.
Edited by B.C. Golematis and V.T. DeVita Jr

These observations confirmed the adverse effects of immunosuppression on both the etiology and aggressiveness of cancer that had been observed in clinical circumstances where immunosuppression was part of treatment, such as in marrow and solid organ transplants. All of this is covered elegantly in this unusual text.

Although over 400 000 cases of human immunodeficiency virus (HIV) infection has been diagnosed in the USA alone by the end of 1994, and 60% have been fatal, this is a mere fraction of the cases that are diagnosed and die of cancer each year in our country. So why the fuss? The fuss is because the statistics are overshadowed by the nature of epidemics in general; they are acutely frightening, especially when they deal with something as central to our existence as human sexuality. Even in the current political turmoil over the appropriate role of government in our private lives most would agree that when the health of the public is threatened, especially by an epidemic as vicious as the AIDS epidemic, the government has an indispensable role to play. It can marshal considerably more resources than any private organization.

We were fortunate we had a model to fall back on at the beginning of the epidemic and this was the second strong link between cancer and AIDS, the US National Cancer Program (NCP) and the AIDS research effort. The NCP itself has been a unique and controversial concept. It served not only as a model for building the entire AIDS research effort as it exists today but also donated many of its building blocks to jump-start the fledgling research program in AIDS. The first money for AIDS research at the National Institutes of Health came from a redirection of money from the National Cancer Institute (NCI) budget, in part by asking Dr Robert Gallo, co-author of the following chapter in this text, to redirect a portion of his laboratory's efforts to the study of this disease. He actually did so reluctantly. Retroviruses had been of interest to cancer researchers for some time, but since the dogma among infectious disease people at the time was that retroviruses did not cause human infectious diseases, most work in retrovirology was conducted in, or supported by, the NCI, and Gallo's lab was a major resource.

The results are now history. When Gallo offered his several strains of viruses to the NCI three years later, what was needed the most was a reliable diagnostic test to help identify those who were infected so we could define the disease and its mode of spread. Speed was essential. The identification of the virus and a supportive cell line, as well as a facility at the NCI's Frederick Cancer Research and Development Center to scale up viral production, allowed the NCI to prepare over 500 liters of viral-infected cells. The press conference that announced the discovery of the virus was a tool to advertise the availability of this resource to industry, and open a competition to contract for the development of a diagnostic test. Because there was so much starting material it took, including Food and Drug Administration (FDA) approval, only nine months to market a test, still a marvel of cooperation between the private and public sector. The rapid availability of a reliable and readily available diagnostic test saved innumerable lives and in many ways made books like this one possible, by giving us the tools to carefully define the natural history of the disease. This remains one of the unsung achievements of the early partnership between cancer and AIDS research.

A related dogma was that viruses could not be eradicated by drugs and so there was no existing research effort of any size to screen for antiviral drugs in the infectious disease community, and none at the US National Institutes of Health. While this same argument had been raised in the case of cancer, it had been overcome by some courageous pioneers at the NCI who gave birth to the NCI's controversial, but now successful, drug development program. Lo and behold, a drug that had initially been designed to be an anticancer drug, and screened in NCI's drug development program, was pulled off the shelf and became the first available treatment tool for patients with AIDS. It was rapidly processed by the NCI and approved by the FDA in 18 months. Because of this success, money was requested and granted to start a parallel program for a drug development program for antiviral agents. While the drugs now available to treat HIV infection are crude, their targets are not, and they are getting sharper every day. Never have we had such precise information on a disease and its causative agent without making significant progress in its treatment. I doubt that AIDS will be an exception.

But how to test new agents? Staff from NCI and the National Institute of Allergy and Infectious Diseases set up a Cooperative Group Program for large-scale AIDS trials modeled after NCI's effort that had been made possible by the resources supplied by the National Cancer Act (NCA). Prior to the creation of the NCP by the NCA in 1971, no resources of any substance were allocated for this type of research. Eventually the program that evolved was separated from NCI, along with the staff to run it, and it has been a major venue for testing anti-AIDS drugs. In fact, it is out of these large studies that we have culled much of the information that has allowed us to characterize the natural history of the disease and the relationship of cancer to AIDS and other complications.

Even the model of the development of infectious diseases in the immunocompromised host had its precedent in the intensively treated cancer patient. *Pneumocystis carinii* pneumonia in adults had first been reported and successfully treated with pentamidine isethionate, and the dosage, schedules, and pharmacokinetics of pentamidine worked out in cancer patients, which was the reason the Center for Disease Control had pentamidine isethionate on hand to respond to the need suddenly presented by homosexual men with AIDS and pneumocystis pneumonia.

A book devoted to cancer and AIDS suggests to me that we have reached an important milestone in this disease. It is a sign of the maturity of the AIDS epidemic that cancer as a defining illness for the diagnosis of AIDS, and AIDS as a complication of the management of non-defining cancers, should be the subject of an entire text. Books like this are, in essence, a coda to the first act of an evolving drama. And the outlines of the remaining acts are clear enough to be composed with some confidence. We know too much about AIDS not to see an ending to this story that may be happier than most expect.

Another lesson is, of course, that it could happen again; it may already have. And like the defense against military aggression, the defense of a nation against threats to the health of its citizens should be imperative to its government. We always will need our own medical smart bombs and cruise missiles on standby.

Cancer in many ways is a larger and much more mature epidemic than AIDS. While it took too long to establish an organized effort to attack it, once it was in place the US NCP, established 25 years ago, provided an excellent model of how to approach these kinds of public health threats. It has been an enormous scientific success and it has been a beacon to the efforts to provide resources to attach problems of importance to the public health without impinging on the freedom of scientists to pursue ideas. Money can't buy ideas, it was said when the NCA was passed. True, but it can put many good scientists to work on a specific problem and they have proven they can generate great ideas. Partly because of the monies supplied by the US NCP, we had a substantial armamentarium of ideas at our disposal at the beginning of the AIDS epidemic.

2

Retroviruses and their Role in Oncogenesis

Sandra Colombini* and Robert C. Gallo†

*National Cancer Institute, National Institutes of Health, Bethesda, Maryland, USA;

†Medical Biotechnology Center, University of Maryland Biotechnology Institute, Baltimore, Maryland, USA

Hematopoietic disorders like leukemia, lymphomas, anemia, and immunodeficiency are widely distributed in the animal world. They not only occur in mammals, but also in birds, fish, and reptiles.

In many cases where the etiology of these diseases, as they naturally occur, is well understood, the primary event is infection with a retrovirus. Retroviruses are enveloped viruses that contain their genetic information in RNA form; to achieve a permanent infection in the host cells the RNA molecules need to be transcribed into DNA by the viral polymerase called reverse transcriptase and the DNA integrated in the host genome. From here, viral progeny can be established that can infect other cells (horizontal transmission). Alternatively, the viral genome can be passively replicated at each cell division (vertical transmission).

Because retroviruses need cells to replicate it is reasonable to hypothesize that they originate from cellular genes. In fact, genetic structures resembling known retroviruses can be found in all mammals. These structures have different degrees of completion and sometimes they can generate retrovirus-like particles and because of these properties they have been called endogenous retroviruses. Endogenous retroviruses are currently believed to have originated from transposing or mobile genetic elements that, like the viral long terminal repeats (LTR), contain repetitive sequences, two of which can enclose genetic elements sufficient for the replication of nucleic acid. It is also believed that retroviruses may play a role in evolution by promoting

AIDS and Malignancies: Current Concepts and Perspectives.
Edited by B.C. Golematis and V.T. DeVita Jr

transfer or amplification of genetic material. Following a random genetic event an infectious retrovirus can be generated which can enter a new species with profound pathological consequences.

Retroviruses were first isolated at the beginning of the century from chicken leukemias by Ellerman and Bang[1] and sarcomas by Rous[2]. Rous actually provided the first demonstration of an oncogenic retrovirus by transmitting disease with filtered cell culture supernatant. Many avian retroviruses have since been described and are all genetically related to each other. The spectrum of diseases that they induce include lymphomas, myeloblastosis, erythroblastosis, and osteopetrosis. Most of them owe their acute oncogenic properties to the acquisition of a cellular gene by genetic recombination; the gene (protooncogene) uncoupled from its cellular regulatory elements and under the control of the viral promoter can directly transform cells. The result is an acutely transforming virus which transforms all infected cells in a polyclonal manner. Rous sarcoma virus (RSV) is of this type.

This transformation mechanism is rare in nature because by acquiring an oncogene the same essential viral information is usually lost and the virus becomes unable to replicate (RSV is an exception). Another important step in the field was achieved by Ludwik Gross, who in the early 1950s demonstrated the viral etiology of leukemia in some inbred strains of laboratory mice[3]. Following his work, Jarrett in Glasgow was able to prove that the causative agent of the naturally occurring feline leukemia in outbred domestic cats was indeed a retrovirus, feline leukemia virus (FeLV)[4]. This was the first demonstration of a retrovirus operating in a natural setting and whose pathogenetic process seems quite different from the previously described ones. In fact, FeLV virus induces disease only after a long incubation period and not in all infected animals, thus behaving like the later discovered bovine leukemia virus (BLV) and finally human T-cell leukemia/lymphotropic virus type I (HTLV-I). The mechanism of transformation by FeLV involves, in some cases, the transduction of an oncogene, but there is also evidence of insertional mutagenesis, a mechanism first described in chicken leukemia, in which transformation is the product of the viral integration in the vicinity of a protooncogene which leads to its dysregulation[5].

These transformation mechanisms involved abundant viral replication which made them readily detectable with the technology available at that time. For this reason (even if a retroviral origin was suspected for a long time because of the clustering of the disease within herds) BLV was not discovered until the late 1960s, when the leukemic lymphocytes could be successfully cultured[6].

In fact, BLV does not replicate or express viral protein *in vivo*, but it does when the leukemic cells are cultured. The discovery that marked a turning point in retroviral research was the one made by Temin and Baltimore in 1970. They determined that the viral RNA genome was reverse transcribed into DNA by the viral polymerase then named reverse transcriptase[7,8].

Because reverse transcriptase is ubiquitous to all retroviruses, from that moment a new retrovirus could be detected by an enzymatic assay whose sensitivity was much higher than that of the techniques previously available. Because of the precedent of the retroviral etiology of many animal leukemias, there was great expectation that by the early 1970s, a comparable human retrovirus would be readily isolated. However, that turned out not to be the case for a number of reasons.

First, all the retroviral research was conducted on the assumption of high viral replication in leukemic cells like the one observed in the animal systems that we described previously. Second, as already mentioned for BLV, retroviruses can be in a latent state during the course of the disease and viral replication can be observed only when the proper target cells can be successfully grown in culture. Since the animal retroviruses could be grown in fibroblast it was wrongly assumed that these were the appropriate target cells. Therefore, despite many efforts, only suggestive evidence could be gathered for the existence of a human retrovirus. These include the detection of apparently exogenous DNA in some human leukemias by Baxt and Spiegelman[9] and the sporadic detection of cell-associated reverse transcriptase-like activity by various laboratories, including our own[10,11].

Coming to the conclusion that it would be necessary to be able to grow the infected cells (hematopoietic cells) in order to isolate a human retrovirus, our laboratory intensified the effort in the direction of isolating a specific growth factor for T-cells and in 1976 successfully accomplished the task of isolation and characterization of T-cell growth factor (interleukin 2 (IL-2)) from media of phytohemagglutinin-stimulated peripheral blood cells[12]. The availability of these two important tools, reverse transcriptase and IL-2, finally led to the isolation of HTLV-I from several cases of cutaneous T-cell lymphomas[13–15] and its clear association with human disease led to the inclusion of retroviruses among human pathogens[16,17].

HTLV-I is the cause of both a hematopoietic malignancy called adult T-cell leukemia/lymphoma (ATLL) and a progressive myelopathy called tropical spastic paraparesis/HTLV-I-associated myelopathy (TSP/HAM)[18,19]. It displays the same characteristic of chronic and acute animal classes of retroviruses[20] (for a recent review see ref.21). In the same way that chronic retroviruses induce T-cell leukemia after a long latency period (20–30 years), it does not integrate in the proximity of an oncogene and the virus seems to be latent in leukemic cells. Like acutely transforming animal retroviruses it can transform *in vitro* T-cells. HTLV-I infection is endemic in some Asian and African countries, as well as in Central America and the Caribbean islands. In the few areas of the USA where it is endemic, it is found mainly in individuals of African–American background. HTLV-I is transmitted sexually, by breast milk and by blood products. Epidemiological evidence suggests that ATLL develops mainly in people infected at birth, indicating that the time of onset of viral infection may be important for the development of the leukemia. ATLL is a mature leukemia/lymphoma most often of $CD4^-$ phenotype and occurs in a very small percentage (2–5%) of HTLV-I infected people in approximately 20–30 years from the time of infection. Clinically, it is an aggressive, rapidly lethal disease whose features include the appearance in the blood of morphologically unique, flower-like T-cells with lobulated nucleoli, extensive peripheral lymphadenopathy, hepatosplenomegaly without thymic enlargement, and frequent skin infiltration. Lytic bone lesions are often present despite the minimal bone marrow involvement. Hypercalcemia occurs in about 50% of patients and attempts to control calcium levels may dominate the acute clinical course. The mechanism underlining this clinical sign appears to be a paraneoplastic syndrome associated with the production of a parathyroid hormone-releasing hormone (PTH-RH)-like hormone.

In its classical presentation, ATLL is a rapidly progressive and usually fatal disease. Average survival beyond the acute episode is approximately six months. The diagnosis of ATLL includes at least four different subtypes: acute, chronic, lymphomatous and smoldering, depending on the extent of the disease. All the leukemia subtypes are characterized by the presence of HTLV-I proviral genome clonally integrated in the DNA of the leukemic T-cells. In fact, the appearance of prevalent T-cell clones carrying the HTLV-I genome in an infected individual is an unfavorable prognosis.

As mentioned before, the virus in the leukemic cells seems to be latent or defective, because expression of viral proteins is missing, suggesting that at the onset of the disease these proteins may not be necessary. If the HTLV-I pathogenetic mechanism and its oncogenicity are still unclear, far less clear is its mechanism in the TSP/HAM syndrome. It has been suggested that HTLV-I can lead to neurological disease by dysregulating cytokine production or by inducing autoimmune phenomena, but these speculations may only reflect the difficulty of demonstrating that HTLV-I can infect and replicate in the cells of the central nervous system.

Shortly after HTLV-I was isolated, HTLV-II was isolated from a patient with an unusual form of hairy T-cell leukemia[22], however, this virus still remains in search of a disease since later studies did not associate HTLV-II etiologically with this form of human leukemia.

In the early 1980s a new epidemic whose characteristics would suggest an infectious agent as a possible cause, acquired immunodeficiency syndrome (AIDS), was clustering with certain subgroups in the general population and it was transmitted with blood products and by sex. Several factors made a retrovirus an appealing candidate. First, it was a T-cell disease, and all human retroviruses to date were T-cell tropic; second, some animal retroviruses, especially FeLV, can cause immunosuppressive disorders; and third, the disease had a rather delayed onset following the presumptive transmission event. Using T-cell culture and reverse transcriptase assay, Barré-Sinoussi *et al.*[23] were able to identify a virus that was later proved to be the AIDS agent.

Subsequent identification of a permissive cell line that would allow viral replication but resist the virus lytic effect by Popovic *et al.*[24], the development of a blood test by Sarngadharan *et al.*[25,26], and frequent isolation of human immunodeficiency virus type 1 (HIV-1) from patients with AIDS by Gallo *et al.*[27] made it possible to characterize such a virus and prove that it was indeed the etiological agent for AIDS. This virus is now known as HIV-1. Using similar techniques, related viruses were identified in African monkeys[28] and in humans in western Africa[29].

The latter virus, called HIV-2, is still associated with an AIDS-like disease but is far less pathogenic than HIV-1. There are currently two groups of human retroviruses distantly related to each other: HTLV-I and HTLV-II belong to the oncornavirus family, and HIV-1 and HIV-2 to the lentivirus family. They share the ability to infect T-cells, but HIV-1 and HIV-2 utilize CD4 as a receptor; therefore, its tropism is restricted to T-helper cells and monocyte/macrophages. The receptor for HTLV-I and HTLV-II is not known but the virus is able to infect a broader spectrum of T-cells.

From the beginning of the AIDS epidemic it was clear that there was a striking association between AIDS disease and a rare tumor previously found mainly in Africa and in males of Mediterranean origin, Kaposi's sarcoma (KS). The epidemic KS (AIDS-KS, as this particular form of KS associated with AIDS is called) affects young individuals, mostly homosexual and bisexual men, and has an aggressive course, often resulting in multicentric lesions with involvement of lymph nodes and viscera. In addition to the AIDS-KS, three different forms of KS are known: the 'classical KS' which affects the skin of the lower extremities of elderly men of Mediterranean and eastern European origin; the 'endemic KS', more virulent than the classical form, is frequent among black males of equatorial Africa and can occur in females and children; and the 'iatrogenic KS', which arises in patients treated with immunosuppressive drugs, particularly recipients of grafts. All forms of KS are characterized by the same histopathology whose typical marks are growth of spindle-shaped cells and angiogenesis. In the early stage, lymphoreticular inflammatory cell infiltration and edema are also present. The iatrogenic KS can occasionally spontaneously regress. This observation, the absence of chromosomal abnormalities in most KS spindle cells, and the fact that early KS resembles a granulation tissue, suggested that KS may not be a real cancer, at least early in the disease. When in 1988 our laboratory succeeded in growing KS spindle cells in long-term culture[30], it was evident that these cells had a complex requirement for cytokines and growth factors to sustain their growth, among them being basic fibroblast growth factor (bFGF), IL-1, oncostatin M, vascular fibroblast growth factor and tumor necrosis factor, which play a crucial role[31]. These factors can be supplied by HIV-infected and HIV-activated mononuclear cells like the ones present in the KS lesions of AIDS patients. In addition, KS spindle cells themselves produce several growth factors suggesting the existence of autocrine and paracrine circuits in KS proliferation. One of these factors, bFGF, is a potent inducer of angiogenesis and it is believed to be partially responsible for the neovascular changes that are the histological signature of KS. Furthermore, the KS spindle cells, when inoculated in nude mice, cause a tumor of mouse origin near the inoculation site which regresses when the spindle cells die. The tumor resembles early KS with blood vessel proliferation, fibroblast, leukocyte infiltration, and spindle cells[32]. All these observations suggested that KS may be the product of cytokine dysregulation. Another interesting element was introduced with the work of Vogel *et al.*, who demonstrated that transgenic mice carrying the HIV transactivator *tat* gene developed lesions similar to human KS[33]. Around the same period, work in our laboratory demonstrated that the Tat protein, which is released by CD4-infected cells, is taken up by KS spindle cells and stimulates their proliferation[34]. In addition, Tat promotes the migration, invasion and adhesion of the same KS spindle cells through the intercellular matrix and cooperates with bFGF in inducing KS-like lesions in nude mice[35]. All this evidence suggested that Tat is one factor responsible for the increased frequency and aggressiveness of KS in the setting of HIV infection. Another is probably the increase in inflammatory cytokines that occurs after HIV infection. As mentioned before, different cell types participate in the KS lesion and whether the tumor is a true malignancy or a polyclonal hyperplasia has been the object of intense speculation. Most studies report that KS spindle cells have a normal karyotype and this, in addition to the fact that the lesion can regress spontaneously in some instances, has favored the notion that KS may not be a true malignancy as indicated above. Furthermore, KS spindle cells, believed to be of endothelial origin, depend on condition media from activated T-cells for their growth in culture, and the lesion they induce in the mice is transient and apparently depends on cytokines released by the injected human KS spindle cells. In 1995 Lunardi-Iskandar *et al.*, in our laboratory, was able to isolate the first malignant KS cell line from a pleural effusion of an AIDS-KS patient. This cell line, KS Y-1, is growth independent of exogenous growth factors, possess an abnormal karyotype and is capable of inducing malignant metastatic tumors in SCID mice[36]. A short while later we showed that KS Y-1 cells, as well as the hyperplastic spindle cells, are killed *in vitro* and *in vivo* by a pregnancy hormone, the β-chain of human chorionic gonadotropin (βhCG)[37]. The βhCG and the β-chain of the luteinizing hormone are 85% homologous. The luteinizing hormone is present cyclically at high levels in non-pregnant females, which could explain why KS affects woman less frequently then males.

This finding has therapeutic implications. KS affects 39% of HIV-1-infected homosexual/bisexual men and the incidence of KS in virtually all HIV-1-infected people is dramatically increased. Several epidemiological findings have suggested from the very beginning of the AIDS epidemic the possible involvement of an additional sexually transmitted infectious agent. Over the course of years many papers have identified this agent with cytomegalovirus, human papillomavirus 16 and others, but further investigations have not confirmed these claims. In 1994 Chang *et al.* utilizing a new technique, representation difference analysis (RDA), were able to detect DNA sequences that identified a new herpesvirus in 98% of the lesions of all forms of KS[38]. This finding, confirmed by laboratories all over the world, may then lead to an easy conclusion: that the new virus is the etiological agent of KS. The assumption is based on the fact that human herpesvirus 8 (HHV-8) sequences are present exclusively in the lesions and in the peripheral blood of KS patients and homosexuals at high risk for KS. The finding, quite unusual in the herpesvirus field (herpesviruses tend to be ubiquitous), has been challenged by numerous investigators. Among them are Peter Rady, who detected viral sequences in benign and malignant skin lesions of organ transplant patients[39], Paolo Monini, who did the same in the cellular component of sperm from normal donors and our laboratory, with the identification of HHV-8 in 15% of normal blood donors.

The true epidemiological prevalence of the virus is still unknown and will be solved only by the establishment of a serological test with sufficient virus (so far unavailable). In the meantime, KS neoplastic tests score negative for viral sequences[36]. Personal communications from various investigators indicate that the virus, although present when cells from a KS lesion are put in culture, is subsequently lost with cell passage. This is inconsistent with the direct transforming capability of the virus itself and suggests instead that HHV-8 needs the particular milieu of factors and cellular components present in the lesion to develop. HHV-8 does provide a link with the second most prevalent malignancy in HIV-1-infected people, B-cell lymphomas (BCL). In fact, HHV-8 has been found in a rare subset of BCL, body cavity-based BCL[40].

BCL became an AIDS-defining condition in 1985. At the present time 3% of AIDS cases have BCL as a first clinical manifestation. However, the incidence of BCL rises dramatically with the progression to AIDS. Some studies have shown that the frequency of BCL can reach 30% after three years of antiretroviral therapy (azidothymidine (AZT) and dideoxyinosine (ddI). Histologically, most of the AIDS-associated BCL cases are classified as high-grade immunoblastic lymphoma, but the non-cleaved Burkitt-like phenotype is also present in a minority of cases. Extranodal localizations, especially in the digestive tract and the brain, occur frequently. Like other non-Hodgkin's lymphomas arising from a background of immunosuppression, the initial lesions are often polyclonal, but later evolve into histological, phenotypic and clinically malignant high-grade monoclonal BCL with a very poor prognosis. We believe that the pathogenesis of these lymphomas is very similar to the one of Burkitt lymphoma in Africa. In both lymphomas,the key element is the association of concomitant immunostimulation and immunodeficiency. Chronic antigenic stimulation is provided in one case by multiple infections and HIV-1 itself, and in the other by holoendemic malaria that is clearly associated with the increase of this tumor in parts of Africa. Immunostimulation leads to a signal for B-cell activation and proliferation; B-cells may be more inclined to become neoplastic because of the 'plasticity' of their DNA, which undergoes constant rearrangement in the synthesis of the immunoglobulin. At the same time, cytotoxic T-cell function is impaired directly by HIV-1 and by plasmodium, so the built-in principal mechanism for immunological surveillance is missing. This constant expansion of the B-cell compartment is thought to increase the risk of disabling genetic events like the *c-myc* translocation that occurs in Burkitt lymphoma determining final malignant transformation.

REFERENCES

1. Ellerman V, Bang O. Experimentelle Keukamie bei Huhnern. *Centralbl Bakteriol* **1** (orig.) 1908; 46: 595–605.
2. Rous P. Transmission of a malignant new growth by means of a cell-free filtrate. *JAMA* 1911; 56: 198–204.
3. Gross L. 'Spontaneous' leukemia developing in C3H mice following inoculation in infancy with AK-leukemic extracts, or AK-embryos. *Proc Soc Exp Biol Med* 1951; 78: 27–39.
4. Jarrett W, Crawford E, Martin W, Davie F. Leukemia in the cat: a virus-like particle associated with leukaemia (lymphosarcoma). *Nature* 1964; 202: 567–568.
5. Hayward WS, Neel BG, Astrin SM. Induction of lymphocytic leukosis by avian leukosis virus: activation of a cellular 'onc' gene by promoter insertion. *Nature* 1981; 290: 475–479.
6. Miller J, Miller L, Olson C, Gillette K. Virus-like particles in phytohemagglutinin-stimulated lymphocyte cultures with reference to bovine lymphosarcoma. *J Natl Cancer Inst* 1969; 43: 1297–1301.
7. Temin H, Mizutani S. RNA-dependent DNA polymerase in virions of Rous sarcoma virus. *Nature* 1970; 226: 1211–1213.
8. Baltimore D, Viral RNA-dependent DNA polymerase. *Nature* 1970; 226: 1209–1211.
9. Baxt WG, Spiegelman S. Nuclear DNA sequences present in human leukemic cells and absent in normal leukocytes. *Proc Natl Acad Sci USA* 1973; 71: 1309–1313.
10. Goodenow RS, Kaplan HS. Characterization of the reverse transcriptase of a type C virus produced by a human lymphoma cell line. *Proc Natl Acad Sci USA* 1979; 76: 4971–4975.
11. Sarngadharan MG, Sarin PS, Reitz MS, Gall RC. Reverse transcriptase activity of human acute leukemic cells: purification of the enzyme, response to AMV 70S RNA, and characterization of the DNA product. *Nature New Biol* 1979; 240: 67–69.
12. Morgan DA, Ruscetti FW, Gallo RC. Selective in vitro growth of T-lymphocytes from normal human bone marrow. *Science* 1976; 193: 1007–1010.
13. Poiesz BJ, Ruscetti FW, Gazdar AF *et al.* Detection and isolation of type C retrovirus particles from fresh and cultured lymphocytes of a patient with cutaneous T-cell lymphoma. *Proc Natl Acad Sci USA* 1980; 77: 7415–7419.
14. Poiesz BJ, Ruscetti FW, Reitz MS *et al.* Isolation of a new type-C retrovirus (HTLV) in primary uncultured cells of a patient with Sezary T-cell leukaemia. *Nature* 1981; 294: 268–271.

15. Gallo RC, Mann DL, Broder S *et al.* Human T-cell leukemia–lymphoma virus (HTLV) is in T- but not B-lymphocytes from a patient with cutaneous T-cell lymphoma. *Proc Natl Acad Sci USA* 1982; 79: 4680–4684.
16. Hinuma Y, Nagata K, Hanaoka M *et al.* Adult T-cell leukemia: antigen in an ATL cell line and detection of antibodies to the antigen in human sera. *Proc Natl Acad Sci USA* 1981; 78: 6476–6480.
17. Robert-Guroff M, Nakao Y, Notake K *et al.* Natural antibodies to the human retrovirus, HTLV, in a cluster of Japanese patients with adult T-cell leukemia. *Science* 1987; 215: 975–978.
18. Gessain A, Barin F, Vernant JC *et al.* Antibodies to human T-lymphotropic virus type I in patients with tropical spastic paraparesis. *Lancet* 1986; ii: 407–410.
19. Osame M, Usuku K, Izumo S *et al.* HTLV-I associated myelopathy: a new clinical entity. *Lancet* 1986; i: 1031–1032.
20. Coffin JM. Structure and classification of retroviruses. In Levy A (ed.) *The Retroviridae 1*. New York: Plenum, 1993.
21. Franchini G. Molecular mechanisms of human T-cell leukemia/lymphotropic virus type I infection. *Blood* 1995; 86: 3619–3639.
22. Kalyanaraman VS, Sarangadharan MG, Miyoshi I *et al.* A new subtype of human T-cell leukemia virus (HTLV-II) associated with a T-cell variant of hairy cell leukemia. *Science* 1982; 218: 571–573.
23. Barré-Sinoussi F, Chermann JC, Rey F *et al.* Isolation of a T-lymphotropic retrovirus from a patient at risk for acquired immune deficiency syndrome. *Science* 1983; 220: 868–871.
24. Popovic M, Sarngadharan MG, Read E, Gallo RC. Detection, isolation and continuous production of cytopathic retroviruses (HTLV-III) from patients with AIDs and pre-AIDS. *Science* 1984; 224: 497–500.
25. Sarngadharan MG, Popovic M, Bruch L *et al.* Antibodies reactive with human T-lymphotropic retroviruses (HTLV-III) in the serum of patients with AIDS. *Science* 1984; 224: 506–508.
26. Schupbach J, Popvic M, Gilden RV *et al.* Serological analysis of a subgroup of human T-lymphotropic retroviruses (HTLV-III) associated with AIDS. *Science* 1984; 224: 503–505.
27. Gallo RC, Salahuddin SZ, Popovic M *et al.* Frequent detection and isolation of cytopathic retroviruses (HTLV-III) from patients with AIDS and at risk for AIDS. *Science* 1984; 224: 500–503.
28. Daniel MD, Letvin NL, King NW *et al.* Serologic identification and characterization of a macaque T-lymphotropic retrovirus closely related to HTLV-III. *Science* 1985; 228: 1201–1203.
29. Clavel F, Guetard D, Brun-Vezinet F *et al.* Isolation of a new human retrovirus from West African patients with AIDS. *Science* 1986; 233: 343–346.
30. Nakamura S, Salahuddin SZ, Biberfeld P *et al.* Kaposi's sarcoma cells: long-term culture with growth factor from retrovirus-infected CD4+ T cells. *Science* 1988; 242: 427–430.
31. Ensoli B, Nakamura S, Salahuddin SZ *et al.* AIDS–Kaposi's sarcoma-derived cells express cytokines with autocrine and paracrine growth effects. *Science* 1989; 243: 223–226.
32. Salahuddin SZ, Nakamura S, Biberfeld P *et al.* Angiogenesis properties of Kaposi's sarcoma-derived cells after long-term culture in vitro. *Science* 1988; 242: 430–433.
33. Vogel J, Hinrichs SH, Reynolds RK *et al.* HIV-1 tat gene induces dermal lesions resembling Kaposi's sarcoma in transgenic mice. *Nature* 1988; 335: 606–611.
34. Ensoli B, Barillari G, Salahuddin SZ *et al.* Tat protein of HIV1 stimulates the

growth of cells derived from Kaposi's sarcoma lesions of AIDS patients. *Nature* 1990; 345: 84–86.
35. Ensoli B, Gendelman R, Markham P *et al.* Synergy between basic fibroblast growth factor and HIV-1 Tat protein in induction of Kaposi's sarcoma. *Nature* 1994; 371: 674–680.
36. Lunardi-Iskandar Y, Gill P, Lam VH *et al.* Isolation and characterization of an immortal neoplastic cell line (KS Y-1) from AIDS-associated Kaposi's sarcoma. *J Natl Cancer Inst* 1995; 87: 974–981.
37. Lunardi-Iskandar Y, Bryant JL, Zeman RA *et al.* Tumorogenesis and metastasis of neoplastic Kaposi's sarcoma cell line in immunodeficient mice blocked by a human pregnancy hormone. *Nature* 1995; 375: 64–68.
38. Chang Y, Ceserman E, Pessin MS *et al.* Identification of herpesvirus-like DNA sequences in AIDS-associated Kaposi's sarcoma. *Science* 1994; 266: 1865–1868.
39. Rady PL, Yen A, Rollefson JL *et al* Herpesvirus-like DNA sequences in non-Kaposi's sarcoma skin lesions of transplant patients. *Lancet* 1995; 345: 1339–1340.
40. Ceserman E, Chang Y, Moore PS *et al.* Kaposi's sarcoma-associated herpesvirus-like DNA sequences in AIDS related body-cavity-based lymphomas. *N Engl J Med* 1995; 332: 1186–1191.

3

Pathogenesis of HIV-1

Jaap Goudsmit

Human Retrovirus Laboratory, Academic Medical Center, Amsterdam, Netherlands

VIRUS–HOST INTERACTION *IN VIVO:* PATHOGENESIS VERSUS VIRULENCE

The pathogenesis and virulence of human immunodeficiency virus (HIV) are two sides of the same coin. We consider the way HIV causes disease as pathogenesis and the frequency and severity of disease caused by HIV as virulence.

How HIV causes acquired immunodeficiency syndrome (AIDS) is still not completely understood, but the natural history of an HIV infection has taught us a lot. HIV-infected individuals with high levels of antigenaemia show the fastest $CD4^+$ cell decline and progress of AIDS most rapidly[1,2], indicating that the excessive production of proteins, being building blocks of the viral particle, is associated with the occurrence of immunodeficiency. AIDS has to be considered the clinical manifestation of severe immunodeficiency. Recently, the groups of David Ho and George Shaw have shown that the quantity of virus produced daily is in the order of 60 million to 1 billion virions[3].

The half-life of cell free virus is approximately two days, indirectly suggesting that new infections produce these viruses and not so much persistently infected cells. The turnover of virus producing CD4 cells has been estimated to be between 50 million and 2 billion a day. In order to raise $CD4^+$ cell numbers as quickly as is seen following effective antiviral therapy with niverapine or protease inhibitors, the $CD4^+$ cell renewal rate must be enormous. This in itself indicates that the level of virus production may be directly related to HIV pathogenesis, when $CD4^+$ cell decline is considered the hallmark of HIV-related immunodeficiency. A single infectious unit appears to represent approximately 10^4–10^6 virions[4,5], indicating the forma-

AIDS and Malignancies: Current Concepts and Perspectives.
Edited by B.C. Golematis and V.T. DeVita Jr

tion of large numbers of defective particles. To date it is unclear whether these defective particles interfere with virus replication and the production of infectious virions. Equally uncertain is whether the ratio of defective and non-defective particles changes in the course of HIV infection and, if so, whether these changes are related to disease progression. It remains remarkable that infectious HIV titres are highest early and late in HIV infection of progressors while the number of particles remains relatively constant[4,6]. Piatak and coworkers clearly indicate that this still might be related to differential sensitivity of the assays and not so much to a proportional increase or decrease of infectious particles[5].

Independently of virus load, virus phenotype has been shown to be a strong predictor of rapid $CD4^+$ cell decline and disease progression[7].

The present review will first focus on the role of different aspects of virus replication, then on the role of the biological phenotype and cell tropism, and lastly on the virological characteristics marking the long-term symptom-free period.

THE ROLE OF HIV PRODUCTION AND CLEARANCE IN HIV PATHOGENESIS AND VIRULENCE

Virus load is generally assessed in the peripheral blood[8,9]. Virus load or virus burden has to be well defined, because there is more and more evidence that different measures of virus load reflect completely different dynamic processes. Firstly, the level of circulating infectious virus can be measured[6]. Subsequently distinction has to be made between reflections of number of infected cells in the peripheral blood, i.e. quantity of proviral DNA[10,11]; reflections of transport to the nucleus[12] and integration, i.e. quantity of circular HIV DNA; active replication in cells of the peripheral blood, i.e. quantity of mRNA[13]; and reflections of total virus production and clearance, i.e. quantity of genomic RNA present in blood[14,15]. Pre-seroconversion genomic RNA (gRNA) levels peak, falling one or two logs in the first months of seroconversion[5,16]. At seroconversion future progressors and non-progressors have indistinguishable levels of virus[17,18], and genomic particle-associated RNA. Although high levels of plasma particle-associated RNA can be detected during all stages of infection, significant differences between progressors and non-progressors occur[4,5]. The levels of infectious virus in plasma is about 10^{-4}–10^{-6} lower than gRNA levels[5,6]. Within the first three years of infection gRNA levels of non-progressors and progressors showing a non-syncytium-inducing (NSI) to syncytium-inducing (SI) virus shift cannot be differentiated, but the CD4 cell numbers distinguish between these two groups. In contrast, gRNA levels decline in the first three years of infection significantly faster in non-progressors than in progressors with stable NSI viruses[4]. The kinetics of this process—stable, high levels of genomic RNA from seroconversion in progressors—strongly indicate that this virus production is not due to replication in cells of the peripheral blood but to replication in the lymphoid organs[19]. This point is corroborated by the temporal kinetics of mRNA[13] and/or circular unintegrated DNA[20,21]. The levels of mRNA[22] and cDNA, as well as total DNA[11], rise and fall with the level of infectious virus recovery[23,24] from the blood, early as well as late in infection. Linear unintegrated DNA appears the dominant form of the HIV genome during the clinical latency phase in between[25,26]. T-cell activation causes the HIV genome in quiescent cells to integrate and to be transcribed and translated[26]. We have to remind ourselves that during this whole non-producer state in the peripheral blood, virus is still produced in lymphoid organs.

During the period of clinical latency, mRNA levels and cDNA levels are low, and following qualitative and quantitative abnormalities of the CD4⁺ cell population the levels of infected cells[27], mRNA[28] and cDNA rise again[21]. These data indicate that during clinical latency the block of virus replication may be pre-integration and that activation of cells leads to integration as well as mRNA production. These processes may, however, be of minor importance since the major reservoir of HIV appears to be in lymphoid organs.

The increase of HIV replication in peripheral blood may occur late in infection and therefore is strongly related to $CD4^+$ cell numbers[29], not by virtue of pathogenetic mechanisms, but by the fact that replication of HIV in peripheral blood is activated late in infection when $CD4^+$ cells are already reduced to abnormal levels. Such virus progeny from blood cells have acquired increased replication competence in peripheral blood mononuclear cells[30].

THE ROLE OF BIOLOGICAL PHENOTYPE IN PATHOGENESIS AND NATURAL HISTORY OF HIV

A general hallmark of lentiviruses appears to be the tropism for cells of the monocyte/macrophage lineage. HIV is not an exception to this rule[31]. All HIV isolates from infected individuals who are newly infected appear to be macrophage tropic, indicating that initial replication of HIV at the port of entry is in cells of the monocyte/macrophage lineage. Such isolates multiply also in both fresh and viably frozen heterologous peripheral blood mononuclear cells, suggesting that these isolates are dual tropic and also multiply in $CD4^+$ T-cells. These viruses, isolated early in HIV infection, lack mostly the ability to enter, multiply and cause cytopathy in transformed $CD4^+$ T-cell lines[32,33], MT2 in particular[34]. However, a shift from monocytotropic to T-cell tropic virus populations can be observed during disease progression[35]. In the

Amsterdam cohort studies over 90% of all viruses isolated at seroconversion were non-MT2 tropic and were therefore designated NSI[2]. Based on the fact that specific non-silent mutations within the third variable domain (V3) of the HIV external envelope glycoprotein gp120 confer the MT2-tropic SI phenotype[35–39], again over 90% of the new infections is of the NSI phenotype. This mainly reflects the phenotypic composition of the donor virus populations[40]. Results obtained by biologically cloning of bulk SI isolates and NSI isolates revealed that bulk SI isolates are heterogeneous and contain 5–100% of viruses with the SI phenotype. Most virus populations with an SI phenotype in bulk cultures contain a majority of NSI biological clones. This contrasts with virus populations with the NSI bulk phenotype that contains generally only NSI biological clones.

Although macrophage tropism[41] strongly overlaps with the NSI phenotype, SI viruses infecting MT2 cells are transmissible[42]. Transmissible SI isolates have been shown to be macrophage tropic, in contrast to SI viruses isolated during late HIV infection. SI transmission, however, appears to be rare and depends on the number of biological virus clones with the SI phenotype within the bulk SI virus population. The rarity of SI virus transmission[43] is related to the dominance of NSI virus clones throughout all phases of HIV infection in the current phase of the epidemic. This appears to be the case for HIV-1 strains circulating in Europe and the USA among homosexual men and intravenous drug users. It remains to be seen if HIV strains of the SI phenotype are inherently less transmissible than HIV strains of the NSI phenotype and, if so, whether this is related to macrophage tropism. SI virus isolation marks low CD4 numbers and AIDS[44]. This is of importance because the shift in virus phenotype from NSI to SI is strongly related to rapid $CD4^+$ cell decline and progression to clinical manifestations or immunodeficiency[7,45,46]. However, one has to realize that only in about 50% of HIV-infected individuals does a shift from NSI to SI viruses occur prior to the first AIDS-defining illness[7,47]. Following the diagnosis of AIDS, NSI-to-SI shifts keep occurring at the same rate as prior to the manifestation of AIDS. Therefore, it may be that the shift from predominantly macrophage-tropic viruses to T-cell-tropic viruses in the circulation may reflect a natural virological endpoint to functional immunodeficiency. Functional immunodeficiency occurs frequently prior to $CD4^+$ cell decline below 400 and the outgrowth of SI viruses. These data suggest that efficiency of entry and replication in macrophages frequently associated with the NSI, non-MT2-tropic phenotype is a major determinant of HIV pathogenesis. Recently, it has been shown that the HIV genes crucial to entry and replication in cells of the macrophage lineage are coding for Vpr[48] as well as the envelope. Both proteins are present in the HIV particle and have been shown to be shed during natural HIV infection. In addition, these proteins may also play a role in replication in $CD4^+$ T-cells. In contrast to cells of the macrophage lineage, HIV replication in $CD4^+$ T-cells requires activation. Vpr is apparently able to rescue HIV from quiescent cells by activating HIV transmission. The level of HIV replication and spread in human lymphoid organs—at the cellular level, macrophages/monocytes—may therefore be the best reflection of HIV virulence.

CONCLUSION

HIV-1 pathogenesis and natural course is heavily influenced by the level of HIV-1 replication reached early in infection and maintained during the symptom-free period. The majority of virus production occurs in the lymphoid organs, primarily in cells of the monocyte/macrophage lineage. If the level of this virus production is high, disease progression is likely to occur. Persistent virus production from monocytes/macrophages in lymphoid organs apparently results, at particular thresholds, in multiple passages in $CD4^+$ T-cells. This may be related to $CD4^+$ T-cell activation by viral proteins such as vpr. In a major group of patients this leads to increasing levels of mRNA and cDNA and in about half of them in an NSI to SI phenotypic switch. Both increased levels of virus replication and changes in cell tropism appear to contribute to disease progression.

From the natural history of HIV, one may conclude that disease progression is far away as long as the following virological characteristics[1,20,49,50] are maintained:

(1) (cytoplasmic?) linear unintegrated DNA in all (or most) DNA^+ cells (about 0.1% of peripheral blood mononuclear cells);
(2) no/little nuclear, integrated or circular unintegrated DNA in any DNA^+ cell (0.4–1% of peripheral blood mononuclear cells);
(3) low/no levels of genomic RNA in serum;
(4) low/no p24 antigen in serum (±acid/triton); high anti-p24 titres;
(5) low/no yield of virus from plasma;
(6) coculture of peripheral blood mononuclear cells yields virus of the non-syncytium-inducing phenotype that is not transmissible to cell lines (MT2).

These observations clearly point to a model of HIV pathogenesis involving direct cytopathicity of HIV for $CD4^+$ cells like T-helper cells and monocyte/macrophages. The direct relationship between virus load and CD4 cell numbers indicates that models of HIV pathogenesis, including autoimmune mechanisms, other indirect effects of HIV on the immune system and cofactors, are unnecessarily complicated. This does in no way mean that HIV-related immune responses do not play a role in HIV pathogenesis and virulence. Preliminary evidence from David Ho's laboratory (personal communication) indicates that sera of long-term asymptomatic individuals are well able to block *in vitro* infection by primary HIV isolates of primary bound mononuclear cells, while sera of progressors lack this capacity. In addition, CTL responses are more vigorous in non-progressors compared to progressors[51–53]. Thus HIV pathogenesis depends on a three-way interaction: the infectivity and replication competence of the virus, the susceptibility of particular cell types for HIV entry and replication, and the vigour of the HIV-specific immune response.

REFERENCES

1. Wolf de F, Lange JMA, Houweling JTM *et al.* Numbers of CD4+ cells and the levels of core antigens of and antibodies to the human immunodeficiency virus as predictors of AIDS among seropositive homosexual men. *J Infect Dis* 1988; 158: 615–622.
2. Keet IPM, Krijnen P, Koot M *et al.* Predictors of rapid progression to AIDS in HIV-1 seroconverters. *AIDS* 1993; 7: 51–57.
3. Gozlan M. Conference review 9th Cent Gardes 1994: AIDS pathogenesis and prevention. *Lancet* 1994; 344: 1287–1288.
4. Jurriaans S, Gemen van B, Weverling GJ *et al.* The natural history of HIV-1 infection: virus load and virus phenotype independent determinants of clinical course? *Virology* 1994; 204: 223–233.
5. Piatak MJ, Saag MS, Yang LC *et al.* High levels of HIV-1 in plasma during all stages of infection determined by competitive PCR. *Science* 1993; 259: 1749–1754.
6. Saag MS, Crain MJ, Decker WD *et al.* High-level viremia in adults and children infected with human immunodeficiency virus relation to disease stage and CD4+ lymphocyte levels. *J Infect Dis* 1991; 164: 72–80.
7. Koot M, Keet RPM, Vos AHV *et al.* Prognostic value of HIV-1 syncytium-inducing phenotype for rate of CD4+ cell depletion and progression to AIDS. *Ann Intern Med* 1993; 118: 681–688.
8. Baltimore D, Feinberg MB. HIV revealed: toward a natural history of the infection. *N Engl J Med* 1989; 321: 1673–1675.
9. Aoki-Sei S, Yarchoan R, Kageyama S *et al.* Plasma HIV-1 viremia in HIV-1 infected individuals assessed by polymerase chain reaction. *AIDS Res Hum Retroviruses* 1992; 8: 1263–1270.
10. Bagasra O, Hauptman SP, Lischner HW *et al.* Detection of human immunodeficiency virus type 1 provirus in mononuclear cells by in situ polymerase chain reaction. *N Engl J Med* 1992; 326: 1385–1391.
11. Jurriaans S, Dekker JT, Ronde de A. HIV-1 viral DNA load in peripheral blood mononuclear cells from seroconverters and long-term infected individuals. *AIDS* 1992; 6: 635–641.
12. Bukrinsky MI, Sharova N, Dempsey MP *et al.* Active nuclear import of human immunodeficiency virus type 1 preintegration complexes. *Proc Natl Acad Sci USA* 1992; 89: 6580–6584.
13. Bagnarelli P, Valenza A, Menzo S *et al.* Dynamics of molecular parameters of human immunodeficiency virus type 1 activity in vivo. *J Virol* 1994; 68: 2495–2502.
14. Bagnarelli P, Menzo S, Manzin, A *et al.* Detection of human immunodeficiency virus type 1 genomic RNA in plasma samples by reverse-transcriptase polymerase chain reaction. *J Med Virol* 1991; 34: 89–95.
15. Holodniy M, Katzenstein DA, Sengupta S *et al.* Detection and quantification of

human immunodeficiency virus RNA in patient serum by use of the polymerase chain reaction. *J Infect Dis* 1991; 163: 862–866.
16. Gemen van B, Kievits T, Schukkink R, Strijp van D *et al.* Quantification of HIV-1 RNA in plasma using NASBA TM during HIV-1 primary infection. *J Virol Methods* 1993; 43: 177–188.
17. Clark SJ, Saag MS, Decker WD *et al.* High titers of cytopathic virus in plasma of patients with symptomatic primary HIV-1 infection. *N Engl J Med* 1991; 324: 954–960.
18. Daar ES, Moudgil T, Meyer RD, Ho DD. Transient high levels of viremia in patients with primary human immunodeficiency virus type 1 infection. *N Engl J Med* 1991; 324: 961–964.
19. Pantaleo G, Graziosi C, Demarest JF *et al.* HIV infection is active and progressive in lymphoid tissue during the clinically latent stage of disease. *Nature* 1993; 362: 355.
20. Bukrinsky MI, Stanwick TL, Dempsey, MP, Stevenson M. Quiescent T lymphocytes as an inducible virus reservoir in HIV-1 infection. *Science* 1991; 254: 423–427.
21. Jurriaans S, Ronde de A, Dekker J *et al.* Increased number of single-LTR HIV-1 DNA junctions correlates with HIV-1 antigen expression and CD4+ cell decline in vivo. *J Med Virol* 1995; 45: 91–98.
22. Graziosi C, Pantaleo G, Butini L *et al.* Kinetics of human immunodeficiency virus type 1 (HIV-1) DNA/RNA synthesis during primary HIV-1 infection. *Proc Natl Acad Sci USA* 1993; 90: 6405–6409.
23. Coombs RW, Collier AC, Allain JP *et al.* Plasma viremia in human immunodeficiency virus infection. *N Engl J Med* 1989; 321: 1626–1631.
24. Ho DD, Moudgil T, Alam M. Quantitation of human immunodeficiency virus type 1 in the blood of infected persons. *N Engl J Med* 1989; 321: 1621–1625.
25. Zack JA, Arrigo SJ, Weitsman SR *et al.* HIV-1 entry into quiescent primary lymphocytes: molecular analysis reveals a labile, latent viral structure. *Cell* 1990; 61: 213–222.
26. Stevenson M, Stanwick TL, Dempsey MP, Lamonica CA. HIV-1 replication is controlled at the level of T cell activation and proviral integration. *EMBO J* 1990; 95: 1551–1560.
27. Schnittman SM, Greenhouse JJ, Psallidopoulos MC *et al.* Increasing viral burden in CD4+ T cells from patients with human immunodeficiency virus (HIV) infection reflects rapidly progressive immunosuppression and clinical disease. *Ann Intern Med* 1990; 113: 438–443.
28. Saksela K, Stevens S, Rubinstein P, Baltimore D. Human immunodeficiency virus type 1 mRNA expression in peripheral blood cells predicts disease progression independently of the numbers of CD4+ lymphocytes. *Proc Natl Acad Sci USA* 1994; 91: 1104–1108.
29. Michael NL, Vahey M, Burke DS, Redfield RR. Viral DNA and mRNA expression correlate with the stage of human immunodeficiency virus (HIV) type 1 infection in humans: evidence for viral replication in all stages of HIV disease. *J Virol* 1992; 66: 310–316.
30. Connor RI, Mohri H, Cao Y, Ho DD. Increased viral burden and cytopathicity correlate temporally with CD4+ T-lymphocyte decline and clinical progression in human immunodeficiency virus type 1 infected individuals. *J Virol* 1993; 67: 1772–1777.
31. Schuitemaker H, Kootstra NA, Goede de REY *et al.* Monocytotropic human immunodeficiency virus type 1 (HIV-1) variants detectable in all stages of HIV-1 infection lack T-cell line tropism and syncytium-inducing ability in primary T-cell culture. *J Virol* 1991; 65: 356–363.

32. Asjö B, Albert J, Karlsson A *et al.* Replicative capacity of human immunodeficiency virus from patients with varying severity of HIV infection. *Lancet* 1986; ii: 660–662.
33. Cheng-Mayer C, Seto D, Tateno M, Levy JA. Biologic features of HIV-1 that correlate with virulence in the host. *Science* 1988; 240: 80–82.
34. Koot M, Vos AHV, Keet RPM *et al.* HIV-1 biological phenotype in long-termed infected individuals evaluated with an MT-2 cocultivation assay. *AIDS* 1992; 6: 49–54.
35. Schuitemaker H, Koot M, Kootstra NA *et al.* Biological phenotype of human immunodeficiency virus type 1 clones at different stages of infection: progression of disease is associated with a shift from monocytotropic to T-cell-tropic virus populations. *J Virol* 1992; 66: 1354–1360.
36. Fouchier RAM, Groenink M, Kootstra NA *et al.* Phenotype associated sequence variation in the third variable domain to the human immunodeficiency virus type 1 gp120 molecule. *J Virol* 1992; 66: 3183–3187.
37. Jong de JJ, Goudsmit J, Keulen W *et al.* Human immunodeficiency viruses type 1 chimeric for the envelope V3 domain are distinct in syncytium formation and replication capacity. *J Virol* 1992; 66: 757–765.
38. Kuiken CL, Jong de JJ, Baan E *et al.* Evolution of the V3 envelope domain in proviral sequences and isolates of human immunodeficiency virus type 1 during transition of the viral biological phenotype. *J Virol* 1992; 66: 4622–4627.
39. Jong de J, Ronde de A, Keulen W *et al.* Minimal requirements for the human immunodeficiency virus type 1 V3 domain to support the syncytium-inducing (SI) phenotype: analysis by single amino acid substitution. *J Virol* 1992; 66: 6777–6780.
40. Roos MTL, Lange JMA, Goede de REY *et al.* Virus phenotype and immune response in primary HIV-1 infection. *J Infect Dis* 1992; 165: 427–432.
41. Chesebro B, Wehrly K, Nishio J, Perryman S. Macrophage-tropic immunodeficiency virus isolates from different patients exhibit unusual V3 envelope sequence heterogeneity in comparison with T-cell-tropic isolates: definition of critical amino acids involved in cell tropism. *J Virol* 1992; 66: 6547–6554.
42. Cornelissen M, Mulder-Kampinga G, Veenstra J *et al.* SI phenotype suppression at seroconversion following intramuscular inoculation of an NSI/SI phenotypically mixed HIV population. Submitted 1994.
43. Zhu T, Mo H, Wang N *et al.* Genotypic and phenotypic characterization of HIV-1 in patients with primary infection. *Science* 1993; 261: 1179–1181.
44. Tersmette M, Goede de REY, Al BJM *et al.* Differential syncytium-inducing capacity of HIV isolates: frequent detection of syncytium-inducing isolates in patients with AIDS and ARC. *J Virol* 1988; 62: 2026–2032.
45. Tersmette M, Gruters RA, Wolfe de F *et al.* Evidence for a role of virulent human immunodeficiency virus (HIV) variants in the pathogenesis of acquired immunodeficiency syndrome: studies on sequential HIV isolates. *J Virol* 1989; 63: 2118–2125.
46. Tersmette M, Lange JMA, Goede de REY *et al.* Association between biological properties of human immunodeficiency virus variants and risk for AIDS and AIDS mortality. *Lancet* 1989; i: 983–985.
47. Schellekens PTA, Tersmette M, Roos MTL *et al.* Biphasic rate of decline during progression to AIDS correlates with HIV phenotype. *AIDS* 1992; 6: 665–669.
48. Levy DN, Refaeli Y, MacGregor RR, Weiner DB. Serum vpr regulates productive infection and latency of human immunodeficiency virus type 1. *Proc Natl Acad Sci USA* 1995; 92: 3621–3625.
49. Wolf de F, Lange JMA, Houweling JTM *et al.* Appearance of predictors of disease progression in relation to development of AIDS. *AIDS* 1989; 3: 563–569.

50. Hogervorst E, Jurriaans S, Wolfe de F *et al.* Predictors for non- and slow progression in human immunodeficiency virus type 1 infection: low viral RNA copy numbers in serum and maintenance of high HIV-1 p24-specific, but not V3-specific antibody levels. *J Infect Dis* 1994; in press.
51. Koup RA, Safrit JT, Cao Y *et al.* Temporal association of cellular immune responses with the initial control of viremia in primary human immunodeficiency virus type 1 syndrome. *J Virol* 1994; 68: 4650–4655.
52. Borrow P, Lewicki H, Hahn BH *et al.* Virus-specific CD8+ cytotoxic T-lymphocyte activity associated with control of viremia in primary human immunodeficiency virus type 1 infection. *J Virol* 1994; 68: 6103–6110.
53. Pantaleo G, Demarest JF, Soudeyns H *et al.* Major expansion of CD8+ T cells with a predominant Vβ usage during the primary immune response to HIV. *Nature* 1994; 370: 463–467.

4

Pathogenesis of HIV-2

Efi Kokkotou and Phyllis J. Kanki

Harvard AIDS Institute, Harvard School of Public Health, Boston, Massachusetts, USA

INTRODUCTION

The human immunodeficiency viruses (HIVs) and simian immunodeficiency viruses (SIVs) constitute a diverse group of complex retroviruses that belong to the subfamily Lentivirinae. HIV-1 and HIV-2 are 40–50% related at a primary nucleotide level and demonstrate significant genetic variability within each virus type[1]. Related non-human primate viruses, SIVs, have been described from a variety of primate species, and are generally more closely related to HIV-2; certain SIVs from African monkeys have been described that are indistinguishable for HIV-2[2]. More recently, a chimpanzee lentivirus, SIVcpz, has been described that is more closely related to HIV-1[3]. Thus, the family of primate immunodeficiency viruses is large, with distinct viruses in a variety of monkeys, apes and humans[4]. Studies of the various viruses found in non-human primates also suggest a wide diversity in pathogenicity. The most developed SIV model for disease is in Asian macaque species, and since SIVs have never been observed in wild Asian macaques, it is likely that infection of this species occurred accidentally in captivity from African monkeys or human origin[5]. It is not known when or how these related viruses moved into different monkey or human populations and how pathogenicity may have been altered by such cross-species transmissions. Suffice it to say, that based on current genetic analyses, the HIVs and SIVs most likely shared a common ancestor at some time in their evolution[4]. Further understanding of the behavior of these viruses *in vivo* may aid us in further defining the evolutionary history of non-human and human immunodeficiency viruses.

HIV-2, the second immunodeficiency virus in humans, was serologically

AIDS and Malignancies: Current Concepts and Perspectives.
Edited by B.C. Golematis and V.T. DeVita Jr

identified in 1985 in healthy registered prostitutes from Senegal[6]. Our group described serological reactivity to all SIV antigens with only cross-reactivity to the Gag and Pol antigens of HIV-1, the prototype acquired immunodeficiency syndrome (AIDS) virus. This strongly indicated infection with a virus more closely related to SIV than to HIV-1. We therefore hypothesized in 1985 that the SIV from African monkeys may have served as a reservoir for infection to humans at some point in time[5,6]. The existence of a second immunodeficiency virus of people, at least partially related to HIV-1, the prototype AIDS virus, suggested to many that the biology of HIV-2 could be easily predicted. However, despite almost a decade of research, the virological similarities of HIV-2 and HIV-1 have not proven to be predictive of the distinctly different biological properties of HIV-2 in people.

HIV-2 and HIV-1 share many important virological characteristics. They have similar genetic structures and genome organization, they exhibit similar cell tropism for CD4-bearing cells and are capable of establishing persistent infection *in vitro* and *in vivo*[7,8]. Like HIV-1, HIV-2 appears to be transmitted by the same routes and infection can be diagnosed with analogous serological or virological assays. Despite these similarities, the epidemiology of HIV-2 appears distinct[9]. For the most part, HIV-2 infection is concentrated in West Africa, where infection appears to have been endemic for quite some time. The transmission of HIV-2 also appears to be significantly slower than that of HIV-1 by both sexual and perinatal routes. Although end-stage HIV-2 disease appears to be similar to HIV-1-induced AIDS, the rate of disease progression is much slower than that of HIV-1, suggesting that some HIV-2-infected individuals may be true long-term non-progressors.

As specific serodiagnostic testing for HIV-2 becomes more common worldwide, clinicians and public health officials will need to be familiar with the distinct biological and clinical characteristics of HIV-2 infection. Further studies are clearly needed to better understand the distinct biological properties of this virus. From the research perspective, a better understanding of the comparative molecular, cellular and host factors involved in HIV-2 and HIV-1 infection should help us acquire the biomedical tools necessary to combat both viruses.

VIROLOGY AND BIOLOGY OF HIV-2

HIV-2s are morphologically similar to HIV-1, with spherical, 100–120 nm virions and a conical electron-dense core[10]. Distinct for HIV-2 and SIV are the prominent protruding envelope projections and the electron-lucent paranucleoid space which is an open ring around the triangular core, compared to HIV-1 where the lucent space extends from the core to the envelope[11]. Despite significant sequence divergence between HIV-1 and HIV-2, the two viruses share many basic virological properties including a similar genomic organization, a common cellular receptor, and similarities in the virus replication cycle and invoked immune response.

Like all retroviruses, HIV-2 encodes Gag (nucleocapsid), Pol (polymerase) and Env (envelope) structural gene products flanked by two long terminal repeat sequences (LTRs). The Gag precursor polyprotein of HIV-2 is translated from the full-length genomic RNA to a 57 kDa protein that is myristylated and cleaved at five cleavage sites to yield six products, p17–p27–p2–p1–p8–p6[12]. The major core protein p27 is slightly larger in HIV-2 than in HIV-1 (p24), whereas the myristylated matrix proteins p17 are of similar size. After a Gag–Pol polyprotein precursor is formed, the complete Pol precursor is cleaved and forms a protein of approximately 180 kDa. This product is in turn cleaved to form p64 (reverse transcriptase/RNaseH), p36 (endonuclease/integrase), and p11 (protease) of HIV-2. The major viral structural proteins are readily distinguished on immunoblots and regularly recognized by HIV-2-positive serum samples[13]. The *gag* and *pol* genes are well conserved among the HIVs and SIVs; the high degree of conservation in these structural genes accounts for the cross-reactivity of HIV-2 sera on HIV-1 Gag and Pol antigens as seen in some serological assays[6,13–15].

In HIV-2 the envelope polyprotein precursor is a heavily glycosylated protein which is cleaved to form the mature (gp120–105) and the transmembrane (gp32–40) envelope proteins[13,16]. Like HIV-1, genetic variation between HIV-2 isolates has been demonstrated, with the most marked variation in the envelope gene[17–22]. The envelope gene demonstrates genetic variation from isolate to isolate with some polymorphism exhibited at a protein level[23].

The gp105 (gp120) of HIV-2 binds to the CD4 molecule on lymphocytes, macrophages and possibly other cells, and is therefore one of the determinants of tissue tropism and pathogenicity[24–26]. In comparison with HIV-1, the binding affinity of HIV-2 gp105 for the CD4 molecule appears to be 10–100-fold less[27]. Different strains of HIV-2 show different abilities to bind to CD4, as well as varying degrees of infectivity and syncytia-inducing ability[28,29]. The possibility that HIV-2 may use a receptor in addition to CD4 has been raised, as some cell lines transfected with the CD4 receptor show different sensitivity to HIV-2 compared with HIV-1[30]. Despite this, HIV-2 can cross-interfere with HIV-1 *in vitro*[31,32]. Interestingly, HIV-2 appears to interfere with HIV-1 infection *in vitro* better than HIV-1's interference with HIV-2[31,32].

Truncation of the transmembrane envelope protein has been observed with isolates of HIV-2 and SIVmac, but not with HIV-1 isolates[33–35]. Interestingly, the transmembrane subunits of lentiviruses normally possess cytoplasmic domains that are much longer than those of other retroviruses. Site-directed mutagenesis studies have shown that the cytoplasmic domain truncation is responsible for enhanced fusion activity[33]. It has been proposed that the cytoplasmic domain of the transmembrane protein modulates fusion activity of the exterior glycoprotein complex in a cell-specific manner, which may regulate viral cytopathicity in selected cell types during natural infection.

Functionally important sites on the external glycoprotein appear conserved between HIV-1 and HIV-2. This includes the CD4-binding domain[36,37], precursor processing[38], fusion[38,39] and principal neutralizing domain at V3[40–42] and at least some cytolytic T-cell epitopes[43]. Unlike HIV-1, envelope-binding activity appears to concentrate in the middle portion of the gp105 molecule, as opposed to the HIV-1 antibody response, which is directed more broadly across most of the gp120 molecule[44–46]. Another important immunogenic domain of the envelope is found in the amino terminus of the transmembrane protein[47,48], which has been used to advantage for a variety of peptide- and recombinant-based type-specific diagnostic assays.

Like other complex retroviruses, HIV-2 possesses a number of accessory genes with variable homology to HIV-1 genes, including *tat, rev, nef, vif* and *vpr*[1,7,17]. Both SIV and HIV-2 possess a *vpx* gene which is absent in HIV-1 and they both lack the *vpu* gene, the unique accessory gene of HIV-1[49–52]. Mutational studies have shown that *vpx* is not required for virus replication, yet may facilitate infection in fresh lymphocytes and monocytes[53,54]. Thus, the Vpx gene product appears to be necessary for efficient viral replication under certain circumstances. Although the general genomic structures of HIV-2 and HIV-1 are similar, the reading frames differ[17,36]. The reading frames for HIV-2 *gag, pol* and *vif* are similar for HIV-1, but the remainder of the open reading frames are different from that of HIV-1. This frame-shift occurs at the site of *vpx*, the unique gene of HIV-2/SIVmac type viruses.

HIV-2 encodes the *vif* gene which, by analogy to HIV-1, is likely to be involved in infectivity in certain cell types[1,55,56]. The *nef* gene, originally considered, on the basis of tissue culture experiments, to encode a negative regulatory element, is now known to encode a protein which actually increases SIV (and presumably HIV-2) replication *in vivo*[57–59]. The product of the *vpr* gene appears to be a virion-associated structural protein which has been shown to modestly increase HIV-1 replication and be critical for macrophage infection[60–62]. Recent data suggests that Vpr may function as a regulator of cellular permissiveness to HIV-1 replication. Serum Vpr from HIV-1-infected patients activated virus expression in latently infected cell lines and in resting peripheral blood mononuclear cells, thus indicating that Vpr may control HIV latency *in vivo*[63]. The distant genetic relatedness of Vpr to Vpx has suggested that the Vpx in HIV-2/SIV results from an ancient duplication of the *vpr* gene[64]. The relevance of this observation to the function of these genes in HIV-2 is still not known.

The Tat protein of HIV-2, like that of HIV-1, acts in *trans* to stimulate viral production and, by analogy to HIV-1, is assumed to be essential for viral replication[1]. The Tat proteins are unusual viral transactivators in that their action is mediated through a site(s) downstream of the RNA initiation site. It is generally believed that the primary role of Tat is to permit the elongation of properly initiated viral transcripts. Whereas the RNA target for HIV-1 Tat has only one stem loop structure, the HIV-2 Tat target sequence has two[65,66]. However, it appears that the distal site may be employed only when the proximal site cannot be used[67]. Functional evidence of Tat activity has been shown for HIV-2 and SIV, similar and cross-reactive with HIV-1 Tat[68,69].

Another regulatory gene of HIV-1 and HIV-2 is the *rev* gene, which exhibits a complex mechanism of action and is required for viral replication[1]. *rev* acts through its RNA target in the *env* gene, the RRE (rev-responsive element), to increase the number of transcripts for the HIV structural genes found in the cytoplasm. *rev* performs this function by increasing the transport of unspliced (structural gene) viral RNA from the nucleus and/or by regulating RNA splicing[70–72]. Interaction of *rev* with the RRE RNA either alone or with additional cellular factors presumably mediates the export of these RNAs from the nucleus to the cytoplasm. In the absence of *rev*, the viral proteins encoded by these mRNAs are not expressed because their respective mRNAs are trapped in the nucleus. While less well studied, HIV-2 Rev appears to function similarly to HIV-1 Rev[71]. Similar to HIV-1 Rev, the HIV-2 Rev is phosphorylated, albeit to a much lesser extent and localized to the nucleus, with marked accumulation in the nucleolus. While HIV-1 Rev can function with both the HIV-1 and HIV-2 RREs, HIV-2 Rev functions only with its own RRE and that of SIV[71,72].

Little is currently known regarding the immunogenicity of HIV-2 regulatory proteins *in vivo*. Our preliminary data suggest that similar to the HIV-1 system they will be less uniformly immunogenic[50,73] (unpublished observations). These less immunoreactive serological markers may not be useful for serodiagnosis but may be useful in certain diagnostic settings such as discriminating virus types or in mother–infant studies where active antibodies may be distinguished from passive.

In general, the regulation of viral gene expression in HIV-2 seems to resemble that observed in HIV-1. However, several differences have been described that may play a role in the differential pathogenicity of these viruses. For example, sequence comparisons of HIV-1 and HIV-2 have demonstrated differences in the LTR structure. Whereas HIV-1 has two NF-kB enhancer binding sites, only one can be identified for HIV-2 or most SIVs[74]. This may be of biological significance, as recent studies of two different strains of SIV with dramatic difference in virulence *in vivo* have demonstrated the duplication of the NF-kB binding sites in the virulent strain[75]. The regulation and response to T-cell activation via the viral LTR also appears to be distinct in HIV-2 as compared to HIV-1[76–79]. Specific and unique elements in the HIV-2 LTR may regulate HIV-2 gene expression independently of the T-cell activation signals or cytokines that would normally modulate HIV-1 gene expression[76,77,80]. Mutational studies of the unique sites in the HIV-2 LTR responsible for inducible enhancer function demonstrate that this function is more readily disrupted in HIV-2 compared with HIV-1[80], perhaps explaining some of the distinct biological properties of the virus.

The *in vitro* behavior of HIV-1 viruses has been used as an indicator of pathogenicity. In contrast to most HIV-1s, HIV-2 isolates demonstrate decreased cell killing, syncytial cell formation, reduced virus replication and differences in interaction with CD4, frequently related to the clinical stage of the HIV-2-infected individual[28,34,81,82]. Studies of HIV-1 *in vitro* growth characteristics have found that isolates from asymptomatic individuals are more likely to demonstrate 'slow–low' growth kinetics versus the 'rapid–high' growth kinetics from AIDS patient isolates. HIV-2 is more difficult to isolate from asymptomatic people than is HIV-1, but when isolated it appears to show the 'slow–low' pattern[82–84]. Similarly, the 'rapid–high' isolates were more likely to be from HIV-2-infected people with advanced stage disease. Adequate studies have not been conducted to determine if changes in envelope sequence are correlated with these *in vitro* properties of HIV-2s. One study that compared HIV-2 cytopathic and fusigenic variants derived from one isolate failed to identify the genetic determinants of this activity[85].

It is now well established that genetic variants of HIV-1 evolve over time in the same individual after infection. As disease develops, HIV-1s that have changed, particularly in the envelope V3 loop, evolve; intra-patient variation can reach greater than 10%[86–88]. These viruses are often associated with higher virus loads in blood and syncytia induction in T-cell lines with 'rapid–high' growth characteristics. Evaluation of intra-patient variation in the V3 region of HIV-2 in asymptomatic and symptomatic individuals followed over time has shown a lower variation when compared to HIV-1[89]. This lower intra-patient variation appears to be a distinct feature of HIV-2 infection that may result from decreased viral burden and also contribute to lower rates of transmission and disease development.

DIAGNOSIS OF HIV-2 INFECTION

The close relationship of HIV-2 to HIV-1 on a genetic and antigenic level has necessitated the development and implementation of type-specific diagnostic assays. Studies of HIV-2 epidemiology and natural history are heavily reliant on accurate diagnosis, which must be type specific in areas of the world where both viruses are prevalent. Cross-reactivity between HIV-1 and HIV-2 is demonstrated particularly in viral structural proteins such as Gag and Pol[6,13–15]. The more specific antibody reactivity to envelope antigens in infected individuals has been used to distinguish between HIV-1 and HIV-2 infection. Currently, combination HIV-1 and HIV-2 enzyme-linked immunosorbent assay (ELISA) screening tests are employed in all US blood banks and most other clinical diagnostic settings[90], and in large part are implemented worldwide. Since the combination screening assays are incapable of distinguishing HIV type, HIV-1 and HIV-2 confirmatory assays must be performed on all ELISA-positive samples in order to obtain a type-specific diagnosis.

According to standard criteria for HIV-2 immunoblot diagnosis established by the World Heath Organization, HIV-2-specific diagnosis requires antibody reactivity to Env/Gag/Pol antigens. In the absence of reactivity to Gag or Pol antigens, the presence of reactivity to both envelope antigens is required (gp105 and transmembrane gp32–40)[91]. A number of recombinant or synthetic peptide-based assays have been developed and evaluated to distinguish virus types with these serological techniques. In most instances, the antigen source for these assays has been derived from HIV type-specific regions such as the amino terminus of the envelope transmembrane protein[46–48] or the carboxy terminus of gp105–120[44,92]. Recently, a newly developed serological assay based on inhibition of type-specific reverse transcriptase has shown promising results as a type-specific assay[93]. However, testing and implementation of these type-specific assays have been difficult. Theoretically, the gold standard for these assays is virus isolation followed by type-specific polymerase chain reaction (PCR) and/or sequence analysis. Numerous limitations exist with performing these types of assays on HIV-2-infected samples, where virus isolation rates from antibody-positive individuals have generally been lower than those of HIV-1[84]. In addition, only limited studies of type-specific HIV PCR have been described, in most cases with less than 100% sensitivity[94–97]. It is also difficult to perform these assays on large numbers of samples as part of routine laboratory diagnosis, particularly in developing countries, where the price per sample often exceeds the budget of many laboratories. Thus, progress in development of cost-effective HIV-specific assays has been hampered and the lack of such assays has delayed our understanding of HIV dual infection, as described below.

The HIV dual antibody profile is characterized by antibodies with equally strong reactivity to the Env antigens of both HIV-1 and HIV-2 by immunoblot and/or radioimmunoprecipitation analysis (RIPA)[13–15,98]. Several possible biological explanations for this phenomenon can be entertained including extensive cross-reactivity by either of the HIVs, dual infection or infection with an intermediate virus. Isolation of both HIV-1 and HIV-2 has been reported from selected HIV-dual cases[99] and PCR evidence of both viruses has ranged from 30% to 80%, in serologically defined dual reactives reported from similar populations[95,96]. It is unclear whether the low and variable rate of concordance between serology and PCR is due to extensive HIV-1 cross-reactivity as suggested, misclassification of samples based on serodiagnosis or insensitivity of the PCR assays.

We have found that appropriate serological testing and PCR amplification can be highly correlated, particularly when serological[100] and PCR assays are well standardized and optimized for sensitivity[101]. We have utilized two sets of nested primers for each HIV type with Southern blot hybridization to confirm the amplified product. With this methodology we had uniform detection of the appropriate proviral HIV in singly infected individuals and in healthy individuals with HIV-dual serological patterns. By contrast, we found that in serologically designated HIV-dual individuals with low $CD4^+$ counts (<400 cells/mm^3), PCR confirmation of HIV-2 was compromised[101]. We would hypothesize that when the CD4 cell population is compromised the differential viral replication properties of the two viruses results in an overabundance of cells with HIV-1 provirus. The prospective evaluation of these superinfected individuals with sequential samples will give us a better understanding of the interaction between HIV-1 and HIV-2.

VIROLOGICAL OR IMMUNOLOGICAL MARKERS OF HIV-2 INFECTION

In general, our understanding of the immune response to HIV-2 is somewhat limited and we draw heavily on data from studies of HIV-1 infection. Although small cross-sectional studies have been performed to evaluate both humoral and cellular immune responses to HIV-2, the correlation of this data with prospectively collected virological and clinical data is still forthcoming. This type of data is, of course, necessary to link particular immune responses to the pathogenesis of the virus.

As with HIV-1, the antibody response to most viral structural proteins occurs shortly after infection and is thought to persist. Similar to HIV-1-infected individuals the antibody response to *pol*-encoded proteins is frequently seen, this being somewhat unique in other retroviral systems. In fact, in HIV-2 infection over 90% of seropositives evaluated in Senegal demonstrated strong antibodies to *gag-*, *pol-* and *env*-encoded antigens[6,13]. As already noted, the cross-reactive response to analogous HIV-1 antigens is significant in highly conserved gene products such as Gag and Pol and less with envelope antigens.

Previously, circulated p24 antigen of HIV-1 has been useful as a marker of virus replication *in vivo*, although this has been somewhat replaced with more direct measurements of virus using PCR technology in recent times. Analogous studies with HIV-2 have not been performed, perhaps because antibodies to p27 are found in the majority of HIV-2-infected sera and therefore it has been assumed that complexing by free circulating p27 is less frequent. Primary infection with HIV-2 has not been described in the literature, another instance where the presence of excess circulating p27 antigen might exist.

HIV-2-neutralizing antibodies have been described[40–42,102,103], and in studies with fresh isolates the broadness of the HIV-2-neutralizing response has been unusual and distinct from the neutralizing antibody response to HIV-1[104]. Virus neutralization studies have shown that a proportion of HIV-2 sera are also capable of cross-neutralizing HIV-1 isolates in addition to HIV-2 isolates[102,103]. The degree of which HIV-1-positive sera can cross-neutralize HIV-2 isolates remains controversial. Cross-reaction between HIV-1 and HIV-2 in antibody-dependent cellular cytotoxicity (ADCC) studies has also been reported[41,105]. Characterization of the neutralizing and ADCC domains in the HIV-2 envelope has been less extensive compared with HIV-1[40,41]. It is still not known whether some of the conserved domains of env will be capable of eliciting a cross-protective response to both viruses.

Cytotoxic T-lymphocyte (CTL) responses against HIV-2 Gag, Pol and Nef proteins have been described in 16 HIV-2-infected and four dually infected individuals from the Gambia of variable health status. After 14 days of culture, CTL responses against Gag or Pol proteins were seen in 18 (90.0%) and 14 (70.0%) of 20 subjects, respectively, whereas a CTL response to Nef protein was seen in five (25%) of the 20 subjects. The specific lysis of the dominant CTL response correlated strongly with HIV-2 proviral load expressed as copies per 10^5 $CD4^+$ cells ($r=-0.674$, $p=0.001$)[106]. HLA-B53-restricted, HIV-2 Gag-specific CTLs did not recognize target cells expressing HIV-1 Gag proteins, suggesting the absence of a cellular cross-protective response[107].

Markers of immune activation such as neopterin and β_2-microglobulin levels are elevated in HIV-2-infected individuals but less so than in HIV-1-infected people[108–110]. Lymphocyte proliferative responses to mitogens and antigens are also less pronounced in HIV-2 infection[111]. Lower and stable plasma tumor necrosis factor α (TNF-α) levels have been found in HIV-2-infected patients with lower viral load and higher $CD4^+$ lymphocyte counts, suggesting a more efficient and appropriate immune response in HIV-2 infection[112]. However, when these measurements were normalized for viral load and/or CD4 counts, the differences between HIV-1 and HIV-2 infection were diminished.

Differences in the rate of HIV-2 transmission and disease development may be due to characteristics of the virus or elicited host response that result in a lower virus burden. Evidence for a lower viral burden in HIV-2-infected individuals has been reported from both virus isolation and PCR studies[84,97,113]. The isolation rate of HIV-2 from peripheral blood mononuclear cells or plasma of asymptomatic HIV-2-infected individuals is lower than the HIV-1 isolation rate[84]. As CD4 T-lymphocyte counts fall, virus isolation becomes equally efficient in the two infections.

Quantitative PCR provides a more reliable measurement of viral burden or load, and preliminary data from studies in The Gambia and Senegal suggests that proviral HIV-2 copies increase with disease development and the drop of CD4 lymphocytes[89,97,101,113]. When compared to HIV-1-infected individuals, the proviral copy number appears to be significantly lower throughout most of the course of HIV-2 infection except in end-stage disease[89,97,101].

GEOGRAPHIC DISTRIBUTION OF HIV-2 INFECTION

Significant HIV-2 has been well documented in most West African countries, although HIV-2 prevalence rates vary greatly between different countries and in different groups sampled[6,8,13,114,115]. The highest rates of HIV-2 infection in the general population have been found in Guinea Bissau, where seroprevalence rates in low-risk populations exceed 10%[13,115]. In Guinea Bissau, The Gambia, Cape Verde and Senegal, the prevalence of HIV-2 infection exceeds that of infection with HIV-1, but HIV-1 infection appears to be increasing[8,23,111,115–119]. In most other countries of West Africa—Burkina Faso, Ghana, Ivory Coast, Nigeria, and Mali—infection with HIV-1 is 3–24 times more prevalent than HIV-2, indicating that HIV-1 will become the predominant HIV type in much of the region[9,114,120–124]. In these regions, the interaction of HIV-1 and HIV-2 at a population level is currently taking place; continual surveillance of the two virus infections will be an important research priority in the region.

Outside of West Africa, in regions of the continent with the highest rates of HIV-1 infection and AIDS, the HIV-2 virus has not reached significant levels[125]. However, Angola and Mozambique are notable exceptions, where early studies indicated significant rates of infection in various cross-sectional surveys[114,126,127]. More recent data from these former Portuguese colonies is not available.

Outside Africa, significant HIV-2 infection has been reported in Portugal, Spain, southwestern India and Brazil, all areas with former colonist ties to Portugal. In Portugal, 10–12% of HIV infections were attributed to HIV-2. Of persons infected with HIV-2, 48% had some link with West Africa or Angola[128,129]. Of 34 cases of HIV-2 infection recognized to date in neighboring Spain, 31 were African immigrants and three had a history of possible heterosexual exposure to HIV-2-infected persons in Africa[130].

HIV-2 infection has been documented in persons originating from the Caribbean, including Cuba[131]. HIV-2 infections were also identified in Cuban soldiers returning from campaigns in Africa, although comprehensive surveillance data has not been published. The epidemiological status of HIV-2 infection in Brazil, which has important links with West Africa and Portugal, has been confusing. Early reports of dual serological reactivity in residents of Brazil were interpreted as indicative of HIV-2 infection[132,133], but subsequent studies showed no evidence of HIV-2 infection in high-risk Brazilian populations[134]. A recent report of hospitalized patients found both monotypic HIV-2 and HIV-dual infections as demonstrated by PCR[135].

HIV-2 infection at significant levels has also been reported in parts of southwestern India[136]. Of the HIV-positive serum samples from patients with sexually transmitted diseases in Bombay, 76% were reactive to HIV-1, 4% to HIV-2, and 20% to both viruses[137]. Goa, a former Portuguese colony, situated south of Bombay on the western coast, has reported 4.9% infection with HIV-2 and 9.8% infection with HIV-1 in sexually transmitted disease (STD) patients surveyed[138]. Further epidemiological data on the prevalence and distribution of HIV-1 and HIV-2 infections in other parts of India are still forthcoming. Significant HIV-2 infection has not been reported in other parts of Asia to date.

The detection and reporting of HIV-2 infection in countries outside of West Africa have been somewhat dependent on when HIV-2 testing was instituted as a public health measure and/or when research studies demonstrated significant rates. France was one of the first countries to institute HIV-2 testing in blood donors, and several HIV-2 cases were identified[139]. Of 75 HIV-2-infected persons studied in Paris, 58 were of African origin, 12 European, and five Caribbean[140]. In a survey from 1988 to 1993 of 15 611 people attending an anonymous test site in Paris, 0.07% HIV-2 infection was found compared to 0.23% HIV-1[141]. To a lesser degree, other European countries have reported sporadic cases of HIV-2 infection in large serosurveys, usually with a link to West Africa[115,142,143]. It is interesting to speculate that the relatively high rates of HIV-2 infection reported in France may be due to significant ties with former colonies in French West Africa.

In North America, only sporadic cases of HIV-2 infection have been reported. Of 17 HIV-2-infected persons detected through case reports by the Centers for Disease Control (CDC), 13 were West Africans[144]. An additional 15 HIV-2 cases were recognized in the USA through serological surveillance but the origins of the infected persons were not identified. Only one HIV-2-infected blood donor has been identified in the USA, indicating that HIV-2 infection is extremely rare in the US blood donor population[145].

Thus, the current data suggests that HIV-2 has been present in certain populations of West Africa for a long time in order to establish endemic infection, and its spread outside of these areas is limited by a low transmission potential. The potential association of HIV-2 geographic distribution with historical colonial ties and current links between diverse parts of the world are of interest. Data collected thus far indicates that areas of the world with significant migration of individuals from HIV-2 endemic areas should be high-priority areas for further surveillance efforts.

TRANSMISSION OF HIV-2

Our current understanding of HIV-2 biology and epidemiology suggests that HIV-2 can be transmitted by the same modes of transmission as HIV-1. Since most West African countries have been afflicted with both HIV-1 and HIV-2 infections, they provide the ideal setting for direct comparison of the behavior of the two viruses in human populations.

Rates of perinatal transmission of HIV-1 have ranged from 13% to 32% in Europe and the USA and from 25% to 48% in developing countries[146]. Although study of HIV-2 perinatal transmission has been more limited, ample data now shows that perinatal transmission of HIV-2 is less frequent than observed with HIV-1 infection. Early studies reported on the isolation of HIV-2 from infants born to HIV-2-infected mothers[147]. A family cluster has been reported in which a mother and two of her children were infected with HIV-2[148]. Cross-sectional studies noted that serological concordance between HIV-2-positive women and their children was rare and pediatric HIV-2 infection extremely uncommon[130,149,150]. All these findings point to the rarity of mother-to-child transmission.

Prospective studies of HIV-2 perinatal transmission have been conducted in Guinea Bissau, Ivory Coast, France and Senegal, all demonstrating extremely low rates of perinatal transmission of HIV-2, ranging from 0% to 3.4%[151–155]. In studies that compared HIV-2 and HIV-1 transmission, the rate of HIV-1 perinatal transmission was 10–20-fold higher than that of HIV-2[152–155].

The predominant route of HIV-2 spread in endemic areas is via heterosexual sex. Incidence trends of both HIV-1 and HIV-2 have been reported in registered female prostitutes in Dakar, Senegal, followed for a nine-year period[156]. Between 1985 and 1994, the overall incidence of HIV-2 was 0.92 per 100 person-years of observation (PYO), and was 1.15 per 100 PYO for HIV-1. Over the nine-year period, the annual incidence of HIV-1 dramatically increased, with a 1.4-fold increased risk per year and over 12–17-fold increase in risk over the entire study period. The incidence of HIV-2 remained stable despite higher HIV-2 prevalence. In this high-risk group, the heterosexual transmission of HIV-2 was significantly slower than that of HIV-1, which strongly suggests differences in the infectivity potential of these two related immunodeficiency viruses. Based on data from the same population, using mathematical modeling techniques, the efficiency of heterosexual transmission of HIV-2 has been estimated to range from five to nine times less than that of HIV-1 per sexual act with an infected partner[157].

Further analysis of the incidence trends of HIV-1 and HIV-2 in this high-risk cohort suggests another intriguing aspect of HIV-2 infection. The low and constant rate of HIV-2 infection in this high-risk population supports the hypothesis that HIV-2 has been in the population for some time and that its spread via sexual transmission is relatively constant. Epidemic curves that have demonstrated low plateau infection rates have been characteristically described in other infectious agents where transmission is inefficient and/or abortive infection can occur[158]. There is evidence supporting both hypotheses in the case of HIV-2 infection. The evidence of slower heterosexual and perinatal transmission of HIV-2 has been discussed previously. Unpublished observations from the same cohort study suggest that there are individuals that despite frequent exposure to HIV-2 remain seronegative. It is possible that some of these high-risk women have been exposed to the virus and somehow managed to clear the infection. Virological and host determinants of the immunity/resistance to HIV-2 infection have yet to be elucidated. Perhaps supportive of this hypothesis is the recent observation that three out of six HIV-negative female prostitutes from The Gambia demonstrated HIV-specific CTLs in the absence of evidence of viral infection by PCR or isolation[159].

Like HIV-1, HIV-2 infection can also be acquired by transfusion of blood or blood products. Currently, most countries have instituted blood bank screening for both HIV-1 and HIV-2. Thus, the risk of transmission by this route is thought to be greatly reduced and almost nil in non-endemic areas of the world.

HIV-2 PATHOGENESIS AND CLINICAL OUTCOME

Although HIV-2 can cause AIDS[160], it is now clear that it has a lower pathogenic potential than HIV-1. Studies of HIV-infected asymptomatic individuals followed over time have been critical to our understanding of HIV pathogenesis in people. The long latency of the HIV viruses has made such prospective studies lengthy and logistically difficult. Studies in Dakar, Senegal, have described the natural history of HIV-2 and HIV-1 over a nine-year period[108,161]. These studies are particularly unique, since the presence of both HIV-2 and HIV-1 in Senegal allowed the measurement and comparison of disease development for both viruses. Among the 103 HIV-2-infected women followed, one AIDS case was observed after 435 PYO. Kaplan–Meier analysis comparing HIV-2 and HIV-1 seroincident women showed a 60% AIDS-free survival for HIV-1 incident women, at five years post infection. In contrast, none of the HIV-2 seroincident women developed AIDS, therefore exhibiting a 100% probability of AIDS-free survival time after five years, a statistically significant difference (log rank test; p value=0.01). These differences in survival probabilities between HIV-2 and HIV-1 were also seen for CDC intravenous disease and $CD4^+$ lymphocyte counts below 400 cells/mm^3 as outcomes[161].

The natural history data suggests that the incubation period to immunological compromise is quite lengthy in HIV-2 infection. Once immunological compromise has occurred the course of HIV-2 infection may be more similar to that of HIV-1. However, prospective studies to address this aspect of the natural history of HIV-2 infection have been lacking[160]. A less aggressive course of HIV-2 infection is suggested by studies in Dakar, Senegal, where HIV-2 is predominant among asymptomatic people yet HIV-1 is more frequent among hospitalized patients with diagnosed AIDS[162]. In cross-sectional studies,similar, although less marked, immunological abnormalities were found in individuals infected with HIV-2 than those infected with HIV-1. $CD4^+$ lymphocyte counts and CD4/CD8 ratios appeared reduced in HIV-2-infected healthy carriers, but less dramatically than for HIV-1-infected carriers[108–110,162]. Similar results were observed with evaluation of delayed-type hypersensitivity as measured by skin test anergy to tuberculin ppd antigen[108,109].

At the population level, a large number of case reports and cross-sectional studies of hospitalized patients have described AIDS associated with HIV-2 infection[160,162,166]. In West African HIV-2 AIDS cases, disease characteristics have included tuberculosis, chronic diarrhea, and *Candida* infections similar to HIV-1-associated AIDS[162–166]. Central nervous system involvement has also been described in HIV-2-infected people[167,168]. The association of HIV-2 with various cancers has been addressed to a limited extent. In cross-sectional studies, rates of HIV-2 infection in patients with lymphoma and Kaposi sarcoma were not elevated compared with healthy population controls (unpublished data).

The conditions in most countries endemic for HIV-2 also favor infection by a variety of other infectious organisms, including tuberculosis, various protozoan parasites, helminths, viruses and bacteria. The reactivation of some of these agents or enhanced susceptibility as a result of HIV-2 immunosuppression is responsible for the spectrum of opportunistic diseases found in HIV-associated AIDS cases. The extreme immunosuppression as a result of prolonged survival with HIV infection, as is the case of HIV-2 infection, suggests a modified natural history for HIV-2, such that patients may survive longer in the terminal stage of HIV infection. In reality, this may not be the case, since people may die from malnutrition and other causes related to low socioeconomic and poor health status before they develop the full spectrum of AIDS pathogenicity.

In an autopsy study reported from the Ivory Coast, the autopsy findings in 294 HIV-infected patients were described[169]. Tuberculosis, bacteremia with a predominance of Gram-negative rods and cerebral toxoplasmosis were responsible for a significant proportion of all HIV-positive deaths. Forty-three cadavers were HIV-2 positive and 40 out of 43 (93%) had died of HIV-related disease. The pathologies in HIV-2-positive cadavers were similar to HIV-1-positive cadavers except for three conditions, including severe multi-organ cytomegalovirus (CMV) infection, multinucleate giant cell encephalitis and intra- or extra-hepatic cholangitis. All three lesions were associated with extreme immunosuppression, suggesting a prolonged survival with HIV infection. This data seems to indicate a modified natural history for HIV-2, such that patients may survive longer in the terminal stage of HIV infection.

HIV-2 PROTECTION FROM HIV-1 INFECTION

The low transmissibility and long AIDS-free survival time of HIV-2 have suggested the possibility that this related but less virulent virus might protect against subsequent infection by HIV-1. During a nine-year period in Dakar, Senegal, the seroincidence of both HIVs was measured in a cohort of female prostitutes[170]. For the 618 women initially HIV seronegative, 61 seroconverted to HIV-1; the overall HIV-1 incidence rate was 2.53/100 PYO. Among 187 women seropositive to HIV-2, seven women seroconverted to an HIV-dually reactive status. Seven of seven were PCR positive for both viruses, and all demonstrated seroconversion to both recombinant env type-specific proteins. The HIV-1 incidence rate in the HIV-2-positive group was 1.07/100 PYO—lower than the incidence rate among the HIV-seronegative group. A multivariate Poisson regression analysis included age, nationality, age at registration, incident gonorrhea, incident HIV-1 infection and calendar year. The multivariate analysis indicated a decrease in risk of HIV-1 infection associated with HIV-2 infection, with an adjusted relative risk of 0.32 (p=0.008), suggesting almost 70% protection. In the reverse analysis, HIV-1 did not show protection from subsequent HIV-2 infection. Further studies are clearly needed to understand the cross-protective mechanisms that may be involved in this interaction: nonetheless, the data suggests a novel mode of inducing HIV-1 immunity.

SUMMARY AND CONCLUSIONS

HIV-2 is a virus endemic to West Africa and regions of the world with close ties to West Africa and its former colonists. Despite its genetic relatedness to HIV-1 and various SIVs, the exact mechanism by which these viruses arose from presumed common ancestors is still only speculative. A number of important virological characteristics of HIV-2 are shared with those of HIV-1 but nonetheless the biology of this virus in people appears to be quite distinct. It is likely that virus and host immune factors play a role in the decreased transmissibility of the virus and the long incubation period to disease. From a biological standpoint, HIV-2 appears to behave as an 'attenuated'-type virus, and thus it is not surprising that it affords significant protection from HIV-1 infection. We still have much to learn about the biology and pathogenesis of HIV-2 infection. It seems clear that this virus infection can be considered a model for the long-term non-progressors seen in a small proportion of HIV-1-infected individuals. Further studies of the differences and cross-reactivities between the two viruses may help us identify correlates of HIV immunity that are so critical for HIV vaccine development. In conclusion, the continued comparative prospective research on HIV-2 and HIV-1 should provide us with important clues in the understanding of HIV pathogenesis and its ultimate control and prevention.

REFERENCES

1. Wong-Staal F. Human immunodeficiency viruses and their replication. In Fields BN, Knipe DM (eds) *Virology*. New York: Raven Press, 1990; pp. 1529–1543.
2. Gao F, Yue L, White AT *et al.* Human infection by genetically diverse SIV_{SM}-related HIV-2 in West Africa. *Nature* 1992; 358: 495–499.
3. Peeters M, Honore C, Huet T *et al.* Isolation and partial characterization of an HIV-related virus occurring naturally in chimpanzees in Gabon. *AIDS* 1989; 3: 625–630.
4. Myers G, Pavlakis GN. Evolutionary potential of complex retroviruses. In Levy J (ed.) *The Retroviridae*. New York: Plenum Press, 1992; pp. 1–37.
5. Essex M, Kanki P. The origins of the AIDS virus. *Sci Am* 1988; 259: 64–71.
6. Barin F, Mboup S, Denis F *et al.* Serological evidence for virus related to simian T-lymphotropic retrovirus III in residents of West Africa. *Lancet* 1986; ii: 1387–1389.
7. Essex M, Kanki P. Human immunodeficiency virus type 2 (HIV-2). In Broder S, Merigan T, Bolognesi D (eds) *Textbook of AIDS Medicine*. Baltimore: Williams & Wilkins, 1994; pp. 873–886.
8. Marlink R. The biology and epidemiology of HIV-2. In Essex M, Mboup S, Kanki P, Kalengayi M (eds) *AIDS in Africa*. New York: Raven Press, 1994; pp. 47–65.
9. Kanki PJ, De Cock KM. Epidemiology and natural history of HIV-2. *AIDS* 1994; 8: S1–9.
10. Hockley DJ, Wood RD, Jacobs PJ, Garrett AJ. Electron microscopy of human immunodeficiency virus. *J Gen Virol* 1988; 69: 2455–2469.
11. Yu Q-C, Ito S, Matsuda Z *et al.* Paranucleoid region of mature virions is a consistent difference between HIV-1 and HIV-2/SIV. *AIDS Res Hum Retroviruses* 1994; 6: 751–761.
12. Henderson LE, Sowder RC, Copeland TD *et al.* Gag precursors of HIV and SIV are cleaved into six proteins found in the mature virions. *J Med Primatol* 1990; 19: 411–419.
13. Kanki PJ, Mboup S, Ricard D *et al.* Human T-lymphotropic virus type 4 and the human immunodeficiency virus in West Africa. *Science* 1987; 236: 827–831.
14. Holzer TJ, Allen RG, Heynen CA *et al.* Discrimination of HIV-2 infection from HIV-1 infection by western blot and radioimmuno-precipitation analysis. *AIDS Res Hum Retroviruses* 1990; 6: 515–524.
15. De Cock KM, Porter A, Kouadia J *et al.* Cross-reactivity on western blots in HIV-1 and HIV-2 infections. *AIDS* 1991; 5: 859–863.
16. Hoxie JA. Hypothetical assignment of intrachain disulfide bonds for HIV-2 and SIV envelope glycoproteins. *AIDS Res Hum Retroviruses* 1991; 7: 495–499.
17. Guyader M, Emerman M, Sonigo P *et al.* Genome organization and transactivation of the human immunodeficiency virus type 2. *Nature* 1987; 326: 662–669.
18. Zagury JF, Franchini G, Reitz M *et al.* Genetic variability between isolates of human immunodeficiency virus (HIV) type 2 is comparable to the variability among HIV type 1. *Proc Natl Acad Sci USA* 1988; 85: 5941–5945.
19. Franchini G, Fargnoli KA, Giombini F *et al.* Molecular and biological characterization of a replication competent human immuno-deficiency type 2 (HIV-2) proviral clone. *Proc Natl Acad Sci USA* 1989; 86: 2433–2437.
20. Kuhnel H, von Briesen H, Dietrich U *et al.* Molecular cloning of two west African human immunodeficiency virus type 2 isolates that replicate well in macrophages: a Gambian isolate, from a patient with neurologic acquired immunodeficiency syndrome, and a highly divergent Ghanian isolate. *Proc Natl Acad Sci USA* 1989; 86: 2383–2387.
21. Hasegawa A, Tsujimoto H, Maki N *et al.* Genomic divergence of HIV-2 from Ghana. *AIDS Res Hum Retroviruses* 1989; 5: 593–604.

22. Boeri E, Giri A, Lillo F *et al.* In vivo genetic variability of the human immunodeficiency virus type 2 V3 region. *J Virol* 1992; 66: 4546–4550.
23. Kanki PJ. Virologic and biologic features of HIV-2. In Wormser GP (ed.) *AIDS and Other Manifestations of HIV Infection*. New York: Raven Press, 1992; pp. 85–93.
24. Sattentau QJ, Clapham PR, Weiss RA *et al.* The human and simian immunodeficiency viruses HIV-1, HIV-2 and SIV interact with similar epitopes on their cellular receptor, the CD4 molecule. *AIDS* 1988; 2: 101–105.
25. Clapham P, Webber JN, Whitby D *et al.* Soluble CD4 blocks and infectivity of diverse strains of HIV and SIV for T-cells and monocytes but not for brain and muscle cells. *Nature* 1989; 337: 368–370.
26. Looney D, Hayashi S, Nicklas M *et al.* Differences in the interaction of HIV-1 and HIV-2 with CD4. *J AIDS* 1990; 3: 619–657.
27. Moore JP. Simple methods for monitoring HIV-1 and HIV-2 gp120 binding to soluble CD4 by enzyme-linked immunosorbent assay: HIV-2 has a 25-fold lower affinity than HIV-1 for soluble CD4. *AIDS* 1990; 4: 297–305.
28. Hoxie JA, Brass LF, Pletcher CH *et al.* Cytopathic variants of an attenuated isolate of human immunodeficiency virus type 2 exhibit increased affinity for CD4. *J Virol* 1991; 65: 5096–5101.
29. Mulligan MJ, Ritter GD Jr, Chaikin MA *et al.* Human immuno-deficiency virus type 2 envelope glycoprotein: differential CD4 interactions of soluble gp120 versus the assembled envelope complex. *Virology* 1992; 187: 233–241.
30. Clapham PR, McKnight A, Weiss RA. Human immunodeficiency virus type 2 infection and fusion of CD4-negative human cell lines: induction and enhancement by soluble CD4. *J Virol* 1992; 66: 3531–3537.
31. Hart AR, Cloyd MW. Interference patterns of human immunodeficiency viruses HIV-1 and HIV-2. *Virology* 1990; 177: 1–10.
32. Le Guern M, Levy JA. Human immunodeficiency virus (HIV) type 1 can superinfect HIV-2-infected cells: pseudotype virions produced with expanded cellular host range. *Proc Natl Acad Sci USA* 1992; 89: 363–367.
33. Mulligan MJ, Yamshchikov GV, Ritter GD Jr *et al.* Cytoplasmic domain truncation enhances fusion activity by the exterior glycoprotein complex of human immunodeficiency virus type 2 in selected cell types. *J Virol* 1992; 66: 3971–3975.
34. Kong LI, Lee SW, Kappes JC *et al.* West African HIV-2-related human retrovirus with attenuated cytopathicity. *Science* 1988; 240: 1525–1529.
35. Johnston PB, Dubay JW, Hunter E. Truncations of the simian immunodeficiency virus transmembrane protein confer expanded virus host range by removing a block to virus entry into cells. *J Virol* 1993; 67: 3077–3086.
36. Kirchhoff F, Jentsch KD, Bachmann B *et al.* A novel proviral clone of HIV-2: biological and phylogenetic relationship to other primate immunodeficiency viruses. *Virology* 1990; 177: 305–311.
37. Franchini G, Gurgo C, Guo HG *et al.* Sequence of simian immuno-deficiency virus and its relationship to the human immuno-deficiency viruses. *Nature* 1987; 328: 539–543.
38. Freed EO, Myers DJ. Identification and characterization of fusion and processing domains of the human immunodeficiency virus type 2 envelope glycoprotein. *J Virol* 1992; 66: 5472–5478.
39. Steffy KR, Kraus G, Looney DJ, Wong-Staal F. Role of the fusogenic peptide sequence in syncytium induction and infectivity of human immunodeficiency virus type 2. *J Virol* 1992; 66: 4532–4535.
40. Robert-Guroff M, Aldrich K, Muldoon R. *et al.* Cross-neutralization of human immunodeficiency virus type 1 and 2 and simian immunodeficiency virus isolates. *J Virol* 1992; 66: 3602–3608.

41. Bjorling E, Broliden K, Bernardi D *et al.* Hyperimmune antisera against synthetic peptides representing the glycoprotein of human immunodeficiency virus type 2 can mediate neutralization and antibody-dependent cytotoxic activity. *Proc Natl Acad Sci USA* 1991; 88: 6082–6086.
42. Bjorling E, Chiodi F, Utter G, Norrby E. Two neutralizing domains in the V3 region of the envelope glycoprotein gp125 of HIV-2 type 2. *J Immunol* 1994; 152: 1952–1959.
43. Nixon DF, Huet S, Rothbard J *et al.* An HIV-1 and HIV-2 cross-reactive cytotoxic T-cell epitope. *AIDS* 1990; 4: 841–845.
44. Huang ML, Essex M, Lee TH. Localization of immunogenic domains in the human immunodeficiency virus type 2 envelope. *J Virol* 1991; 65: 5073–5079.
45. Mannervik M, Putkonen P, Ruden U *et al.* Identification of B-cell antigenic sites on HIV-2 gp125. *J AIDS* 1992; 5: 177–187.
46. Zuber M, Samuel KP, Lautenberger JA *et al.* Bacterially-produced HIV-2 env polypeptides specific for distinguishing HIV-2 from HIV-1 infections. *AIDS Res Hum Retroviruses* 1990; 6: 525–534.
47. Norrby E, Putkonen P, Bottiger B *et al.* Comparison of linear antigenic sites in the envelope proteins of human immunodeficiency virus (HIV) type 2 and type 1. *AIDS Res Hum Retroviruses* 1991; 7: 279–285.
48. Gnann JW Jr, McCormick JB, Mitchell S *et al.* Synthetic peptides immunoassay distinguishes HIV type 1 and HIV type 2 infections. *Science* 1987; 237: 1346–1349.
49. Henderson LE, Sowder RC, Copeland TD *et al.* Isolation and characterization of a novel protein (X-ORF product) from SIV and HIV-2. *Science* 1988; 241: 199–201.
50. Yu XF, Ito S, Essex M, Lee TH. A naturally immunogenic virion-associated protein specific for HIV-2 and SIV. *Nature* 1988; 335: 262–265.
51. Matsuda Z, Chou MJ, Matsuda M *et al.* Human immunodeficiency virus type 1 has an additional coding sequence in the central region of the genome. *Proc Natl Acad Sci USA* 1988; 85: 6968–6972.
52. Kappes JC, Morrow CD, Lee SW *et al.* Identification of a novel retroviral gene unique to human immunodeficiency virus type 2 and simian immunodeficiency virus SIVMAC. *J Virol* 1988; 62: 3501–3505.
53. Yu XF, Yu QC, Essex M, Lee TH. The vpx gene of simian immunodeficiency virus facilitates efficient viral replication in fresh lymphocytes and macrophage. *J Virol* 1991; 65: 5088–5091.
54. Kappes JC, Conway JA, Lee SW *et al.* Human immunodeficiency virus type 2 vpx protein augments viral infectivity. *Virology* 1991; 184: 197–209.
55. Lee TH, Coligan JE, Allan JS *et al.* A new HTLV-III/LAV protein encoded by a gene found in cytopathic retroviruses. *Science* 1986; 231: 1546–1549.
56. Gabuzda DH, Lawrence K, Langhoff E *et al.* Role of vif in replication of human immunodeficiency virus type 1 in CD4+ T lymphocytes. *J Virol* 1992; 66: 6489–6495.
57. Allan JS, Coligan JE, Lee TH *et al.* A new HTLV-III/LAV encoded antigen detected by antibodies from AIDS patients. *Science* 1985; 230: 810–813.
58. Cheng-Meyer C, Iannello P, Shaw K *et al.* Differential effects of nef on HIV replication: implications for viral pathogenesis in the host. *Science* 1989; 246: 1629–1632.
59. Kestler HW III, Ringler DJ, Mori K *et al.* Importance of the nef gene for maintenance of high virus loads and for development of AIDS. *Cell* 1991; 65: 651–662.
60. Yuan X, Matsuda Z, Matsuda M *et al.* Human immunodeficiency virus vpr gene encodes a virion-associated protein. *AIDS Res Hum Retroviruses* 1990; 6: 1265–1271.

61. Ogawa K, Shibata R, Kiyomasu T *et al.* Mutational analysis of the human immunodeficiency virus vpr open reading frame. *J Virol* 1989; 63: 4110–4114.
62. Hattori N, Michaels F, Fargnoli K *et al.* The human immunodeficiency virus type 2 vpr gene is essential for productive infection of human macrophages. *Proc Natl Acad Sci USA* 1990; 87: 8080–8084.
63. Levy DN, Refaeli Y, MacGregor RR, Weiner DB. Serum vpr regulates productive infection and latency of human immunodeficiency virus type 1. *Proc Natl Acad Sci USA* 1994; 91: 10873–10877.
64. Tristem M, Marshall C, Karpas A *et al.* Origin of vpx in lentiviruses. *Nature* 1990; 347: 341–342.
65. Arya SK. Human and simian immunodeficiency retroviruses: activation and differential transactivation of gene expression. *AIDS Res Hum Retroviruses* 1988; 4: 175–186.
66. Berkhout B, Gatignol A, Silver J, Jeang KT. Efficient trans-activation by the HIV-2 Tat protein requires a duplicated TAR RNA structure. *Nucleic Acids Res* 1990; 18: 1839–1846.
67. Chang YN, Jeang KT. The basic RNA-binding domain of HIV-2 Tat contributes to preferential trans-activation of TAR2-containing LTR. *Nucleic Acids Res* 1992; 20: 5465–5472.
68. Fenrick R, Melim MH, Hauber J *et al.* Functional analysis of the tat trans activator of human immunodeficiency virus type 2. *J Virol* 1989; 63: 5006–5012.
69. Arya SK, Beaver B, Jagodzinski L *et al.* New human and simian HIV-related retroviruses possess functional transactivator tat gene. *Nature* 1987; 328: 548–550.
70. Malim MH, Hauber J, Le S-Y *et al.* The HIV-1 Rev trans-activator acts through a structured target sequence to activate nuclear export of unspliced viral mRNA. *Nature* 1989; 338: 254–257.
71. Dillon PJ, Nelbock P, Perkins A, Rosen CA. Structural and functional analysis of the human immunodeficiency virus type 2 rev protein. *J Virol* 1991; 65: 445–449.
72. Lewis N, William J, Rekosh D, Hammarskjold M-L. Identification of a cis-acting element in human immunodeficiency virus type 2 HIV-2 that is responsive to the HIV-1 rev and human T-cell leukemia virus types I and IIrex proteins. *J Virol* 1990; 64: 1690–1697.
73. Yu XF, Matsuda M, Essex M, Lee TH. Open reading frame vpr of simian immunodeficiency virus encodes a virion-associated protein. *J Virol* 1990; 64: 5688–5693.
74. Arya S, Gallo C. Human immunodeficiency virus type 2 long terminal repeat: analysis of regulatory elements. *AIDS* 1988; 85: 9753–9757.
75. Courgnaud V, Laure F, Fultz PN *et al.* Genetic differences accounting for evolution and pathogenicity of simian immunodeficiency virus from a sooty mangabey after cross-species transmission to a pig-tailed macaque. *J Virol* 1992; 66: 414–419.
76. Markovitz D, Hannibal M, Perz V *et al.* Differential regulation of human immunodeficiency viruses (HIVs): specific regulatory element of HIV-2 responds to stimulation of the T-cell antigen receptor. *Proc Natl Acad Sci* 1990; 87: 9098–9102.
77. Tong-Starksen S, Welsh T, Peterlin M. Differences in transcriptional enhancers of HIV-1 and HIV-2 response to T-cell activation signals. *J Immunol* 1990; 145: 4348–4354.
78. Arya SK. Human immunodeficiency virus type 2 (HIV-2) gene expression: downmodulation by sequence elements downstream of the transcriptional initiation site. *AIDS Res Hum Retroviruses* 1991; 7: 1007–1014.
79. Hannibal MC, Markovitz DM, Clark N, Nabel GJ. Differential activation of human immunodeficiency virus type 1 and 2 transcription by specific T-cell activation signals. *J Virol* 1993; 67: 5035–5040.

80. Markovitz DM, Smith MJ, Hilfinger J *et al.* Activation of the human immunodeficiency virus type 2 enhancer is dependent on purine box and kappa B regulatory elements. *J Virol* 1992; 66: 5479–5484.
81. Castro BA, Barnett SW, Evans LA *et al.* Biologic heterogeneity of human immunodeficiency virus type 2 (HIV-2) strains. *Virology* 1990; 178: 527–534.
82. Albert J, Naucler A, Bottiger B *et al.* Replicative capacity of HIV-2, like HIV-1, correlates with severity of immunodeficiency. *AIDS* 1990; 4: 291–295.
83. Schulz TF, Whitby D, Hoad JG *et al.* Biological and molecular variability of human immunodeficiency virus type 2 isolates from The Gambia. *J Virol* 1990; 64: 5177–5182.
84. Simon F, Matheron S, Tamalet C *et al.* Cellular and plasma viral load in patients infected with HIV-2. *AIDS* 1993; 7: 1411–1417.
85. Kumar P, Hui HX, Kappes JC *et al.* Molecular characterization of an attenuated human immunodeficiency virus type 2 isolate. *J Virol* 1990; 64: 890–901.
86. Fenyo EM, Albert J, Asjo B. Replicative capacity, cytopathic effect and cell tropism of HIV. *AIDS* 1989; 3(Suppl. 1):S5–12.
87. Tersmette M, De Goede RE, Al BJ *et al.* Differential syncytium-inducing capacity of human immunodeficiency virus isolates: frequent detection of syncytium-inducing isolates in patients with acquired immunodeficiency syndrome (AIDS) and AIDS-related complex. *J Virol* 1988; 62: 2026–2032.
88. Schuitemaker H, Koot M, Kootstra NA *et al.* Biological phenotype of human immunodeficiency virus type 1 clones at different stages of infection: progression of disease is associated with a shift from monocytotropic to T-cell-tropic virus population. *J Virol* 1992; 66: 1354–1360.
89. Sankalé J-L, Sallier de la Tour R, Renjifo B *et al.* Intra-patient variability of the human immunodeficiency virus Type-2 (HIV-2) envelope V3 loop. *AIDS Res Hum Retroviruses* 1995; 11: 617–623.
90. Parkman PD. *Recommendations for the prevention of human immunodeficiency virus (HIV) transmission by blood and blood products* (Memorandum to all registered blood establishments). Bethesda, MD: Food and Drug Administration, Center for Biologics Evaluation and Research, 1990.
91. Anonymous, AIDS: recommendations for interpretation of HIV-2 western blot results. *Who Weekly Epidemiol Rec* 1990; 65: 74–75.
92. Baillou A, Barin F, Leonard G *et al.* Competitive enzyme-immunoassays using native viral antigens to discriminate between HIV-1 and HIV-2 infections. *J Virol Methods* 1990; 29: 81–89.
93. Urabe T, Sano K, Nakano T *et al.* Differentiation between human immunodeficiency virus type 1 (HIV-1) and HIV-2 isolates by nonradioisotopic reverse transcriptase-typing assay. *J Clin Microbiol* 1994; 32: 1870–1875.
94. Grankvist O, Bredberg-Raden U, Gustafsson A *et al.* Improved detection of HIV-2 DNA in clinical samples using a nested primer-based polymerase chain reaction. *J AIDS* 1990; 5: 286–293.
95. Peeters M, Gershy-Damet GM, Fransen K *et al.* Virological and polymerase chain reaction studies of HIV-1/HIV-2 dual infection in Cote d'Ivoire. *Lancet* 1992; 340: 339–340.
96. Rayfield M, De Cock K, Heyward W *et al.* Mixed human immunodeficiency virus (HIV) infection in an individual: demonstration of both HIV type 1 and type 2 proviral sequence by using polymerase chain reaction. *J Infect Dis* 1988; 158: 1170–1176.
97. Berry N, Ariyoshi K, Jobe O *et al.* HIV type 2 proviral load measured by quantitative polymerase chain reaction correlates with CD4+ lymphopenia in HIV type 2-infected individuals. *AIDS Res Hum Retroviruses* 1994; 10: 1031–1037.

98. Tedder RS, O'Connor T, Hughs A *et al.* Envelope cross-reactivity in western blot for HIV-1 and HIV-2 may not indicate dual infection. *Lancet* 1988; ii: 927–930.
99. Evans LA, Moreau J, Odehouri K *et al.* Simultaneous isolation of HIV-1 and HIV-2 from an AIDS patient. *Lancet* 1988; ii: 1389–1391.
100. Gueye-Ndiaye A, Clark RJ, Samuel KP *et al.* Cost-effective diagnosis of HIV-1 and HIV-2 by recombinant-expressed env peptide (566/966) dot blot analysis. *AIDS* 1993; 7: 475–481.
101. Dieng-Sarr A, Mboup S, Kanki PJ *et al.* Dual HIV infection in most individuals with serologic profiles reactive to HIV-1 and HIV-2. Submitted.
102. Weiss RA, Clapham PR, Weber JN *et al.* HIV-2 antisera cross-neutralize HIV-1. *AIDS* 1987; 2: 95–100.
103. Bottiger B, Karlsson A, Andreasson PA *et al.* Cross-neutralizing antibodies against HIV-1 (HTLV-IIIB and HTLV-IIIRF) and HIV-2 (SBL-6669 and a new isolate SBL-K135). *AIDS Res Hum Retroviruses* 1989; 5: 525–533.
104. Fenyo EM. Antigenic variation of primate lentirviruses in humans and experimentally infected macaques. *Immunol Rev* 1994; 140: 131–146.
105. Norley SG, Mikschy U, Werner A *et al.* Demonstration of cross-reactive antibodies able to elicit lysis of both HIV-1- and HIV-2-infected cells. *J Immunol.* 1990; 145: 1700–1705.
106. Ariyoshi K, Cham F, Berry N *et al.* HIV-2-specific cytotoxic T-lymphocyte activity is inversely related to proviral load. *AIDS* 1995; 9: 555–559.
107. Gotch F, McAdam SN, Allsopp CEM *et al.* Cytotoxic T cells in HIV-2 seropositive Gambians. *J Immunol* 1993; 151: 3361–3369.
108. Marlink R, Ricard D, Mboup S *et al.* Clinical, hematologic, and immunologic cross-sectional evaluation of individuals exposed to human immunodeficiency virus type 2 (HIV-2). *AIDS Res Hum Retroviruses* 1988; 4: 137–148.
109. Kestens L, Brattegaard K, Adjorlolo G *et al.* Immunological comparison of HIV-1-, HIV-2 and dually-reactive women delivering in Abidjan, Cote d'Ivoire. *AIDS* 1992; 6: 803–807.
110. Whittle H, Egboga A, Todd J *et al.* Clinical and laboratory predictors of survival in Gambian patients with symptomatic HIV-1 or HIV-2 infection. *AIDS* 1992; 6: 685–689.
111. Pepin J, Dunn D, Gaye I *et al.* HIV-2 infection among prostitutes working in The Gambia: association with serological evidence of genital ulcer diseases and generalized lymphadenopathy. *AIDS* 1991; 5: 69–75.
112. Chollet-Martin S, Simon F, Matheron S *et al.* Comparison of plasma cytokine levels in African patients with HIV-1 and HIV-2 infection. *AIDS* 1994; 8: 879–884.
113. Korber B, Kanki P, Barin F *et al.* Genetic and antigenic variability in different HIV-2 viral isolates. *IVth International Conference on AIDS and Associated Cancers in Africa*, Marseille, October 1989 (Abstract 329).
114. Denis F, Barin F, Gershey-Damet G *et al.* Prevalence of human T-lymphotropic retroviruses type III (HIV) and type IV in Ivory Coast. *Lancet* 1987; i: 408–411.
115. De Cock KM, Brun-Vezinet F. Epidemiology of HIV-2. *AIDS* 1989; 3: S89–95.
116. Kanki P, Mboup S, Marlink R *et al.* Prevalence and risk determinants of human immunodeficiency virus type 2 (HIV-2) and human immunodeficiency virus type 1 (HIV-1) in West African female prostitutes. *Am J Epidemiol* 1992; 136: 895–907.
117. Del Mistro A, Chotard J, Mali AJ *et al.* HIV-1 and HIV-2 seroprevalence rates in mother–child pairs living in The Gambia, West Africa. *J AIDS* 1992; 5: 19–24.
118. Harrison L, Da Silva APJ, Gayle H *et al.* Risk factors for HIV-2 infection in Guinea–Bissau. *J AIDS* 1991; 4: 1155–1160.
119. Mabey DC, Tedder RS, Hughes AS *et al.* Human retroviral infections in The Gambia: prevalence and clinical features. *Br Med J* 1988; 296: 83–86.

120. Ankrah TC, Roberts MA, Antwi P *et al.* The African AIDS case definition and HIV serology in medical in-patients at Komfo Anokye Teaching Hospital, Kumasi, Ghana. *West Afr J Med* 1994; 13: 98–101.
121. Olaleye OD, Bernstein L, Ekweozor CC *et al.* Prevalence of human immunodeficiency virus types 1 and 2 infections in Nigeria. *J Infect Dis* 1993; 167: 710–714.
122. Kline RL, Dada A, Blattner W, Quinn TC. Diagnosis and differentiation of HIV-1 and HIV-2 infection by two rapid assays in Nigeria. *J AIDS* 1994; 7: 623–626.
123. Maiga YI, Sissoko Z, Maiga MA. Etude de la séroprevalence de l'Infection à VIH dans les 7 régions économiques du Mali (Abstract). *VIIIth International Conference on AIDS and Associated Cancers in Africa/VIIIth African Conference on Sexually Transmitted Diseases*, Marrakech, December 1993.
124. Koffi K, Gershey-Damet GM, Peeters M *et al.* Rapid spread of HIV infections in Abidjan, Ivory Coast, 1987–1990. *Eur J Clin Microbiol Infect Dis* 1992; 11: 271–273.
125. Kanki PJ, Allan J, Barin F *et al.* Absence of antibodies to HIV-2/HTLV-4 in six central African nations. *AIDS Res Hum Retroviruses* 1987; 3: 317–322.
126. Saal F, Sidibe S, Alves-Cardoso E *et al.* Anti HIV-2 serological screening in Portuguese populations native from or having had close contact with Africa. *AIDS Res Hum Retroviruses* 1987; 3: 341–342.
127. Santos-Ferreira MO, Cohen T, Lourenco MH *et al.* A study of seroprevalence of HIV-1 and HIV-2 in six provinces of People's Republic of Angola: clues to the spread of HIV infection. *J AIDS* 1990; 3: 780–786.
128. Mota-Miranda A, Gomes MH, Sarmento R *et al.* HIV-2 infection in the north of Portugal (Abstract). *IXth International Conference on AIDS*, Berlin, June 1993.
129. Centro de vigilancia epidemioloca das doencas transmissiveis sindrome de immunodeficiencia adquirida. A situacao em Portugal em 30 de Junho de 1992. In Machado Caetano J, Bandeira Costa J, Champalimaud J *et al.* (eds) Lisbon: Instituto Nacional de Saude, 1992.
130. Soriano V, Gutierrez M, Fernandez JL *et al.* HIV-2 infection in Spain: report of the first 34 cases. *AIDS* 1992; 6: 1222–1223.
131. Martin R, Machedo F, Menedez J, Zamora F. Study for the detection of antibodies and follow-up of seropositive subjects to HIV and AIDS patients (Abstract). *IXth International Conference on AIDS*, San Francisco, June 1990.
132. Veronesi R, Mazza CC, Santos Ferreira MO, Lourenco MH. HIV-2 in Brazil. *Lancet* 1987; ii: 402.
133. Cortes E, Detels R, Aboulafia D *et al.* HIV-1, HIV-2, and HTLV-1 infection in high-risk groups in Brazil. *N Engl J Med* 1989; 320: 9538.
134. Hendry RM, Parks DE, Campos Mello DLA *et al.* Lack of evidence for HIV-2 infection among at-risk individuals in Brazil. *J AIDS* 1991; 4: 623–627.
135. Pieniazek D, Peralta JM, Ferreira JA *et al.* Identification of mixed HIV-1/HIV-2 infections in Brazil by polymerase chain reaction. *AIDS* 1991; 5: 1293–1299.
137. Pfutzner A, Dietrich U, Von Eichel U *et al.* HIV-1 and HIV-2 infections in a high-risk population in Bombay, India: evidence for the spread of HIV-2 and presence of a divergent HIV-1 subtype. *J AIDS* 1992; 5: 972–977.
138. Rubsamen-Waigmann H, Maniar J, Gerte S *et al.* High proportion of HIV-2 and HIV-1/2 double-reactive sera in two Indian states, Maharashtra and Goa: first appearance of an HIV-2 epidemic along with an HIV-1 epidemic outside of Africa. *Int J Med Microbiol Virol Parasitol Infect Dis* 1994; 280: 398–402.
140. Matheron S, Simon F, Sassi G *et al.* Infection HIV-2 chez l'adulte: étude de cohorte; Paris 1986–1993 (Abstract). *VIIIth International Conference on AIDS and Associated Cancers in Africa/VIIIth African Conference on Sexually Transmitted Diseases*, Marrakech, December 1993.

141. Mazeron MC, Cerboni J, Alain S *et al.* Prevalence of HIV infections among patients attending a Parisian anonymous testing center between 1988 and 1993. *Pathol Biol (Paris)* 1994; 42: 530–532.
142. Kanki P, Marlink R, Siby T *et al.* Biology of HIV-2 infection in West Africa. In Papas TS (ed.) *Gene Regulation and AIDS*. Houston: Portfolio, 1990; pp. 255–271.
143. Smallman-Raynor M, Cliff A. The spread of human immunodeficiency virus type 2 into Europe: a geographical analysis. *Int J Epidemiol* 1991; 20: 480–489.
144. O'Brien TR, George JR, Holmberg SD. Human immunodeficiency virus type 2 infection in the United States: epidemiology, diagnosis, and public health implications. *JAMA* 1992; 267: 2775–2779.
145. Centers for Disease Control. Surveillance for HIV-2 infection in blood donors: United States, 1987–1989. *MMWR* 1990; 39: 829.
146. Mofenson LM. Epidemiology and determinants of vertical HIV transmission. *Semin Pediatr Infect Dis* 1994; 5: 252–258.
147. Matheron S, Courpotin C, Simon F *et al.* Vertical transmission of HIV-2. *Lancet* 1990; 335: 1103–1104.
148. Gnaore E, De Cock KM, Gayle H *et al.* Prevalence mortality from HIV type 2 in Guinea Bissau, West Africa. *Lancet* 1989; ii: 513.
149. Poulsen AG, Kvinesdal BB, Aaby P *et al.* Lack of evidence of vertical transmission of human immunodeficiency virus type 2 in a sample of the general population in Bissau. *J AIDS* 1992; 5: 25–30.
150. Gayle H, Gnaore E, Adjorlolo G *et al.* HIV-1 and HIV-2 infection in children in Abidjan, Cote D'Ivoire. *J AIDS* 1992; 5: 513–517.
151. Andreasson PA, Dias F, Naucler A *et al.* A prospective study of vertical transmission of HIV-2 in Bissau, Guinea-Bissau. *AIDS* 1993; 7: 989–993.
152. Adjorlolo-Johnson G, De Cock KM, Ekpini E *et al.* Prospective comparison of mother-to-child transmission of HIV-1 and HIV-2 in Abidjan, Ivory Coast. *JAMA* 1994; 272: 481–486.
153. Anonymous. Comparison of vertical human immunodeficiency virus type 2 and human immunodeficiency virus type 1 transmission in the French prospective cohort. The HIV Infection in Newborns French Collaborative Study Group. *Pediatr Infect Dis J* 1994; 13: 502–506.
154. Ngagne-Mbay, Diouf A, Kebe F *et al.* Histoire naturelle de la transmission verticale VIH1 et VIH2 à Dakar (Abstract). *VIIIth International Conference on AIDS and Associated Cancers in Africa/VIIIth African Conference on Sexually Transmitted Diseases*, Marrakech, December 1993.
155. Abbott RC, Ndour-Sarr A, Diouf A *et al.* Risk determinants for HIV infection and adverse obstetrical outcomes in pregnant women in Dakar, Senegal. *J AIDS* 1994; 7: 711–717.
156. Kanki PJ, Travers K, Mboup S *et al.* Slower heterosexual spread of HIV-2 than HIV-1. *Lancet* 1994; 343: 943–946.
157. Donnelly C, Leisenring W, Kanki P *et al.* Comparison of transmission rates of HIV-1 and HIV-2 in a cohort of prostitutes in Senegal. *Bull Math Biol* 1993; 55: 731–741.
158. Anderson RM, May RM. Vaccination and herd immunity to infectious disease. *Nature* 1985; 318: 323–329.
159. Rowland-Jones S, Sutton J, Ariyoshi K *et al.* HIV-specific cytotoxic T-cells in HIV-exposed but uninfected Gambian women. *Nature Med* 1995; 1: 59–64.
160. Romieu I, Marlink R, Kanki P *et al.* HIV-2 link to AIDS in West Africa. *J AIDS* 1990; 3: 220–230.
161. Marlink R, Kanki P, Thior I *et al.* Reduced virulence of HIV-2 compared to HIV-1. *Science* 1994; 265: 1587–1590.

162. Le Guenno BM, Barabe P, Griffet PA *et al.* HIV-2 and HIV-1 AIDS cases in Senegal: clinical patterns and immunological perturbations. *J AIDS* 1991; 4: 421–427.
163. Clavel F, Guetard D, Brun-Vezinet F *et al.* Isolation of a new human retrovirus from West African patients with AIDS. *Science* 1986; 233: 343–346.
164. Saimot AG, Coulaud JP, Mechali D *et al.* HIV-2/LAV-2 in Portuguese man with AIDS (Paris, 1978) who had served in Angola in 1968–74. *Lancet*. 1987; i: 688.
165. Naucler A, Albino P, Da Silva AP *et al.* HIV-2 infection in hospitalized patients in Bissau, Guinea Bissau. *AIDS* 1991; 5: 301–304.
166. De Cock KM, Odehouri K, Colebunders R *et al.* A comparison of HIV-1 and HIV-2 infections in hospitalized patients in Abidjan, Cote d'Ivoire. *AIDS* 1990; 4: 443–448.
167. Schneider J, Luke W, Kirchhoff F *et al.* Isolation and characterization of HIV-2 obtained from a patient with predominantly neurological defects. *AIDS* 1990; 4: 455–457.
168. Dwyer DE, Matheron S, Bakchine S *et al.* Detection of human immunodeficiency virus type 2 in brain tissue. *J Infect Dis* 1992; 166: 888–891.
169. Lucas SB, Hounnou A, Peacock A *et al.* The mortality and pathology of HIV infection in a West African city. *AIDS* 1993; 7: 1569–1579.
170. Travers K, Mboup S, Marlink R *et al.* Natural protections against HIV-1 infection provided by HIV-2. *Science* 1995; 268: 1612–1615.

5

The Biology of AIDS

George N. Pavlakis

ABL-Basic Research Program, NCI-FCRDC, Frederick, Maryland, USA

Acquired immunodeficiency syndrome (AIDS) is caused by the human immunodeficiency virus type 1 (HIV-1), a retrovirus identified 12 years ago[1,2]. Soon after, it was shown that HIV-1 is similar to other lentiviruses[3,4]. Lentiviruses are exogenous, non-oncogenic retroviruses causing chronic active infections leading to diseases with long incubation periods. These viruses usually infect cells of the immune system (macrophages, T-cells) and cause cytopathic effects such as syncytia and cell death in permissive cells. Lentiviral infections are not usually cleared by the immune system.

Due to intense studies of the last decade, HIV-1 has emerged as the prototype lentivirus, for which we have the most detailed information. The accumulated knowledge makes HIV-1 the most studied virus in the history of mankind. This has made HIV-1 an important scientific tool, and has implications for the understanding of the biology and pathogenesis of AIDS, other viral diseases, as well as the function of the immune system.

As a retrovirus, HIV has all the characteristics of this large group of viruses (Figure 5.1). It possesses a dimeric RNA genome, which is identical in nucleotide sequence to the viral mRNA. This RNA genome is transcribed by the viral enzyme reverse transcriptase (RNA-dependent DNA polymerase) into DNA (proviral DNA), which is transported to the nucleus of the infected cell and is integrated into the host genome. This is a unique property of retroviruses, which allows them to remain associated with the host genome. After integration, the DNA provirus has all the characteristics of cellular genes and is transcribed back to RNA using the cellular machinery. There-

AIDS and Malignancies: Current Concepts and Perspectives.
Edited by B.C. Golematis and V.T. DeVita Jr published 1996 John Wiley & Sons Ltd.

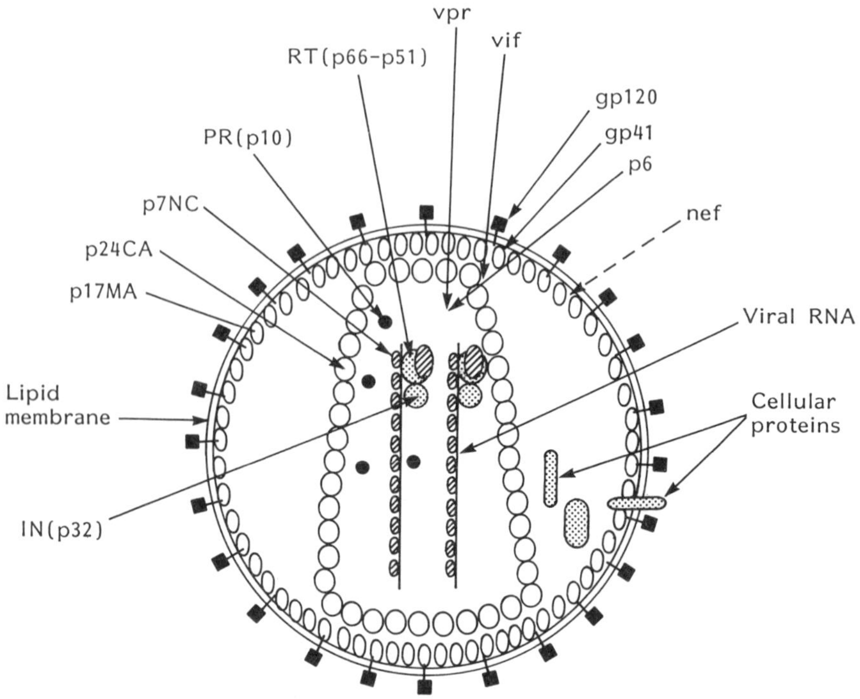

Figure 5.1 *HIV-1 virion structure*

fore, the study of HIV biology is closely associated to the study of gene expression and regulation of the human host. In this chapter we will outline the genome organization and life cycle of HIV-1, and the multiple interactions with the host, which eventually lead to viral pathogenesis and AIDS.

GENOME ORGANIZATION

The genome organization of lentiviruses reflects their needs. Compared to the other retroviruses, the lentiviruses have more genes and are able to regulate their own expression via viral factors. In addition, they carry genes (named accessory genes) that modify the host cell in specific ways. The genomic organization of HIV-1, the prototype lentivirus, is compared to the oncoretrovirus murine leukemia virus (MuLV) in Figure 5.2.

The viral genome found in the integrated state (DNA provirus) is flanked by the long terminal repeats (LTR) containing the signals for transcription initiation and polyadenylation. The three invariable structural genes encoding the components of the virion and the viral enzymes necessary for

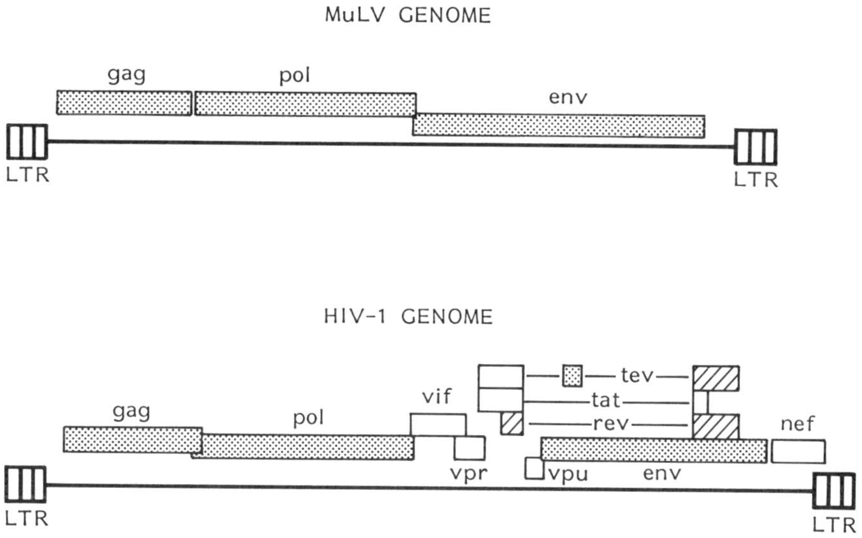

Figure 5.2 *Genomic organization of HIV-1 lentivirus and of type C MuLV oncoretrovirus*

retroviral replication (gag, pol, and env) are arranged similarly to all other retroviruses.

The two regulatory proteins, Tat and Rev, found in all lentiviruses, promote transcriptional and post-transcriptional activation of viral gene expression, respectively, and are essential for viral propagation. The accessory proteins Nef, Vif, Vpr and Vpu are dispensable in many instances *in vitro*, but are important for virus replication or pathogenicity *in vivo*. It appears that most and probably all accessory gene products are included in the virion, in contrast to the regulatory proteins Tat and Rev, which have not been found in the virion. The role of these proteins in the virion is not known. One hypothesis is that they do not have any structural role but they act early after infection to modify the newly infected cell. Alternatively, or in addition, they may modify the virion in ways that improve infectivity.

VIRAL mRNA EXPRESSION

To express the different viral proteins, HIV-1 generates several mRNAs from the genomic mRNA through alternative splicing[5–12]. The mRNAs are distinguished in three size groups: genomic (unspliced), intermediate (singly spliced) and small (multiply spliced) mRNAs (Figure 5.3). For regulatory purposes, these mRNAs can be divided into two groups: the unspliced and the intermediate-spliced mRNAs that contain the Rev responsive element

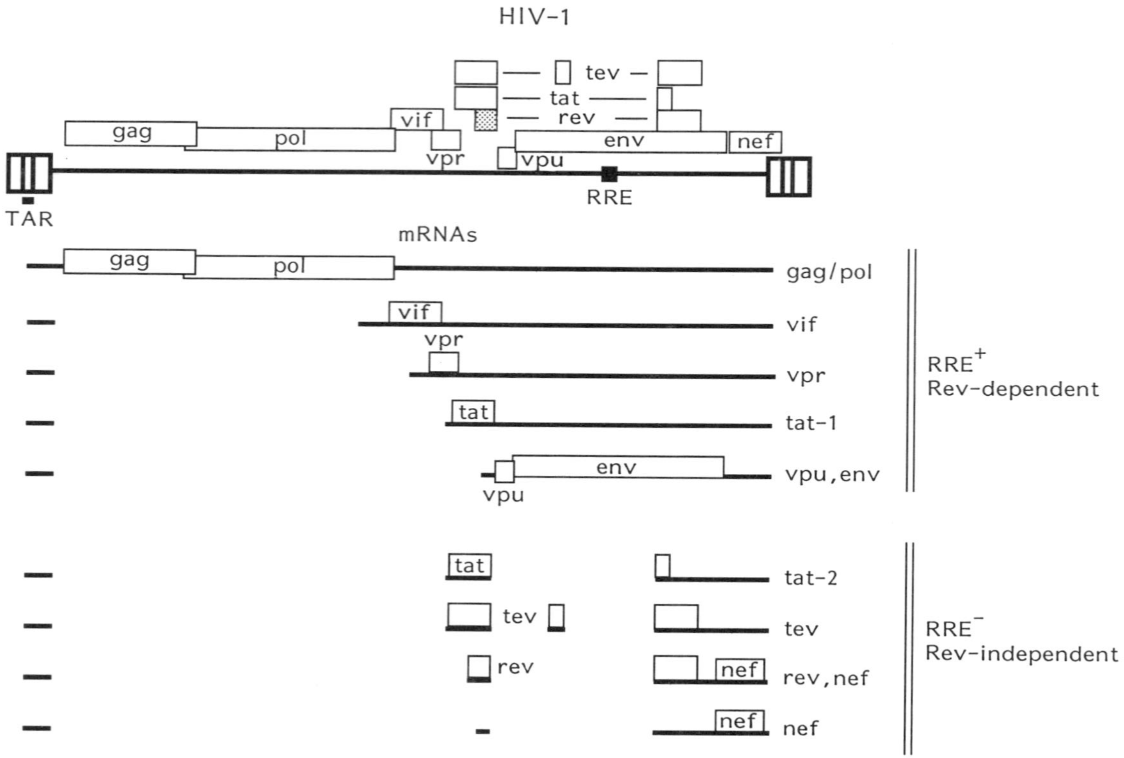

Figure 5.3 *Representative types of mRNAs produced by HIV-1. The mRNAs are distinguished in three size classes (unspliced, partially spliced or intermediate, and multiply spliced) and two functional groups, according to Rev regulation (Rev-dependent and Rev-independent)*

(RRE), and the multiply spliced mRNAs that lack the RRE. The unspliced (encoding Gag/Pol) and the intermediate-spliced mRNAs (encoding Vif, Vpr, and Vpu/Env) cannot be expressed in the absence of the viral Rev protein. Therefore, Rev is essential for HIV-1 replication[13,14]. In contrast, there is no restriction for expression of the multiply spliced mRNAs encoding Tat, Rev, and Nef. Rev binds to RRE and regulates expression of the RRE-containing viral mRNAs at the post-transcriptional level. This is the only essential role of Rev in the viral life cycle in cultured cells, since Rev regulation can be replaced by cellular analogs interacting with other post-transcriptional control elements [15,16]. The total number of individual HIV-1 mRNAs is more than 30. All these differentially spliced mRNAs encode viral proteins. Analysis of expression of isolated mRNAs has identified the mRNAs producing each protein and has led to the discovery of both monocistronic and bicistronic messages[11]. HIV-1 and the other lentiviruses use several strategies to express many proteins (in the case of HIV-1 at least 11) from one primary transcript: alternative splicing, ribosomal frame-shifting and bicistronic mRNAs. It is interesting that production of the abundant HIV-1 Env protein is directed by bicistronic vpu/env mRNAs where env is the second or third reading frame[11,17].

The expression of HIV-1 Env is coordinated with expression of Vpu. This accessory protein is important for Env trafficking. Therefore, the mRNA organization reflects the necessities of the viral life cycle.

HIV-1 LIFE CYCLE, VIRUS–CELL INTERACTIONS

The mature HIV-1 virion infects human cells primarily by binding to the CD4 receptor. CD4 is an important surface marker in lymphocytes and monocytes. Alternative HIV-1 receptors have been found, and accessory molecules for viral entry in addition to the CD4 receptor have been postulated. Binding of Env to the CD4 leads to fusion of the viral and plasma membranes and to internalization of the virus core. This process does not take place in mouse cells even when engineered to express the human CD4 receptor, indicating that additional factors are required for viral internalization.

CD4 contributes to T-cell recognition of foreign antigens in the context of class II major histocompatibility complex (MHC) determinants. Specific activation of T-cells by antigen presentation induces the CD4-TCR cointernalization. CD4 is associated with tyrosine protein kinase $p56^{lck}$. Signal transduction through the CD4 receptor involves the activation of $p56^{lck}$. CD4 interaction with Env leads to CD4 dysregulation. The importance of the Env–CD4 interaction for HIV is underscored by the multiple mechanisms that lead to CD4 modulation. HIV-1 has developed multiple mechanisms for CD4 downregulation, involving Env, Vpu, and Nef proteins.

Virus internalization leads in turn to reverse transcription in the cytoplasm.

Reverse transcription takes place within a ribonucleoprotein particle that contains, in addition to the viral RNA and the viral enzymes reverse transcriptase and integrase, several other HIV-1 proteins including p17gag and Vpr. These additional proteins are considered important for the import of the viral DNA into the cell nucleus. This is an active process in lentiviruses, while the other retroviruses require the elimination of nuclear membrane during mitosis to obtain access to the nuclear DNA. One important property of lentiviruses is that they can infect non-dividing cells. This property is unique among retroviruses and is considered important for virus transmission to the host via non-dividing cells in the vaginal and rectal mucosa.

After nuclear import, the viral DNA integrates into the host chromosome by the aid of the viral integrase, and from this point on behaves as a cellular gene using mostly cellular factors for its transcription and translation. Another characteristic difference between the lentiviruses and most other retroviruses is that two conserved viral regulatory factors, Tat and Rev, participate in the regulation of viral expression at the transcriptional and post-transcriptional level, respectively. The transcription of HIV-1 is governed by factors sensitive to the activation state of the lymphoid cells, primarily NF-kB. It has been shown that HIV-1 may stay dormant in resting T-cells, although the importance of the latent stage in the virus life cycle and pathogenicity is debated. After transcription, the viral mRNAs encoding the regulatory proteins Tat and Rev, as well as Nef, are expressed efficiently. This leads to a great transactivation of the viral promoter by Tat and to the transport and efficient expression of the unspliced and partially spliced mRNAs by Rev.

Expression of the viral structural proteins at high levels leads to particle formation at the plasma membrane. Two molecules of viral unspliced RNA are incorporated per virion. The maturing particle buds through the plasma membrane and is released to the medium. During assembly the viral components interact in an orderly and specific way with each other and with several cellular proteins. Among them are molecular chaperones such as cyclophilin A, which interacts with Gag and is incorporated in the virion. Several other cellular proteins have been found in purified virions, whose role remains to be determined.

HIV-1 AND MALIGNANCIES

Many AIDS patients develop malignancies of various types. To date, the precise role of HIV-1 infection in the generation of these malignancies is not fully elucidated. Clearly, the development of immunodeficiency is a major mechanism for the development of malignancies due to the inability of the immune system to eliminate them. In addition, other viral infections clearly participate in the development of malignancies in AIDS patients. Recently, the identification of a candidate etiological agent for Kaposi's sarcoma (KS) has generated much interest[18,19]. This agent, a new gamma human herpesvirus (HHV-8 or KSHV), has been found in KS patients, while it remains to be determined whether infection by this virus is widespread in the human population. The recent development of culture systems for this herpesvirus will aid the development of diagnostic and therapeutic modalities. To date, HIV-8 is implicated in the development of KS, Castleman's disease, and body cavity-based B lymphoma (primary effusion lymphoma[20–22].

FUNCTIONS OF VIRAL PROTEINS

Gag Proteins

The core viral particle of HIV-1 is formed by the Gag precursor $Pr55^{gag}$, a self-associating protein capable of assembling into virion-like particles without the requirement of any other viral factors. In addition to Gag precursor, a Gag–pol fusion protein ($Pr160^{gag\text{-}pol}$) is produced by ribosomal frame-shifting and is incorporated in the virion. $Pr160^{gag\text{-}pol}$ contains the precursors for the mature viral enzymes reverse transcriptase (RT), integrase (IN), and protease (PR). The viral PR is activated after assembly by dimerization and the Gag precursor is cleaved into four proteins (matrix ($p17^{MA}$), capsid ($p24^{CA}$), nucleocapsid ($p7^{NC}$), and $p6^{gag}$) and two small peptides, $p1^{gag}$ and $p2^{gag}$ (Figure 5.4).

In addition to the viral protease, cellular enzymes also interact with Gag. Proteolytic cleavage, myristylation, and phosphorylation of the Gag precursor are essential steps in the viral life cycle. An essential myristyl group (Myr) is attached to the amino group of Gly2 of the Gag precursor by cellular enzymes. $p17^{MA}$ and $p24^{CA}$ are phosphorylated by cellular kinases. $p7^{NC}$ binds two zinc ions to form the two zinc fingers of the NC domain, which are necessary for protein–RNA interactions. Gag interacts with additional cellular factors, which are essential for formation of infectious virions, such as cyclophilin A[23], a peptidyl-prolyl *cis–trans* isomerase thought to play a role in immune regulation. Mutation of the cyclophilin A binding domain results in non-infectious viral particles[24,25]. Cyclosporin and cyclosporin analogs disrupt the binding of cyclophilin A to Gag and inhibit HIV-1 replication. In contrast, a cyclosporin analog was shown to be inactive against SIVmac, which does not incorporate cyclophilin A[25].

Mature Gag Proteins

Matrix

Matrix (MA) is responsible for the association of Gag with the plasma membrane due to myristylation, and it also plays a role in the transport of the

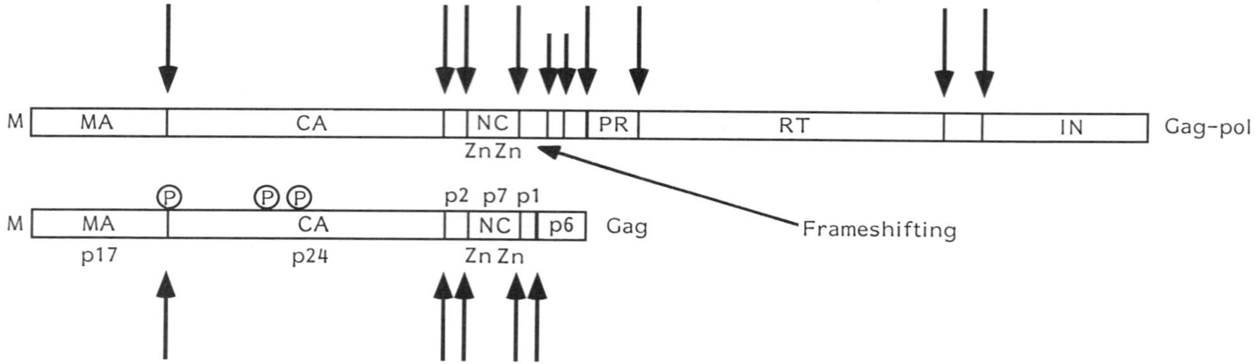

Figure 5.4 *Organization and protease cleavage of the HIV-1 gag/pol polyproteins*

pre-integration complex to the nucleus[26]. A nuclear localization signal (NLS) has been proposed within the MA protein[27]. The MA protein detected in the nucleus is phosphorylated, whereas the MA protein in the virion is not. The phosphorylation of MA at the C-terminal Tyr residue occurs during or after the viral infection and is proposed to be a regulator of nuclear transport and integration of the viral genome[28].

A specific functional interaction between the MA protein and the env cytoplasmic tail has been proposed, since virion incorporation of envelope glycoproteins with long but not short cytoplasmic tails was blocked by specific, single amino acid substitutions in the MA protein[29,30].

Capsid

The capsid (CA) domain of all retroviruses contains a major homology region (MHR) that is required for efficient viral replication and particle production. Several amino acids within the MHRs of all primate lentiviruses are completely conserved. The results of several mutagenesis experiments indicate that specific residues within the MHR are required both for particle assembly and for the correct assembly of the viral core.

Nucleocapsid

The nucleocapsid (NC) domain of the Gag precursor is directly involved in the viral nucleic acid binding. NC contains two copies of a zinc binding sequence (Cys$(X)_2$ Cys$(X)_4$ His$(X)_4$ Cys) referred to as a retroviral CCHC zinc finger. The basic residues confer a nucleic acid binding property to the domain and the CCHC zinc fingers contribute to the specificity for the viral RNA. Disruption of either of the two zinc fingers in the NC domain resulted in non-infectious particles with reduced levels of packaged viral genome[31–33]. Deletion of the zinc fingers also eliminated virus particle formation[34]. NC protein may be involved in annealing of the $tRNA^{lys3}$ to PBS on the viral RNA. These activities may also have implications in strand transfer reactions that occur after the first strong stop synthesis of the proviral DNA[35] to complete the synthesis of the provirus for subsequent integration. The NC protein has also been shown to catalyze the formation of the genomic RNA dimer found in virion particles[36]. Processing may be essential for appropriate NC function[37]. HIV-1 Gag polyprotein and processed NC protein bind specifically to viral RNA containing the encapsidation (psi) signal, as detected by RNA mobility shift assays[38,39]. The psi site comprises four independent stem–loops spanning the major splice donor site and the *gag* start codon of HIV-1[40], although the sequences between the 5 splice donor site and the *gag* start codon may not be required for efficient packaging[41,42].

p6gag

p^{6gag} is the site of Gag interaction with Vpr. This is responsible for the virion incorporation of Vpr[43]. Vpr blocks cells in the G2 phase of the cell cycle and may promote nuclear localization of the pre-integration complex.

p1 and p2

The role of the p1 peptide is not known. p2 sequences were shown to modulate the rates of Gag processing[44,45].

Env

The HIV-1 Env precursor gp160 is cleaved intracellularly into gp120 and gp41 by a cellular protease between Arg511 and Ala512. A membrane-bound processing protease for the gp160 precursor has been identified[46]. The surface glycoprotein gp120 binds CD4, leading to conformational changes and membrane fusion assisted by the N terminus of gp41. The part of Env interacting with the CD4 has been identified within four non-contiguous regions of gp120[47]. Env is a heavily glycosylated protein. N-linked glycans are necessary for the creation, but not the maintenance, of a bioactive conformation, and drug-induced alteration of the glycosylation pattern can lead to impaired virus infectivity[48]. It has been predicted that only few areas of the polypeptide chain such as the CD4 binding site and the V3 loop are exposed, due to extensive glycosylation. HIV Env also interacts with the viral core. The $p17^{MA}$ protein is most likely the site of interaction of the HIV Env with the core virion particle. The functional Env protein is a multimer (tetramer). Multimerization appears to be essential for function and alters the immune response against Env. Multimerization of Env glycoproteins is mediated by the ectodomain of the transmembrane glycoprotein gp41. Sequence comparisons among HIV-1 isolates showed significant diversity primarily in the gp120 coding region of *env*, in five discrete regions named hypervariable regions (V1–V5)[49–51]. The regions between the variable regions are more conserved and were named constant (C1–C5). Immunization with purified Env proteins leads to neutralizing antibodies binding to the V3 hypervariable region, a loop of 33–35 amino acids confined by a conserved disulfide bond (V3 loop). This region has been named the principal neutralizing determinant (PND) of HIV-1[52,53]. In contrast, immunization with oligomeric Env generates a large proportion of antibodies to conformational epitopes in both gp120 and gp41, many of which may be absent from monomeric Env. Few monoclonal antibodies (MAbs) derived from mice immunized with oligomeric Env recognize the V3 loop. Today, the role of V3 loop PND in natural infection is questioned, and accumulating evidence suggests that oligomeric Env may be a better immunogen.

The range of cell types in which different isolates of HIV-1 are able to establish a productive infection varies. The Env glycoprotein gp120 has been shown to be responsible for the difference in cell tropism in many cases, but, clearly, other viral factors also contribute to tropism. The region of Env involved in the determination of cell tropism includes sequences that encode the V3 loop of gp120. Control of cell tropism by a part of Env including the V3 loop has been suggested to be a general phenomenon, which applies to many different HIV-1 isolates[54].

Interactions between gp120 and CD4 are responsible for the entry of HIV-1 into host cells in most cases. HIV-1 replication is commonly followed by the disappearance or downmodulation of cell surface CD4. This process potentially renders cells less susceptible to reinfection by HIV-1, as well as by other viruses that use CD4 as a receptor. Removal of CD4 from the cell surface is mediated by several different viral proteins that act at various stages through the course of the viral life cycle. At the cell surface, gp120 triggers cellular pathways leading to CD4 internalization. In addition, Vpu degrades CD4 intracellularly, via the formation of intracellular Vpu–CD4 complexes. Thirdly, Nef is also able to internalize the membrane-bound CD4. These mechanisms contribute to the depletion of CD4 at the cell surface.

Protease

The aspartic protease responsible for processing of the HIV-1 Gag/Pol polyproteins is expressed as the first part of *pol* open reading frame. It is active as a dimer, which is formed after Gag and Gag–Pol multimerization and contains two identical subunits of approximately 10 kDa[55–57]. The appropriate activation of PR is essential for virus maturation. The cellular aspartic proteases are monomers with distinct characteristics. Inhibition of HIV protease results in non-infectious particles, thus making protease an ideal target for antiviral intervention[57,58]. Elucidation of the tertiary structure of HIV-1 PR[59–61] has aided the rational design and development of protease inhibitors. Antiviral activity of protease inhibitors has been demonstrated *in vitro*, as well as in several clinical trials. To date, saquinavir (Invirase, Hoffman-La Roche), indinavir (Merck), ritonavir (Abbott Laboratories), and nelfinavir (Agouron) have demonstrated antiretroviral activity in patients. Other candidates are also in development (KNI-272 (Kyoto/National Cancer Institute), U-96988 and U-103107 (Upjohn)). These drugs in combination with nucleoside analogs are expected to revolutionize the clinical management of AIDS patients. The problems remaining to be solved with protease drugs is their low bioavailability and very high cost.

Reverse Transcriptase, RNase H

RT and the associated RNase H activity reside in the middle part of the Pol precursor. Proteolytic processing of $Pr160^{gag\text{-}pol}$ by the viral protease[62] results in the production of p66, which dimerizes and is further cleaved at the C-terminal part of one p66 subunit to produce a tightly associated p66–p51 heterodimer with full enzymatic activity. RT binds specifically to $tRNA^{lys3}$, which is preferentially encapsidated and subsequently hybridized to the primer-binding site (pbs).

RT possesses three enzymatic activities: RNA-dependent DNA polymerase, DNA-dependent DNA polymerase, and ribonuclease H (RNase H). The first enzymatic activity uses RNA primers with 3′-OH ends to initiate DNA synthesis. The RNase H activity is responsible for the cleavage of the RNA strand in the produced RNA–DNA hybrid. The synthesis of the minus-strand starts at the pbs by the tRNA primer, while the synthesis of the plus-strand starts also with an RNA primer at the polypurine tract (PPT) next to the U3 region.

Absence of a 3'-exonuclease proofreading activity in RT results in high error rates. The combined error rate during virus replication results in about one error in 10^4 nucleotides; therefore, every genomic RNA molecule of approximately 10^4 nucleotides contains one misincorporation.

RT has been the first target for anti-HIV-1 intervention[63], due to the development of several nucleoside analog inhibitors of RT with widespread clinical utility. The nucleoside analogs that have been approved for clinical use or are at various stages of clinical development include AZT (zidovudine, Retrovir), ddI (didanosine, Videx), ddC (zalcitabine, Hivid), d4T (stavudine, Zerit), and 3TC (lamivudine). These nucleoside analogs inhibit elongation at the active site of RT after phosphorylation to nucleotide triphosphates. Major problems with these drugs are their toxicity, due in part to the inhibition of cellular polymerases, and the rapid development of HIV-1 resistance. Multiple RT mutations have been shown to confer resistance to AZT, including mutations at amino acids 41, 67, 70, 215, and 219. Many mutations have been observed *in vitro*[64–66] and *in vivo*[67–70].

Non-nucleoside inhibitors of RT have also been developed, such as nevirapine, tetrahydro-imidazo [4,5,1,-jk] [1,4] benzodiazepin-2(IH)-thione (TIBO), and L697661[71–73]. These specific inhibitors interact with the same region of the enzyme, at amino acids 181–188, which is distinct from, but functionally and spatially related to, the substrate (dNTP) binding site. High-level resistance against non-nucleoside inhibitors develops after single point mutations in RT (Tyr181 to Cys)[74,75].

Integrase

IN is a 31 kDa protein produced from the C-terminal part of the $Pr160^{gag-pol}$. IN is responsible for the integration of the proviral DNA into the host nuclear DNA. It cleaves the ends of the linear viral RNA, leaving 3' recessed termini that may slow self-ligation and favor integration of the linear two-LTR DNA. It also cleaves the cellular DNA randomly and joins the viral DNA to the chromosome. These activities have been reconstituted and studied extensively *in vitro*.

HIV-1 IN contains domains similar to other retroviral integrases: an N-terminal HH-CC zinc finger, a centrally located region with the conserved catalytic motif (D, D-35-E), and a DNA binding domain implicated in the 3' DNA processing activity and integration[76].

IN is an important component of the pre-integration complex. Association of IN but not RT or MA proteins with viral DNA was stable in the presence of detergents[77]. The domains involved in the integration of IN with the viral DNA substrate have also been studied[78,79].

IN acts as a multimer involving sequences that map to the catalytic center. A stable complex of IN and viral DNA is formed in the presence of Mn^{2+} and requires the complete IN protein[80,81]. The crystal structure of IN has been determined and suggested that IN belongs to a superfamily of polynucleotidyl transferases including RNase H and the Holiday junction resolvase RuvC[82,83].

Integration is an obligate step in productive HIV-1 infection of activated peripheral blood mononuclear cells (PBMCs) and primary human macrophages. Integration of the HIV-1 provirus is essential not only for productive infection of T-cells but also for virus passage in both cultured peripheral blood lymphocytes and macrophages[84,85]. Similarly, SIVmac attenuated by mutation of *int* established a transient infection of permissive cells, resulting in the expression of viral antigen from episomal viral DNA over a limited period of time[86].

Tat

Tat is an essential regulatory protein for HIV-1 replication[87,88]. Two forms of Tat are produced by HIV-1, two-exon (Tat-2)[89–91] and one-exon (Tat-1). Tat is localized primarily in the nucleolus and is a transcriptional activator of HIV expression[91–96]. It binds to the nascent leader of HIV-1 mRNAs soon after RNA synthesis and affects the HIV enhancer-promoter[97–100]. The binding site for Tat on the viral mRNA was named TAR. The core TAR element was mapped to the first 44 nucleotides of mRNA[100,101], which forms a stable stem–loop structure[102]. Tat binds directly to a bulge region of the TAR element[95,98,99,103–109]. The nucleotide sequence of the bulge, UCU, is critical for Tat binding[95,98]. Cellular factors have also been shown to bind to *trans*-activation response (TAR) or to Tat and some cooperate with Tat in promoter activation[110–116]. Factor(s) produced by the human chromosome 12 contribute to the binding of Tat to TAR[117–120]. Experiments using hybrid equine infectious anemia virus (EIAV)/HIV-1 Tat proteins further suggested that cofactors necessary for transactivation are present in limited amounts[121].

Tat may increase transcription initiation or elongation via increased processivity of the polymerase complex, or alternatively, via the suppression of specific termination events[98,122–129].

All known lentiviruses contain transcriptional activators, although the mechanism of transcriptional activation may vary. Comparisons of Tat proteins from different lentiviruses and numerous mutagenesis studies have shown that Tat contains distinct conserved functional domains. Tat contains an 'activation domain', and an arginine-rich basic domain, which are necessary for activation of transcription, specific binding to TAR RNA, and nuclear localization. The RNA binding domain (amino acids 49–72) contains a basic RKKRRQRRR motif. These amino acids are responsible for RNA binding and for nuclear localization of the protein.

Tat-defective HIV-1 clones do not replicate except after special treatment[130,131] (A. Valentin, M. Korneyeva, and G. N. Pavlakis, unpublished data). Tat has been found in the medium of many infected cell cultures, suggesting that it may have an extracellular role[132–134]. Tat has also been implicated as a cofactor in KS development[131].

Rev

Rev is the second essential regulatory viral protein[14,135] of HIV-1. Rev is a small positively charged protein of approximately 116 amino acids. In the absence of Rev, most of the viral mRNAs are multiply spliced, whereas the production of the structural proteins is very low and no virions are formed[135–140]. Rev regulates expression of a subset of viral mRNAs at the post-transcriptional level by binding to RRE[141–146], a unique RNA element located in the *env* coding region of HIV-1[136–140,147–149]. This interaction promotes the transport, stability, and translation of unspliced and partially spliced HIV mRNAs[136,137,139,140,150–153].

Rev is localized primarily in the nucleolus[137,154,155] and shuttles between the nucleolus and the cytoplasm[156–159]. Inhibition of nuclear transport eliminates Rev function.

Rev can be replaced by post-transcriptional control elements of the type D simian retroviruses[15,16]. Therefore, Rev is only required for the post-transcriptional regulation of the unspliced and partially spliced mRNAs[16]. The reason Rev/RRE is necessary for virus propagation is that it counteracts inhibitory/instability regions (INS or CRS), which prevent RNA expression[138,149,153,160]. Multiple, independently acting INS/CRS sequences were found on the viral RNA[138,160–163]. Mutation of the INS sequences within *gag* resulted in Rev-independent expression[163] and viral particle formation in the absence of any HIV regulatory factors (R. Schneider and G. N. Pavlakis, unpublished).

Vif

The *vif* gene encodes a 23 kDa protein, which affects the infectivity of virus particles. The *vif* open reading frame (ORF) overlaps with the 3' part of *pol*

ORF. There is significant conservation among *vif* ORFs in all lentiviruses[4] except for EIAV[164]. Vif is expressed from partially spliced mRNAs and is regulated by Rev protein[12,165]. Vif is highly basic, predominantly cytoplasmic, is associated with the cytoplasmic side of cellular membrane[155,167] and a small quantity is incorporated in the virion. In sucrose density gradients, Vif cosediments with capsid proteins even after detergent treatment of virus preparations, suggesting that Vif is associated with the inner core of HIV particles[168]. A soluble cytosolic form of Vif may also exist.

Vif is required for HIV-1 replication in certain T-cell lines such as CEM and H9 as well as in peripheral blood T-lymphocytes, but it is not required for replication in the SupT1, C8166, or Jurkat T-cell lines. In most cell lines *vif(−)* mutant proviruses have lower replicating capacity. In PBMCs, they replicate at low levels only after cell-mediated infection; however, cell-free infection is not possible[169].

The mechanism of function of Vif is still under investigation. A recent suggestion is that it affects virus particle maturation. It was shown that, in the absence of Vif, the cone-shaped virus core has different morphological appearance[170]. The viral protein content of *vif(−)* virions recovered from restrictive cells, but not from permissive cells, was abnormal[171,172], consistent with the conclusion that the processing of the capsid proteins was affected[171]. It has been reported that no viral DNA synthesis was detectable after acute infection of target cells with phenotypically *vif(−)* virions[171]. Therefore, Vif is required for proper assembly of the virion and for efficient Env-mediated infection of target cells. Failure to infect target cells is due to a defect in the formation of the viral particle in either PBMCs or non-permissive cell lines[173,174].

Vif(−) virions were severely impaired in their ability to complete the synthesis of viral DNA, once they were internalized in the target cell[175]. The impaired reverse transcription may be the result of defects in virus maturation in the non-permissive producer cell. The observation that *vif(−)* virions do not complete viral cDNA synthesis after infection led to an alternative proposal suggesting that Vif stimulates efficient nucleocapsid internalization or activation of reverse transcription after infection[175,176]. Vif must be present in the producing cell and not the recipient cell for appropriate function[177].

Vif colocalizes with the intermediate filament vimentin[168]. Treatment of cells with drugs affecting the structure of vimentin filaments affect the localization of Vif, indicating a close association of Vif with this cytoskeletal component. The association of Vif with vimentin can cause the collapse of the intermediate filament network into a perinuclear aggregate. Analysis of Vif in vimentin-negative cells revealed significant staining of the nucleus and the nuclear membrane in addition to diffuse cytoplasmic staining.

Vif is highly phosphorylated on Ser and Thr. The C terminus of Vif is required for the stable association of Vif with membranes and is also essential for Vif function. The highly conserved regions at residues 103–115 and

142–150 are also important for Vif function[166]. Mutant viruses containing substitutions in either Cys114, Cys133, or both residues displayed a *vif(–)* infection phenotype[178]. All lentiviral Vif proteins contain at least one of two short, highly conserved sequence motifs, SL(I/V)X4YX9Y and SLQXLA.

Vpr

Vpr is a 96-amino acid (14 kDa) protein,which mediates cell growth arrest at G2 phase of the cell cycle in infected cells, and possibly the nuclear import of pre-integration complexes. Other proposed functions for Vpr include trans-activation of cellular genes, and induction of cellular differentiation. Vpr is incorporated into the virion via an interaction with the $p6^{gag}$ part of the $Pr55^{gag}$ precursor[179–182]. The minimal viral genetic information necessary for Vpr incorporation in the virion was mapped within the $Pr55^{gag}$ polyprotein precursor. Incorporation of Vpr requires the expression but not the processing of Gag products and is independent of the presence of Pol and Env. Vpr detected in the cell is localized to the nucleus[183,184]. It is produced by both multiply spliced (Rev-independent), and singly spliced (Rev-dependent) mRNAs[185], suggesting that Vpr is present early after infection. Additional evidence for an important role of Vpr in viral replication comes from experiments showing that a *vpr(–)* molecular clone reverted to wild-type in three of five animals, indicating the Vpr is important for replication *in vivo*[186].

Retroviral integration requires cell division. In contrast, HIV-1 and the other lentiviruses can integrate their genome in non-dividing cells by transporting the pre-integration complex into the nucleus. Vpr, together with $p17^{MA}$, promote nuclear localization of viral nucleic acids in non-dividing cells. Introduction of combinations of $p17^{MA}$ and Vpr mutations in HIV-1 molecular clones attenuated nuclear localization of viral nucleic acids in non-dividing cells and viral replication in monocyte-derived macrophages[183]. None of the mutants abolished infectivity in primary human monocyte-derived macrophages[187], suggesting that the nuclear transport is a rather complex process.

Viruses that contain an intact *vpr* gene are unable to establish a chronic infection of T cells, whereas viruses with a mutated *vpr* gene can readily establish such long-term cultures[188,189]. Expression of Vpr in the absence of any other viral information arrests the cells in G2/M phase[189,190]. Vpr can directly inhibit cell proliferation and induce cell differentiation of the human rhabdomyosarcoma cell line TE671[191]. Cell differentiation may be the result of cell cycle inhibition. Vpr shows some sequence similarity to Sac1p, a protein with functions relating to the yeast cytoskeleton[192].

Several cellular proteins interacting with Vpr have been identified. Important for the role of Vpr in G2 arrest is the binding of type-2A protein phosphatase (PP2A), an enzyme important for the regulation of the G2/M transition. Vpr results in increased phosphorylation of cdc2, inhibiting the enzyme and causing arrest at G2. Vpr binds in addition to Uracil-DNA glycosylase (UNG), an enzyme participating in excision repair. It is interesting that the non-primate lentiviruses encode a viral dUTPase to maintain low incorporation of dUTP into DNA. The primate lentiviruses may maintain a low misincorporation via the interaction of Vpr to UNG. A 41 kDa cytosolic protein also interacts with Vpr *in vitro*[193]. Vpr induced nuclear translocation of this protein, as did glucocorticoid receptor (GR)-II-stimulating steroids. Vpr and the Vpr-binding protein coimmunoprecipitated with the human GR as part of an activated receptor complex. In addition, a 200 kDa protein (RIP) was found to bind to Vpr. Vpr nuclear localization seemed to correlate with Vpr interaction with RIP[194].

HIV-2 and SIV express in addition a protein similar to Vpr, named Vpx, a virion protein which is probably the result of a gene duplication. Recent experiments suggest that SIV Vpr may be responsible for cell cycle arrest, while Vpx may promote infection of non-dividing cells.

Vpu

Vpu is a 16 kDa (81-amino acid) type I integral membrane protein[195] with at least two different biological functions: (a) degradation of CD4 in the endoplasmic reticulum, and (b) enhancement of virion release from the plasma membrane of HIV-1-infected cells. Vpu is found only in HIV-1 and SIVcpz. It is produced by the bicistronic *vpu/env* mRNAs and is positively regulated by Rev[11]. Vpu probably possesses an N-terminal hydrophobic membrane anchor and a hydrophillic moiety[196]. It is phosphorylated by casein kinase II at positions Ser52 and Ser56 within a predicted α-helix–turn-α-helix motif[197,198].

The presence of Vpu releases Env from Env–CD4 complexes trapped in the endoplasmic reticulum. Coexpression of Vpu and CD4 results in the degradation of CD4 in the endoplasmic reticulum[199–201]. Vpu acts on CD4 in the absence of Env or any other viral protein. Vpu-mediated degradation of CD4 depends on the presence of specific sequences located between amino acids 402 and 420 and in the CD4 cytoplasmic domain. Vpu specifically binds to the cytoplasmic tail of CD4[199]. Binding is an early critical event triggering the multistep process leading to CD4 degradation[202]. The amino acid residues in the CD4 cytoplasmic tail that are important for degradation are also necessary for Vpu binding. Sequences on Vpu critical for CD4 downregulation were localized to the hydrophilic C-terminal domain[203]. Vpu phosphorylation is important for function, since unphosphorylated Vpu was unable to induce degradation of CD4.

A second apparent function of Vpu appears to enhance virion release from the infected cells. This function of Vpu may be related to the multimerization of Vpu and potential ion channel-forming capacity[195]. A structural homology of Vpu with the influenza M2 membrane protein has been noted. M2 forms ion channels and may modulate the pH of intracellular compartments. Enhancement of virion release by wild-type Vpu was efficiently blocked when Vpu was artificially retained in the endoplasmic reticulum, suggesting that the two biological functions of Vpu are independent, occur at different sites within the cell, and exhibit different sensitivities to phosphorylation[204].

Nef

Nef is an approximately 27 kDa myristylated protein produced by an ORF located at the 3' end of the primate lentiviruses. Nef is predominantly cytoplasmic and is associated with the plasma membrane via a myristyl residue. Nef has also been found associated with the cytoskeleton in some experiments. Its association with the virion is suspected. Nef is not preferentially accumulated in the virion, but its membrane localization may result in virion incorporation.

The *nef* genes of HIV and SIV are dispensable *in vitro*, but are required for efficient viral replication and pathogenicity *in vivo*. Nef is necessary for the maintenance of high virus loads and for the development of AIDS in macaques[205]. *Nef(−)* SIV replicates at lower levels, and does not cause disease. In addition, it protected the animals from disease after superinfection with wild-type virus[206]. A *nef(+)* HIV-1 molecular clone induced severe depletion of human thymocytes in immunodeficient (scid) mice containing human lymphoid tissues (scid-hu) within six weeks of infection, whereas a *nef(−)* HIV-1 did not[207].

Nef downregulates CD4, the primary viral receptor, by inducing CD4 endocytosis, resulting in its degradation in lysosomes[208–210]. CD4 downregulation is strongly enhanced by the association of Nef with cell membranes through myristylation. A region containing the 20 membrane-proximal residues of the CD4 cytoplasmic domain are sufficient to confer Nef sensitivity. Within this region, a leucine–leucine motif is crucial for CD4 response to Nef. The portion of the cytoplasmic domain required for the downregulation of CD4 by Nef overlaps with the binding site of $p56^{lck}$, but the cysteine residues that are essential for the association of CD4 with $p56^{lck}$ are not required. CD4 downregulation by Nef was also found in cells not producing $p56^{lck}$.

Expression of the Nef protein in transgenic mice perturbs development of $CD4^+$ T-cells in the thymus and elicits depletion of peripheral $CD4^+$ T-cells. The effects of Nef depend on the specific clone expressed. For example, thymic T-cells expressing Nef of HIV-$1_{NL4\text{-}3}$ showed altered activation responses. In contrast, Nef protein of the HIV-1_{HXB3} isolate did not have an overt effect on T-cells when expressed in transgenic animals. The differential effects of the two HIV-1 *nef* alleles in transgenic mice correlated with downregulation of CD4 expression on thymic T-cells[211]. The analysis of Nef variants demonstrated the variability in both sequence and function found in *nef* genes.

In addition to CD4, recent evidence suggests that Nef also binds to another surface molecule, CD69.

Nef has also been shown to increase the viral growth in primary cells and the infectivity of produced virions. The two functions of Nef may be related, since downregulation of CD4 may promote the production of HIV-1 that has greater infectivity. Many studies indicate that optimal infectivity of HIV-1 *in vitro* requires an intact *nef* gene[212–217]. Nef confers a positive growth advantage, which becomes readily discernible in the primary cell setting of virus induction through T-cell activation[218].

A serine kinase activity is associated with Nef in human T-lymphocytes[219]. This kinase has been identified as PAK65 or a closely related molecule. Recent experiments show that proline-rich (PxxP) motifs in HIV-1 Nef bind to SH3 domains of a subset of Src kinases and are required for the enhanced growth of *nef(+)* viruses but not for the downregulation of CD4. Nef PxxP motifs show specific binding to biotinylated SH3 domains of Hck and Lyn, but not to those of other tested Src family kinases or less-related proteins. Endogenous Hck of monocytic U937 cells can be specifically precipitated by matrix-bound HIV-1 Nef but not by mutants lacking PxxP. These experiments suggest that CD4 downregulation and promotion of viral growth are two distinct functions of Nef, since intact Nef PxxP motifs are dispensable for Nef-induced CD4 downregulation but are required for the higher *in vitro* replicative potential of *nef(+)* viruses[220]. An additional cellular protein interacting with Nef, human β-COP, has been detected. This protein is a major coat component of non-clathrin-coated vesicles. Nef and β-COP interacted *in vitro* and were found to be physically associated in HIV-1-infected cells by coimmunoprecipitation[221].

ACKNOWLEDGEMENTS

I thank B.K. Felber for critical discussions, and A. Arthur for editing. Research was sponsored by the National Cancer Institute, DHHS, under contract with ABL.

REFERENCES

1. Barré-Sinoussi F, Cherman JC, Rey F *et al.* Isolation of a T-lymphotropic retrovius from a patient at risk for acquired immune deficiency syndrome (AIDS). *Science* 1983; 220: 868–871.
2. Gallo RC, Salahuddin SZ, Popovic M *et al.* Frequent detection and isolation of

cytopathic retroviruses (HTLV-III) from patients with AIDS and at risk for AIDS. *Science* 1984; 224: 500–503.
3. Gonda MA, Wong-Staal F, Gallo RC *et al.* Sequence homology and morphogenic similarity of HTLV-III and visna virus, a pathogenic lentivirus. *Science* 1985; 227: 173–177.
4. Sonigo P, Alizon M, Staskus K *et al.* Nucleotide sequence of the visna lentivirus: relationship to the AIDS virus. *Cell* 1985; 42: 369–382.
5. Arya SK, Gallo RC. Three novel genes of human T-cell lymphotropic virus type III: immune reactivity of their products with sera from acquired immune deficiency syndrome patients. *Proc Natl Acad Sci USA* 1986; 83: 2209–2213.
6. Benko DM, Schwartz S, Pavlakis GN, Felber BK. A novel human immunodeficiency virus type 1 protein, *tev*, shares sequences with *tat*, *env*, and *rev* proteins. *J Virol* 1990; 64: 2505–2518.
7. Muesing MA, Smith DH, Cabradilla CD *et al.* Nucleic acid structure and expression of the human AIDS/lymphadenopathy retrovirus. *Nature (London)* 1985; 313: 450–458.
8. Purcell DFJ, Martin MA. Alternative splicing of human immunodeficiency virus type 1 mRNA modulates viral protein expression, replication, and infectivity. *J Virol* 1993; 67: 6365–6378.
9. Salfeld J, Gottlinger H, Sia R *et al.* A tripartite HIV-1 tat-env-rev fusion protein. *EMBO J* 1990; 9: 965–970.
10. Schwartz S, Felber BK, Benko DM *et al.* Cloning and functional analysis of multiply spliced mRNA species of human immunodeficiency virus type 1. *J Virol* 1990; 64: 2519–2529.
11. Schwartz S, Felber BK, Fenyö EM, Pavlakis GN. Env and Vpu proteins of human immunodeficiency virus type 1 are produced from multiple bicistronic mRNAs. *J Virol* 1990; 64: 5448–5456.
12. Schwartz S, Felber BK, Pavlakis GN. Expression of human immunodeficiency virus type-1 vif and vpr mRNAs is Rev-dependent and regulated by splicing. *Virology* 1991; 183: 677–686.
13. Feinberg MB, Jarrett RF, Aldovini A *et al.* HTLV-III expression and production involve complex regulation at the levels of splicing and translation of viral RNA. *Cell* 1986; 46: 807–817.
14. Sodroski J, Goh WC, Rosen C *et al.* A second post-transcriptional trans-activator gene required for HTLV-III replication. *Nature* 1986; 321: 412–417.
15. Bray M, Prasad S, Dubay JW *et al.* A small element from the Mason–Pfizer monkey virus genome makes human immunodeficiency virus type 1 expression and replication Rev-independent. *Proc Natl Acad Sci USA* 1994; 91: 1256–1260.
16. Zolotukhin AS, Valentin A, Pavlakis GN, Felber BK. Continuous propagation of RRE(–) and Rev(–)RRE(–) human immunodeficiency virus type 1 molecular clones containing a *cis*-acting element of simian retrovirus type 1 in human peripheral blood lymphocytes. *J Virol* 1994; 68: 7944–7952.
17. Felber BK, Pavlakis GN. Molecular biology of HIV-1: positive and negative regulatory elements important for virus expression. *AIDS* 1993; 7(suppl.): S51–S62.
18. Chang Y, Cesarman E, Pessin MS *et al* Identification of herpesvirus-like DNA sequences in AIDS-associated Kaposi's sarcoma. *Science* 1994; 266: 1865–1869.
19. Moore PS, Gao SJ, Dominguez G *et al.* Primary characterization of a herpesvirus agent associated with Kaposi's sarcoma. *J Virol* 1996; 70: 549–558.
20. Cesarman E, Chang Y, Moore PS *et al.* Kaposi's sarcoma-associated herpesvirus-like DNA sequences in AIDS-related body-cavity-based lymphomas. *N Engl J Med* 1995; 332: 1186–1191.

21. Cesarman E, Moore PS, Rao PH *et al.* In vitro establishment and characterization of two acquired immunodeficiency syndrome-related lymphoma cell lines (BC-1 and BC-2) containing Kaposi's sarcoma-associated herpesvirus-like (KSHV) DNA sequences. *Blood* 1995; 86: 2708–2714.
22. Soulier J, Grollet L, Oksenhendler E *et al.* Kaposi's sarcoma-associated herpes-virus-like DNA sequences in multicentric Castleman's disease. *Blood* 1995; 86: 1276–1280.
23. Luban J, Bossolt KL, Franke EK *et al.* Human immunodeficiency virus type 1 Gag protein binds to cyclophilins A and B. *Cell* 1993; 73: 1067–1078.
24. Franke EK, En Hui Yuan H, Luban J. Specific incorporation of cyclophilin A into HIV-1 virions. *Nature (London)* 1994; 372: 359–362.
25. Thali M, Bukovsky A, Kondo E *et al.* Functional association of cyclophilin A with HIV-1 virions. *Nature (London)* 1994; 372: 363–365.
26. Bukrinksy MI, Sharova N, Dempsey MP *et al.* Active nuclear import of human immunodeficiency virus type 1 preintegration complexes. *Proc Natl Acad Sci USA* 1992; 89: 6580–6584.
27. Bukrinsky MI, Haggerty S, Dempsey MP *et al.* A nuclear localization signal within HIV-1 matrix protein that governs infection of non-dividing cells. *Nature* 1993; 365: 666–669.
28. Gallay P, Swingler S, Aiken C, Trono D. HIV-1 infection of nondividing cells: C-terminal tyrosine phosphorylation of the viral matrix protein is a key regulator. *Cell* 1995; 80: 379–388.
29. Dorfman T, Mammano F, Haseltine WA, Gottlinger HG. Role of the matrix protein in the virion association of the human immunodeficiency virus type 1 envelope glycoprotein. *J Virol* 1994; 68: 1689–1696.
30. Freed EO, Martin MA. Virion incorporation of envelope glycoproteins with long but not short cytoplasmic tails is blocked by specific, single amino acid substitutions in the human immunodeficiency virus type 1 matrix. *J Virol* 1995; 69: 1984–1989.
31. Aldovini A, Young RA. Mutations of RNA and protein sequences involved in human immunodeficiency virus type 1 packaging result in production of noninfectious virus. *J Virol* 1990; 64: 1920–1926.
32. Dorfman T, Luban J, Goff SP *et al.* Mapping of functionally important residues of a cysteine–histidine box in the human immunodeficiency virus type 1 nucleocapsid protein. *J Virol* 1993; 67: 6159–6169.
33. Gorelick RJ, Nigida JSM, Bess JJW *et al.* Noninfectious human immunodeficiency virus type 1 mutants deficient in genomic RNA. *J Virol* 1990; 64: 3207–3211.
34. Spearman P, Wang JJ, Vander Heyden N, Ratner L. Identification of human immunodeficiency virus type 1 Gag protein domains essential to membrane binding and particle assembly. *J Virol* 1994; 68: 3232–3242.
35. Darlix JL, Vincent A, Gabus C *et al.* Trans-activation of the 5' to 3' viral DNA strand transfer by nucleocapsid protein during reverse transcription of HIV-1 RNA. *CR Acad Sci III* 1993; 316: 763–771.
36. Darlix JL, Gabus C, Nugeyre MT *et al.* Cis elements and trans-acting factors involved in the RNA dimerization of the human immunodeficiency virus HIV-1. *J Mol Biol* 1990; 216: 689–699.
37. Fu W, Gorelick RJ, Rein A. Characterization of human immunodeficiency virus type 1 dimeric RNA from wild-type and protease-defective virions. *J Virol* 1994; 68: 5013–5018.
38. Berkowitz RD, Goff SP. Analysis and binding elements in the human immodeficiency virus type 1 genomic RNA and nucleocapsid protein. *Virology* 1994; 202: 233–246.

39. Dannull J, Surovoy A, Jung G, Moelling K. Specific binding of HIV-1 nucleocapsid protein to PSI RNA in vitro requires N-terminal zinc finger and flanking basic amino acid residues. *EMBO J* 1994; 13: 1525–1533.
40. Clever J, Sassetti C, Parslow TG. RNA secondary structure and binding sites for gag gene products in the 5′ packaging signal of human immunodeficiency virus type 1. *J Virol* 1995; 69: 2101–2109.
41. Lee PP, Linial ML. Efficient particle formation can occur if the matrix domain of human immunodeficiency virus type 1 Gag is substituted by a myristylation signal. *J Virol* 1994; 68: 6644–6654.
42. Luban J, Goff SP. Mutational analysis of *cis*-acting packaging signals in human immunodeficiency virus type 1 RNA. *J Virol* 1994; 68: 3784–3793.
43. Krausslich HG, Facke M, Heuser AM *et al.* The spacer peptide between human immunodeficiency virus capsid and nucleocapsid proteins is essential for ordered assembly and viral infectivity. *J Virol* 1995; 69: 3407–3419.
44. Kondo E, Mammano F, Cohen EA, Gottlinger HG. The p6gag domain of human immunodeficiency virus type 1 is sufficient for the incorporation of Vpr into heterologous viral particles. *J Virol* 1995; 69: 2759–2764.
45. Pettit SC, Moody MD, Wehbie RS *et al.* The p2 domain of human immunodeficiency virus type 1 Gag regulates sequential proteolytic processing and is required to produce fully infectious virions. *J Virol* 1994; 68: 8017–8027.
46. Kido H, Kamoshita K, Fukutomi A, Katunuma N. Processing protease for gp160 human immunodeficiency virus type 1 envelope glycoprotein precursor in human T4+ lymphocytes: purification and characterization. *J Biol Chem* 1993; 268: 13406–13413.
47. Lasky LA, Nakamura G, Smith DH *et al.* Delineation of a region of the human immunodeficiency virus type 1 gp120 glycoprotein critical for interaction with the CD4 receptor. *Cell* 1987; 50: 975–985.
48. Fenouillet E, Gluckman JC, Jones IM. Functions of HIV envelope glycans. *Trends Biochem* 1994; 19: 65–70.
49. Meyerhans A, Cheynier R, Albert J *et al.* Temporal fluctuations in HIV quasispecies in vivo are not reflected by sequential HIV isolations. *Cell* 1989; 58: 901–910.
50. Modrow S, Hahn BH, Shaw GM *et al.* Computer-assisted analysis of envelope protein sequences of seven human immunodeficiency virus isolates: prediction of antigenic epitopes in conserved and variable regions. *J Virol* 1987; 61: 570–578.
51. Wong-Staal F, Shaw GM, Hahn BH *et al.* Genomic diversity of human T-lymphotropic virus type III (HTLV-III). *Science* 1985; 229: 759–762.
52. Javaherian K, Langlois AJ, McDanal C *et al.* Principal neutralizing domain of the human immunodeficiency virus type 1 envelope protein. *Proc Natl Acad Sci USA* 1989; 86: 6768–6772.
53. Rusche JR, Javaherian K, McDanal C *et al.* Antibodies that inhibit fusion of human immunodeficiency virus-infected cells bind a 24-amino acid sequence of the viral envelope, gp120. *Proc Natl Acad Sci USA* 1988; 85: 3198–3202.
54. Cann AJ, Churcher MJ, Boyd M *et al.* The region of the envelope gene of human immunodeficiency virus type 1 responsible for determination of cell tropism. *J Virol* 1992; 66: 305–309.
55. Copeland TD, Oroszlan S. Genetic locus, primary structure, and chemical synthesis of human immunodeficiency virus protease. *Gene Anal Tech* 1988; 5: 109–115.
56. Debouck C, Gorniak JG, Strickler JE *et al.* Human immunodeficiency virus protease expressed in *Escherichia coli* exhibits autoprocessing and specific maturation of the gag precursor. *Proc Natl Acad Sci USA* 1987; 84: 8903–8906.
57. Kohl NE, Emini EA, Schleif WA *et al.* Active human immunodeficiency virus

protease is required for viral infectivity. *Proc Natl Acad Sci USA* 1988; 85: 4686–4890.
58. Kaplan AH, Manchester M, Swanstrom R. The activity of the protease of human immunodeficiency virus type 1 is initiated at the membrane of infected cells before the release of viral proteins and is required for release to occur with maximum efficiency. *J Virol* 1994; 68: 6782–6786.
59. Navia M, Fitzgerald PM, McKeever BM *et al.* Three-dimensional structure of aspartyl protease for HIV-1. *Nature (London)* 1989; 337: 615–620.
60. Weber IT, Miller M, Jaskolski M *et al.* Molecular modelling of the HIV-1 protease and its substrate binding site. *Science* 1989; 243: 928–931.
61. Wlodawer A, Miller M, Jaskolski M *et al.* Conserved folding in retroviral proteases: crystal structure of a synthetic HIV-1 protease. *Science* 1989; 245: 616–621.
62. di Marzo Veronese F, Copeland TD, DeVico AL *et al.* Characterization of highly immunogenic p66/p51 as the reverse transcriptase of HTLV-II/LAV. *Science* 1986; 231: 1289–1291.
63. Broder S, Mitsuya H, Yarchoan R, Pavlakis GN. Antiretroviral therapy in AIDS. *Ann Intern Med* 1990; 113: 604–618.
64. Gu Z, Gao Q, Fang H *et al.* Identification of a mutation of codon 65 in the IKKK motif of reverse transcriptase that encodes human immunodeficiency virus resistance to 2',3'-dideoxycytidine and 2',3'-dideoxy-3'-thiacytidine. *Antimicrob Agents Chemother* 1994; 38: 275–281.
65. Larder BA. Interactions between drug resistance mutations in human immunodeficiency virus type 1 reverse transcriptase. *J Gen Virol* 1994; 75: 951–957.
66. Larder BA, Kellam P, Kemp SD. Convergent combination therapy can select viable multidrug-resistant HIV-1 in vitro. *Nature* 1993; 365: 451–453.
67. Kellam P, Boucher CA, Tijnagel JM, Larder BA. Zidovudine treatment results in the selection of human immunodeficiency virus type 1 variants whose genotypes confer increasing levels of drug resistance. *J Gen Virol* 1994; 75: 341–351.
68. Kellam P, Larder BA. Retroviral recombination can lead to linkage of reverse transcriptase mutations that confer increased zidovudine resistance. *J Virol* 1995; 69: 669–674.
69. Najera I, Richman DD, Olivares I *et al.* Natural occurrence of drug resistance mutations in the reverse transcriptase of human immunodeficiency virus type 1 isolates. *AIDS Res Hum Retroviruses* 1994; 10: 1479–1488.
70. Richman DD. Emergence of mutant HIV reverse transcriptase conferring resistance to AZT. *J Enzym Inhib* 1992; 6: 55–64.
71. de Clercq E. HIV-1-specific RT inhibitors: highly selective inhibitors of human immunodeficiency virus type 1 that are specifically targeted at the viral reverse transcriptase. *Med Res Rev* 1993; 13: 229–258.
72. de Clercq E. New developments in the chemotherapy of lentivirus (human immunodeficiency virus) infections: sensitivity/resistance of HIV-1 to non-nucleoside HIV-1-specific inhibitors. *Ann NY Acad Sci* 1994; 724: 438–456.
73. Debyser Z, Pauwels R, Andries K, de Clercq E. Specific HIV-1 reverse transcriptase inhibitors. *J Enzym Inhib* 1992; 6: 47–53.
74. Balzarini J, Karlsson A, Perez-Perez MJ *et al.* HIV-1-specific reverse transcriptase inhibitors show differential activity against HIV-1 mutant strains containing different amino acid substitutions in the reverse transcriptase. *Virology* 1993; 192: 246–253.
75. Balzarini J, Karlsson A, Sardana VV *et al.* Human immunodeficiency virus 1 (HIV-1)-specific reverse transcriptase (RT) inhibitors may suppress the replication of specific drug-resistant (E138K)RT HIV-1 mutants or select for highly resistant (Y181C→C181I)RT HIV-1 mutants. *Proc Natl Acad Sci USA* 1994; 91: 6599–6603.

76. Engelman A, Bushman FD, Craigie R. Identification of discrete functional domains of HIV-1 integrase and their organization within an active multimeric complex. *EMBO J* 1993; 12: 3269–3275.
77. Bukrinsky MI, Sharova N, McDonald TL *et al.* Association of integrase, matrix, and reverse transcriptase antigens of human immunodeficiency virus type 1 with viral nucleic acids following acute infection. *Proc Natl Acad Sci USA* 1993; 90: 6125–6129.
78. Bushman FD, Craigie R. Integration of human immunodeficiency virus DNA: adduct interference analysis of required DNA sites. *Proc Natl Acad Sci USA* 1992; 89: 3458–3462.
79. Drelich M, Haenggi M, and Mous J. Conserved residues Pro-109 and Asp-116 are required for interaction of the human immunodeficiency virus type 1 integrase protein with its viral DNA substrate. *J Virol* 1993; 67: 5041–5044.
80. Vink C, Lutzke RA, Plasterk RH. Formation of a stable complex between the human immunodeficiency virus integrase protein and viral DNA. *Nucleic Acids Res* 1994; 22: 4103–4110.
81. Vink C, Oude Groeneger AM, Plasterk RH. Identification of the catalytic and DNA-binding region of the human immunodeficiency virus type I integrase protein. *Nucleic Acids Res* 1993; 21: 1419–1425.
82. Dyda F, Hickman AB, Jenkins TM *et al.* Crystal structure of the catalytic domain of HIV-1 integrase: similarity to other polynucleotidyl transferases. *Science* 1994; 266: 1981–1986.
83. Yang W, Steitz TA. Recombining the structures of HIV integrase, RuvC and RNase H. *Structure* 1995; 3: 131–134.
84. Engelman A, Englund G, Orenstein JM *et al.* Multiple effects of mutations in human immunodeficiency virus type 1 integrase on viral replication. *J Virol* 1995; 69: 2729–2736.
85. Englund G, Theodore TS, Freed EO *et al.* Integration is required for productive infection of monocyte-derived macrophages by human immunodeficiency virus type 1. *J Virol* 1995; 69: 3216–3219.
86. Vogel M, Cichutek K, Norley S, Kurth R. Self-limiting infection by int/nef-double mutants of simian immunodeficiency virus. *Virology* 1993; 193: 115–123.
87. Dayton AI, Sodroski JG, Rosen CA *et al.* The trans-activator gene of the human T-cell lymphotrophic virus type III is required for replication. *Cell* 1986; 44: 941–947.
88. Fisher AG, Feinberg MB, Josephs SF *et al.* The transactivator gene of HTLV-III is essential for virus replication. *Nature (London)* 1986; 320: 367–371.
89. Arya SK, Guo C, Josephs SF, Wong-Staal F. Trans-activator gene of human T-lymphotrophic virus type III (HTLV-III). *Science* 1985; 229: 69–73.
90. Sodroski J, Patarca R, Rosen C *et al.* Location of the trans-activating region of the genome of human T-cell lymphotrophic virus type III. *Science* 1985; 229: 74–77.
91. Wright CM, Felber BK, Paskalis H, Pavlakis GN. Expression and characterization of the *trans*-activator of HTLV-III/LAV virus. *Science* 1986; 234: 988–992.
92. Cullen BR. Trans-activation of human immunodeficiency virus occurs via a bimodal mechanism. *Cell* 1986; 46: 973–982.
93. Hauber J, Malim MH, Cullen BR. Mutational analysis of the conserved basic domain of human immunodeficiency virus tat protein. *J Virol* 1989; 64: 1181–1187.
94. Peterlin BM, Luciw PA, Barr PJ, Walker MD. Elevated levels of mRNA can account for the trans-activation of human immunodeficiency virus. *Proc Natl Acad Sci USA* 1986; 83: 9734–9738.
95. Roy S, Delling U, Chen C-H *et al.* A bulge structure in HIV-1 TAR RNA is required for tat binding and tat-mediated trans-activation. *Genes Dev* 1990; 4: 1365–1373.

96. Ruben S, Perkins A, Purcell R *et al.* Structural and functional characterization of human immunodeficiency virus tat protein. *J Virol* 1989; 63: 1–8.
97. Berkhout B, Silverman RH, Jeang K-T. Tat trans-activates the human immunodeficiency virus through a nascent RNA target. *Cell* 1989; 59: 273–282.
98. Dingwall C, Ernberg I, Gait M *et al.* HIV-1 Tat protein stimulates transcription by binding to a U-rich bulge in the stem of the TAR RNA structure. *EMBO J* 1990; 9: 4145–4153.
99. Dingwall C, Ernberg I, Gait MH *et al.* Human immunodeficiency virus 1 tat protein binds trans-activation-responsive region (TAR) RNA in vitro. *Proc Natl Acad Sci USA* 1989; 86: 6925–6929.
100. Rosen CA, Sodroski JG, Haseltine WA. The location of cis-acting regulatory sequences in the human T cell lymphotropic virus type III (HTLV-III/LAV) long terminal repeat. *Cell* 1985; 41: 813–823.
101. Hauber J, Cullen BR. Mutational analysis of the *trans*-activation-responsive region of the human immunodeficiency virus type 1 long terminal repeat. *J Virol* 1988; 62: 673–679.
102. Muesing MA, Smith DH, Capon DJ. Regulation of mRNA accumulation by a human immunodeficiency virus trans-activator protein. *Cell* 1987; 48: 691–701.
103. Berkhout B, Jeang KT. Detailed mutational analysis of TAR RNA: critical spacing between the bulge and loop recognition domains. *Nucleic Acids Res* 1991; 19: 6169–6176.
104. Calnan B, Tidor B, Biancalana S *et al.* Arginine-mediated RNA recognition: the arginine fork. *Science* 1991; 252: 1167–1176.
105. Karn J, Dingwall C, Finch J *et al.* RNA binding by the tat and rev proteins of HIV-1. *Biochimie* 1991; 73: 9–16.
106. Puglisi J, Tan R, Calnan B *et al.* Conformation of the TAR RNA–arginine complex of NMR spectroscopy. *Science* 1992; 257: 76–80.
107. Rabbitts P, Forster A, Stinson M, Rabbitts TH. Truncation of exon 1 from the c-myc gene results in prolonged c-myc mRNA stability. *EMBO J* 1985; 4: 3727–3733.
108. Roy S, Parkin NT, Rosen C *et al.* Structural requirements for trans-activation of HIV-1 LTR-directed gene expression by Tat: importance of base pairing, loop sequence, and bulges in the TAR region. *J Virol* 1990; 64: 1402–1406.
109. Weeks KM, Ampe C, Schultz SC *et al.* Fragments of the HIV-1 tat protein specifically bind TAR RNA. *Science* 1990; 249: 1281–1285.
110. Gatignol A, Buckler-White A, Berkhout B, Jeang K-T. Characterization of a human TAR-RNA-binding protein that activates the HIV-1 LTR. *Science* 1991; 251: 1597–1600.
111. Gatignol A, Kumar A, Rabson A, Jeang K-T. Identification of cellular proteins that bind to the human immunodeficiency virus type 1 trans-activation-responsive TAR element RNA. *Proc Natl Acad Sci USA* 1989; 86: 7828–7832.
112. Gaynor R, Soultanaks E, Kuwabara M *et al.* Specific binding of a HeLa cell nuclear protein to RNA sequences in the human immunodeficiency virus transactivating region. *Proc Natl Acad Sci USA* 1989; 86: 4858–4862.
113. Marciniak RA, Garcia-Blanco MA, Sharp PA. Identification and characterization of a HeLa nuclear protein that specifically binds to the trans-activation-response (TAR) element of human immunodeficiency virus. *Proc Natl Acad Sci USA* 1990; 87: 3624–3628.
114. Sheline C, Milocco L, Jones K. Two distinct nuclear transcription factors recognize loop and bulge residues of the HIV-1 TAR RNA hairpin. *Genes Dev* 1991; 5: 2508–2520.
115. Wu F, Garcia J, Sigman D, Gaynor R. *tat* regulates binding of the human

immunodeficiency virus *trans*-activating region RNA loop-binding protein TRP-185. *Genes Dev* 1991; 5: 2128–2140.
116. Yu L, Zhang Z, Loewenstein PM *et al.* Molecular cloning and characterization of a cellular protein that interacts with the human immunodeficiency virus type 1 Tat transactivator and encodes a strong transcriptional activation domain. *J Virol* 1995; 69: 3007–3016.
117. Alonso A, Cujec TP, Peterlin BM. Effects of human chromosome 12 on interactions between Tat and TAR of human immunodeficiency virus type 1. *J Virol* 1994; 68: 6505–6513.
118. Alonso A, Derse D, Peterlin B. Human chromosome 12 is required for optimal interactions between Tat and TAR of human immunodeficiency virus type 1 in rodent cells. *J Virol* 1992; 66: 4617–4621.
119. Hart CE, Ou CY, Galphin JC. Human chromosome 12 is required for elevated HIV-1 expression in human-hamster hybrid cells. *Science* 1989; 246: 488–490.
120. Newstein M, Stanbridge J, Casey G, Shank PR. Human chromosome 12 encodes a species-specific factor which increases human immunodeficiency virus type 1 tat-mediated trans activation in rodent cells. *J Virol* 1990; 64: 4565–4567.
121. Carroll R, Peterlin B, Derse D. Inhibition of human immunodeficiency virus type 1 Tat activity by coexpression of heterologous trans activators. *J Virol* 1992; 66: 2000–2007.
122. Drysdale CM, Pavlakis GN. Rapid activation and subsequent downregulation of the human immunodeficiency virus type 1 promotor in the presence of Tat: possible mechanisms contributing to latency. *J Virol* 1991; 65: 3044–3051.
123. Feinberg M, Baltimore D, Frankel A. The role of Tat in the human immunodeficiency virus life cycle indicates a primary effect on transcriptional elongation. *Proc Natl Acad Sci USA* 1991; 88: 4045–4049.
124. Jeang KT, Berkhout B. Kinetics of HIV-1 long terminal repeat trans-activation: use of intragenic ribozyme to assess rate-limiting steps. *J Biol Chem* 1992; 267: 17891–17899.
125. Kato H, Sumimoto H, Pognonec P *et al.* HIV-1 Tat acts as a processivity factor in vitro in conjunction with cellular elongation factors. *Genes Dev* 1992; 6: 655–666.
126. Kessler M, Mathews M. Premature termination and processing of human immunodeficiency virus type 1-promoted transcripts. *J Virol* 1992; 66: 4488–4496.
127. Laspia M, Rice A, Mathews M. HIV-1 tat protein increases transcriptional initiation and stabilizes elongation. *Cell* 1989; 59: 283–292.
128. Marciniak RA, Calnan BJ, Frankel AD, Sharp PA. HIV-tat protein trans-activates transcription in vitro. *Cell* 1990; 63: 791–802.
129. Rice AP, Mathews MB. Transcriptional but not translational regulation of HIV-1 by the tat gene product. *Nature (London)* 1988; 332: 551–553.
130. Luznik L, Kraus G, Guatelli J *et al.* Tat-independent replication of human immunodeficiency viruses. *J Clin Invest* 1995; 95: 328–332.
131. Sadaie MR, Tschachler E, Valerie K *et al.* Activation of *tat*-defective human immunodeficiency virus by ultraviolet light. *New Biol* 1990; 2: 479–486.
132. Buonaguro L, Barillari G, Chang HK *et al.* Effects of the human immunodeficiency virus type 1 Tat protein on the expression of inflammatory cytokines. *J Virol* 1992; 66: 7159–7167.
133. Ensoli B, Barillari G, Salahuddin SZ *et al.* Tat protein of HIV-1 stimulates growth of cells derived from Kaposi's sarcoma lesions of AIDS patients. *Proc Natl Acad Sci USA* 1990; 87: 3479–3483.
134. Ensoli B, Buonaguro L, Barillari G *et al.* Release, uptake, and effects of extracellular human immunodeficiency virus type 1 Tat protein on cell growth and viral transactivation. *J Virol* 1993; 67: 277–287.

135. Feinberg MB, Jarrett RF, Aldovini A *et al.* HTLV-III expression and production involve complex regulation at the levels of splicing and translation of viral RNA. *Cell* 1986; 46: 807–817.
136. Emerman M, Vazeux R, Peden K. The rev gene product of the human immunodeficiency virus affects envelope-specific RNA localization. *Cell* 1989; 57: 1155–1165.
137. Felber BK, Hadzopoulou-Cladaras M, Cladaras C *et al.* rev protein of human immunodeficiency virus type 1 affects the stability and transport of the viral mRNA. *Proc Natl Acad Sci USA* 1989; 86: 1495–1499.
138. Hadzopoulou-Cladaras M, Felber BK, Cladaras C *et al.* The *rev (trs/art)* protein of human immunodeficiency virus type 1 affects viral mRNA and protein expression via a *cis*-acting sequence in the *env* region. *J Virol* 1989; 63: 1265–1274.
139. Hammarskjöld ML, Heimer J, Hammarskjöld B *et al.* Regulation of human immunodeficiency virus *env* expression by the *rev* gene product. *J Virol* 1989; 63: 1959–1966.
140. Malim MH, Hauber J, Le S-Y *et al.* The HIV-1 *rev trans*-activator acts through a structured target sequence to activate nuclear export of unspliced viral mRNA. *Nature (London)* 1989; 338: 254–257.
141. Bartel D, Zapp M, Green M, Szostak J. HIV-1 Rev regulation involves recognition of non-Watson–Crick base pairs in viral RNA. *Cell* 1991; 67: 529–536.
142. Cook KS, Fisk GJ, Hauber J *et al.* Characterization of HIV- REV protein: binding stoichiometry and minimal RNA substrate. *Nucleic Acids Res* 1991; 19: 1577–1583.
143. Daly TJ, Cook KS, Gray GS *et al.* Specific binding of HIV-1 recombinant Rev protein to the Rev-responsive element in vitro. *Nature* 1989; 342: 816–819.
144. Heaphy S, Dingwall C, Ernberg I *et al.* HIV-1 regulator of virion expression (Rev) protein binds to an RNA stem–loop structure located within the Rev response element region. *Cell* 1990; 60: 685–693.
145. Holland SM, Ahmad N, Maitra RK *et al.* Human immunodeficiency virus Rev protein recognizes a target sequence in Rev-responsive element RNA within the context of RNA secondary structure. *J Virol* 1990; 64: 5966–5975.
146. Holland SM, Chavez M, Gerstberger S, Venkatesan S. A specific sequence with a bulged guanosine residue(s) in a stem–bulge–stem structure of Rev-responsive element RNA is required for trans activation by human immunodeficiency virus type 1 Rev. *J Virol* 1992; 66: 3699–3706.
147. Cochrane A, Chen C-H, Rosen CA. Specific interaction of the human immunodeficiency virus Rev protein with a structured region in the env mRNA. *Proc Natl Acad Sci USA* 1990; 87: 1198–1202.
148. Dayton AI, Terwilliger EF, Potz J *et al.* Cis-acting sequences responsive to the *rev* gene product of the human immunodeficiency virus. *J AIDS* 1988; 1: 441–452.
149. Rosen CA, Terwilliger E, Dayton A *et al.* Intragenic cis-acting *art* gene-responsive sequences of the human immunodeficiency virus. *Proc Natl Acad Sci USA* 1988; 86: 2071–2075.
150. Arrigo SJ, Chen ISY. Rev is necessary for translation but not cytoplasmic accumulation of HIV-1 *vif, vpr,* and *env/vpu* 2 RNAs. *Genes Dev* 1991; 5: 808–819.
151. D'Agostino DM, Felber BK, Harrison JE, Pavlakis GN. The Rev protein of human immunodeficiency virus type 1 promotes polysomal association and translation of *gag/pol* and *vpu/env* mRNA. *Mol Cell Biol* 1992; 12: 1375–1386.
152. Lawrence JB, Cochrane AW, Johnson CV *et al.* The HIV-1 Rev protein: a model system for coupled RNA transport and translation. *New Biol* 1991; 3: 1220–1232.
153. Schwartz S, Felber BK, Pavlakis GN. Distinct RNA sequence in the *gag* region of human immunodeficiency virus type 1 decrease RNA stability and inhibit expression in the absence of Rev protein. *J Virol* 1992; 66: 150–159.

154. Cochrane A, Kramer R, Ruben S *et al.* The human immunodeficiency virus *rev* protein is a nuclear phosphoprotein. *Virology* 1989; 171: 264–266.
155. Cullen BR, Hauber J, Campbell K *et al.* Subcellular localization of the human immunodeficiency virus *trans*-acting *art* gene product. *J Virol* 1988; 62: 2498–2501.
156. D'Agostino DM, Ciminale V, Pavlakis GP, Chieco-Bianchi L. Intracellular trafficking of the human immunodeficiency virus type 1 Rev protein: involvement of continued rRNA synthesis in nuclear retention. *AIDS Res Hum Retroviruses* 1995; 11: 1063–1071.
157. Kalland KH, Szilvay AM, Brokstad KA *et al.* The human immunodeficiency virus type 1 Rev protein shuttles between the cytoplasm and nuclear compartments. *Mol Cell Biol* 1994; 14: 7436–7444.
158. Meyer BE, Malim MH. The HIV-1 Rev *trans*-activator shuttles between the nucleus and the cytoplasm. *Genes Dev* 1994; 8: 1538–1547.
159. Richard N, Iacampo S, Cochrane A. HIV-1 Rev is capable of shuttling between the nucleus and cytoplasm. *Virology* 1994; 204: 123–131.
160. Cochrane AW, Jones KS, Beidas S *et al.* Identification and characterization of intragenic sequences which repress human immunodeficiency virus structural gene expression. *J Virol* 1991; 65: 5305–5313.
161. Maldarelli F, Martin MA, Strebel K. Identification of posttranscriptionally active inhibitory sequences in human immunodeficiency virus type 1 RNA: novel level of gene regulation. *J Virol* 1991; 65: 5732–5743.
162. Nasioulas G, Zolotukhin AS, Tabernero C *et al.* Elements distinct from the human immunodeficiency virus type 1 splice sites are responsible for the Rev dependence of the env mRNA. *J Virol* 1994; 68: 2986–2993.
163. Schwartz S, Campbell M, Nasioulas G *et al.* Mutational inactivation of an inhibitory sequence in human immunodeficiency virus type-1 results in Rev-independent *gag* expression. *J Virol* 1992; 66: 7176–7182.
164. Oberste MS, Gonda MA. Conservation of amino-acid sequence motifs in lentivirus Vif proteins. *Virus Genes* 1992; 6: 95–102.
165. Garrett ED, Tiley LS, Cullen BR. Rev activates expression of the human immunodeficiency virus type 1 vif and vpr gene products. *J Virol* 1991; 65: 1653–1657.
166. Goncalves J, Jallepalli P, Gabuzda DH. Subcellular localization of the Vif protein of human immunodeficiency virus type 1. *J Virol* 1994; 68: 704–712.
167. Michaels FH, Hattori N, Gallo RC, Franchini G. The human immunodeficiency virus type 1 (HIV-1) vif protein is located in the cytoplasm of infected cells and its effect on viral replication is equivalent to HIV-2. *AIDS Res Hum Retroviruses* 1993; 9: 1025–1030.
168. Karczewski MK, Strebel K. Cytoskeleton association and virion incorporation of the human immunodeficiency virus type 1 Vif protein. *J Virol* 1996; 70: 494–507.
169. Fan L, Peden K. Cell-free transmission of Vif mutants of HIV-1. *Virology* 1992; 190: 19–29.
170. Hoglund S, Ohagen A, Lawrence K, Gabuzda D. Role of vif during packing of the core of HIV-1. *Virology* 1994; 201: 349–355.
171. Borman AM, Quillent C, Charneau P *et al.* Human immunodeficiency virus type 1 Vif– mutant particles from restrictive cells: role of Vif in correct particle assembly and infectivity. *J Virol* 1995; 69: 2058–2067.
172. Sakai H, Shibata R, Sakuragi J *et al.* Cell-dependent requirement of human immunodeficiency virus type 1 Vif protein for maturation of virus particles. *J Virol* 1993; 67: 1663–1666.
173. Blanc D, Patience C, Schulz TF *et al.* Transcomplementation of VIF- HIV-1

mutants in CEM cells suggests that VIF affects late steps of the viral life cycle. *Virology* 1993; 193: 186–192.

174. Courcoul M, Patience C, Rey F *et al.* Peripheral blood mononuclear cells produce normal amounts of defective Vif– human immunodeficiency virus type 1 particles which are restricted for the preretrotranscription steps. *J Virol* 1995; 69: 2068–2074.
175. von Schwedler U, Song J, Aiken C, Trono D. Vif is crucial for human immunodeficiency virus type 1 proviral DNA synthesis in infected cells. *J Virol* 1993; 67: 4945–4955.
176. Sova P, Volsky DJ. Efficiency of viral DNA synthesis during infection of permissive and nonpermissive cells with vif-negative human immunodeficiency virus type 1. *J Virol* 1993; 67: 6322–6326.
177. Gabuzda DH, Lawrence K, Langhoff E *et al.* Role of vif in replication of human immunodeficiency virus type 1 in CD4+ T lymphocytes. *J Virol* 1992; 66: 6489–6495.
178. Ma XY, Sova P, Chao W, Volsky DJ. Cysteine residues in the Vif protein of human immunodeficiency virus type 1 are essential for viral infectivity. *J Virol* 1994; 68: 1714–1720.
179. Cohen EA, Dehni G, Sodroski JG, Haseltine WA. Human immunodeficiency virus vpr product is a virion-associated regulatory protein. *J Virol* 1990; 64: 3097–3099.
180. Lavallee C, Yao XJ, Ladha A *et al.* Requirement of the Pr55gag precursor for incorporation of the Vpr product into human immunodeficiency virus type 1 viral particles. *J Virol* 1994; 68: 1926–1934.
181. Paxton W, Connor RI, Landau NR. Incorporation of Vpr into human immunodeficiency virus type 1 virions: requirement for the p6 region of gag and mutational analysis. *J Virol* 1993; 67: 7229–7237.
182. Yuan X, Matsuda Z, Matsuda M *et al.* Human immunodeficiency virus vpr gene encodes a virion-associated protein. *AIDS Res Hum Retroviruses* 1990; 6: 1265–1271.
183. Heinzinger NK, Bukrinsky MI, Haggerty SA *et al.* The Vpr protein of human immunodeficiency virus type 1 influences nuclear localization of viral nucleic acids in nondividing host cells. *Proc Natl Acad Sci USA* 1994; 91: 7311–7315.
184. Wang JJ, Lu Y, Ratner L. Particle assembly and Vpr expression in human immunodeficiency virus type 1-infected cells demonstrated by immunoelectron microscopy. *J Gen Virol* 1994; 75: 2607–2614.
185. Neumann M, Saltarelli M, Harrison J *et al.* Splicing variability in HIV-1 revealed by quantitative RNA-PCR. *AIDS Res Hum Retroviruses* 1994; 10: 1527–1538.
186. Lang SM, Weeger M, Stahl HC *et al.* Importance of vpr for infection of rhesus monkeys with simian immunodeficiency virus. *J Virol* 1993; 67: 902–912.
187. Freed EO, Englund G, and Martin MA. Role of the basic domain of human immunodeficiency virus type 1 matrix in macrophage infection. *J Virol* 1995; 69: 3949–3954.
188. Levy DN, Refaeli Y, Weiner DB. Extracellular Vpr protein increases cellular permissiveness to human immunodeficiency virus replication and reactivates virus from latency. *J Virol* 1995; 69: 1243–1252.
189. Rogel ME, Wu LI, Emerman M. The human immunodeficiency virus type 1 vpr gene prevents cell proliferation during chronic infection. *J Virol* 1995; 69: 882–888.
190. Fritz CC, Zapp ML, Green MR. A human nucleoporin-like protein that specifically interacts with HIV Rev. *Nature* 1995; 376: 530–533.
191. Levy DN, Fernandes LS, Williams WV, Weiner DB. Induction of cell differenti-

ation by human immunodeficiency virus 1 vpr. *Cell* 1993; 72: 541–550.
192. Cleves AE, Novick PJ, Bankaitis VA. Mutations of the SAC1 gene suppress defects in yeast golgi and yeast actin function. *J Cell Biol* 1989; 109: 2939–2950.
193. Refaeli Y, Levy DN, Weiner DB. The glucocorticoid receptor type II complex is a target of the HIV-1 vpr gene product. *Proc Natl Acad Sci USA* 1995; 92: 3621–3625.
194. Zhao LJ, Mukherjee S, Narayan O. Biochemical mechanism of HIV-1 Vpr function. Specific interaction with a cellular protein. *J Biol Chem* 1994; 269: 15577–15582.
195. Maldarelli F, Chen MY, Willey RL, Strebel K. Human immunodeficiency virus type 1 Vpu protein is an oligomeric type I integral membrane protein. *J Virol* 1993; 67: 5056–5061.
196. Henklein P, Schubert U, Kunert O *et al.* Synthesis and characterization of the hydrophilic C-terminal domain of the human immunodeficiency virus type 1-encoded virus protein U (Vpu). *Pept Res* 1993; 6: 79–87.
197. Schubert U, Henklein P, Boldyreff B *et al.* The human immunodeficiency virus type 1 encoded Vpu protein is phosphorylated by casein kinase-2 (CK-2) at positions ser52 and Ser56 within a predicted alpha-helix–turn–alpha-helix-motif. *J Mol Biol* 1994; 236: 16–25.
198. Schubert U, Schneider T, Henklein P *et al.* Human-immunodeficiency-virus-type-1-encoded Vpu protein is phosphorylated by casein kinase II. *Eur J Biochem* 1992; 204: 875–883.
199. Willey RL, Buckler-White A, Strebel K. Sequences present in the cytoplasmic domain of CD4 are necessary and sufficient to confer sensitivity to the human immunodeficiency virus type 1 Vpu protein. *J Virol* 1994; 68: 1207–1212.
200. Willey RL, Maldarelli F, Martin MA, Strebel K. Human immunodeficiency virus type 1 Vpu protein induces rapid degradation of CD4. *J Virol* 1992; 66: 7193–7200.
201. Willey RL, Maldarelli F, Martin MA, Strebel K. Human immunodeficiency virus type 1 protein regulates the formation of intracellular gp160–CD4 complexes. *J Virol* 1992; 66: 226–234.
202. Bour S, Schubert U, Strebel K. The human immunodeficiency virus type 1 Vpu protein specifically binds to the cytoplasmic domain of CD4: implications for the mechanism of degradation. *J Virol* 1995; 69: 1510–1520.
203. Chen MY, Maldarelli F, Karczewski MK *et al.* Human immunodeficiency virus type 1 Vpu protein induces degradation of CD4 in vitro: the cytoplasmic domain of CD4 contributes to Vpu sensitivity. *J Virol* 1993; 67: 3877–3884.
204. Schubert U, Strebel K. Differential activities of the human immunodeficiency virus type 1-encoded Vpu protein are regulated by phosphorylation and occur in different cellular compartments. *J Virol* 1994; 68: 2260–2271.
205. Kestler HW, Ringler DJ, Mori K *et al.* Importance of the nef gene for maintenance of high virus loads and for development of AIDS. *Cell* 1991; 65: 651–662.
206. Daniel MD, Kirchoff F, Czajak SC *et al.* Protective effects of a live-attenuated SIV vaccine with a deletion of the *nef* gene. *Science* 1992; 258: 1938–1941.
207. Jamieson BD, Aldrovandi GM, Planelles V *et al.* Requirement of human immunodeficiency virus type 1 nef for in vivo replication and pathogenicity. *J Virol* 1994; 68: 3478–3485.
208. Garcia JV, Alfano J, Miller AD. The negative effect of human immunodeficiency virus type 1 Nef on cell surface CD4 expression is not species specific and requires the cytoplasmic domain of CD4. *J Virol* 1993; 67: 1511–1516.
209. Garcia JV, Miller AD. Serine phosphorylation-independent downregulation of cell-surface CD4 by nef. *Nature* 1991; 350: 508–511.
210. Aiken C, Konner J, Landau NR *et al.* Nef induces CD4 endocytosis: requirement for a critical dileucine motif in the membrane-proximal CD4 cytoplasmic

domain. *Cell* 1994; 76: 853–864.
211. Skowronski J, Parks D, Mariani R. Altered T cell activation and development in transgenic mice expressing the HIV-1 nef gene. *EMBO J* 1993; 12: 703–713.
212. Chowers MY, Spina CA, Kwoh TJ *et al.* Optimal infectivity in vitro of human immunodeficiency virus type 1 requires an intact nef gene. *J Virol* 1994; 68: 2906–2914.
213. de Ronde A, Klaver B, Keulen W *et al.* Natural HIV-1 NEF accelerates virus replication in primary human lymphocytes. *Virology* 1992; 188: 391–395.
214. Miller MD, Warmerdam MT, Gaston I *et al.* The human immunodeficiency virus-1 nef gene product: a positive factor for viral infection and replication in primary lymphocytes and macrophages. *J Exp Med* 1994; 179: 101–113.
215. Miller MD, Warmerdam MT, Page KA *et al.* Expression of the human immunodeficiency virus type 1 (HIV-1) *nef* gene during HIV-1 production increases progeny particle infectivity independently of gp160 or viral entry. *J Virol* 1995; 69: 579–584.
216. Zazopoulos E, Haseltine WA. Mutational analysis of the human immunodeficiency virus type 1 Eli Nef function. *Proc Natl Acad Sci USA* 1992; 89: 6634–6638.
217. Zazopoulos E, Haseltine WA. Effect of nef alleles on replication of human immunodeficiency virus type 1. *Virology* 1993; 194: 20–27.
218. Spina CA, Kwoh TJ, Chowers MY *et al.* The importance of nef in the induction of human immunodeficiency virus type 1 replication from primary quiescent CD4 lymphocytes. *J Exp Med* 1994; 179: 115–123.
219. Sawai ET, Baur A, Struble H *et al.* Human immunodeficiency virus type 1 Nef associates with a cellular serine kinase in T lymphocytes. *Proc Natl Acad Sci USA* 1994; 91: 1539–1543.
220. Saksela K, Cheng G, Baltimore D. Proline-rich (PxxP) motifs in HIV-1 Nef bind to SH3 domains of a subset of Src kinases and are required for the enhanced growth of Nef+ viruses but not for a down-regulation of CD4. *EMBO J* 1995; 14: 484–491.
221. Benichou S, Bomsel M, Bodeus M *et al.* Physical interaction of the HIV-1 Nef protein with beta-COP, a component of non-clathrin-coated vesicles essential for membrane traffic. *J Biol Chem* 1994; 269: 30073–30076.

6

Carcinogenesis and the Immune System

Manousos M. Konstantoulakis*
Mathios Konstantoulakis†
Panayiotis P. Peveretos*
Basil C. Golematis*
*Athens Medical School, Hippokration Hospital, Athens, Greece;
†Athens Medical Centre, Athens, Greece

INTRODUCTION

Acquired immunodeficiency syndrome (AIDS) is a fatal disease involving the immune system. It is estimated that by the year 2000 the number of people infected with the human immunodeficiency viruses (HIV-1, HIV-2) will be around 100 million or approximately 2% of the world's present population.

There is little doubt that the basic cause of AIDS, accepted by most scientists, is infection with the HIV viruses replicating continuously and that this infection alone will over time cause profound immune dysfunction[1]. No other specific pathogen is necessary although it is likely that other infections may hasten the immune deficiency. There is of course the opposite extreme opinion of Duesberg, who believes that at least the American cases of AIDS are the result of recreational and anti-HIV drugs[2]. His views were somewhat supported by the implication that herpesviruses may be a cause of Kaposi's sarcoma in people without AIDS. In between these beliefs, there are several investigators who believe that HIV is there and plays a significant role, but it is not the whole story[3]. It is our belief that disease development is initiated by the HIV viruses and that step by step the dysfunction of the immune system progresses through various events and finally the full-blown disease appears. The development of various neoplasms is caused not only by the immune

AIDS and Malignancies: Current Concepts and Perspectives.
Edited by B.C. Golematis and V.T. DeVita Jr

deficiency but also by mutations of cells of the lymphatic system and the appearance of autoimmune phenomena that themselves favour the development of neoplasia.

Soon after infection many patients experience a rapidly growing virus load that peaks as specific immunity against HIV comes into force. Then as the specific immunity becomes active the viral burden is suppressed to very low levels for a few or as many as 15 years[3]. The commonly accepted view that during the clinically asymptomatic phase of HIV infection the virus is also microbiologically inactive was challenged after Pantaleo[4], Embretson *et al.*[5], reported that HIV infection is active during the incubation period and the clinically latent stage of the disease. The infection progresses in the lymphoid tissue and there is a massive covert infection of T-helper lymphocytes and macrophages. As a result, during the asymptomatic years there is a slow but steady decline in the number of circulating T-helper lymphocytes that expresses CD4. After a period that may be a few months or many years the immune system ceases to control the replication of the HIV population, the viral burden rises again and the full-blown disease appears, with the opportunistic infections and neoplasms[6].

The most prevalent theories for the propagation of the virus to such levels as to cause disease are the following[7]:

1. HIV's rate of growth increases because of activation of the $CD4^+$ lymphocytes due to immune stimulation by other pathogens.
2. There is evolution of more virulent strains of HIV.
3. Antigenic diversity of the HIV population renders its replication uncontrollable by the immune system.
4. HIV evolves escape mutants.
5. The pool of precursor memory T-lymphocytes specific to HIV is exhausted.
6. Antigen-presenting cells are slowly destroyed.

DEVELOPMENT OF IMMUNE DEFICIENCY

The most important immunological change which follows HIV infection is the depletion of $CD4^+$ lymphocytes. Asymptomatic patients usually have >500 $CD4^+$ cells while, when the number falls to <50 cells/μl, patients already suffer from AIDS and mortality is much increased. There is in the first stages of infection a subtle decline in T-helper function which is independent of the decline in the $CD4^+$ cell counts[8,9].

These investigators examined the function of T-helper lymphocytes by their responsiveness to recall antigens, to 'allo' antigens and to phytohaemagglutinin (PHA). Thirty per cent only of the asymptomatic HIV-infected people had normal responses to all three antigens, while 40% had lost the ability to respond to any antigen and 11% responded to PHA only. According to Shearer and Clerici[9] only 10% of the asymptomatic individuals who respond to the three antigens will develop AIDS in the coming three years but at least 50% of those remain unresponsive to all antigens despite normal $CD4^+$ numbers. According to the model of Miedema *et al.*[10] for AIDS pathogenesis, in the first stage when an individual is infected, a mixture of HIV clones is transmitted. Virulent, high-expressing HIV clones are suppressed by cellular and humoral immune mechanisms. The low-expressing variants persist in a state of latency. This population of low-grade infected cells steadily grows, generating increasingly more virulent variants[11]. In the second stage, the continuous generation of more virulent HIV variants may be responsible for an increased memory. In the third stage, loss of antigen-presenting cell function may contribute to the breakdown of the immune system, leading to the overt replication of highly virulent HIV variants with rapid decline of $CD4^+$ and emergence of the disease (AIDS).

Another mechanism proposed for the loss of T-cell function and of $CD4^+$ depletion is programmed cell death or apoptosis. Activated-induced T-cell death can account for the above abnormalities. The hypothesis advanced by Ameisen and Capron[12] is that inappropriate induction of a form of programmed cell death in mature T-cells is involved in the pathogenesis of AIDS. Programmed cell death may contribute to the massive loss of $CD4^+$ cells that occurs during HIV progression. Programmed cell death induced both in HIV-positive and -negative persons could be prevented by type 1 cytokines (interleukin 1 (IL-1), IL-2, IL-12, interferon γ (IFN-γ)) and promoted by type two cytokines (IL-4, IL-5, IL-6, IL-10). In any case, viral infections in general exploit to various degrees the cells and interactions of the immune system to propagate themselves, which is what happens to people infected with HIV. The virus resides preferentially in $CD4^+$ T-lymphocytes and other cells of the immune system. The activated T-cells are much more hospitable to growing viruses than are resting T-cells. In addition, type 2 cytokines produced by T-cells when type 1 response is lost can actually stimulate the virus in the CD^+ T-cells[13]. Tumour necrosis factor α (TNF-α) and its soluble receptor, which are found at high circulating levels, also promote replication of HIV via activation of the NF-$\kappa\beta$ transcription factor[14].

Another possible mechanism for the decrease in $CD4^+$ T-lymphocytes during the long subclinical phase of infection is autoimmunity. High-resolution electron microscopy has shown that the HIV virion consists of a double layer of lipid molecules similar to the membranes surrounding human cells. These layers contain several proteins, the so-called class I and class II histocompatibility complex molecules, which in their normal location are important in controlling the immune response. The virion also contains several other proteins whose function is still not completely understood. These are the gp120, gp41 and the matrix proteins p17 and p24, which contain the genetic material of the virus. It is possible that gp120 and gp41 have an additional role in enhancing the immune dysregulatory effect of the killer T-cells and antibody-producing B-cells.

AUTOIMMUNE PHENOMENA IN AIDS

Patients infected with HIV and presenting with AIDS may exhibit, in addition to impaired cell-mediated immunity due to qualitative and quantitative $CD4^+$ T-cell defects, abnormalities in B-cell function and the presence of autoreactive T-cells. This results in polyclonal hypergammaglobulinaemia with increases in immunoglobulin G (IgG), IgM and IgD, especially in the early course of the disease[15,16]. However, despite the evidence of polyclonal B-cell activation, B-lymphocytes have reduced responses *in vitro* to mitogens and various other antigens. In addition, HIV-positive patients not infrequently exhibit autoimmune phenomena and disorders. Since the first description of pancytopenia accompanying AIDS in 1983[17] many cases of cytopenias related to HIV and AIDS have appeared in the literature. A high percentage of these cytopenias may be autoimmune in origin. Cytopenias in AIDS may be partially due to the presence of autoantibodies against lymphocytes and neutrophils, as already mentioned. The antilymphocyte antibodies are directed against non-polymorphic determinants of the major histocompatibility complex (MHC) class II molecules[18], while antineutrophil antibodies seem to be non-specific and increase in quantity as the disease progresses, worsening the neutropenia[19].

Autoimmune haemolytic anaemia is rather rare although the direct Coombs test is positive in 20% of the patients who have hypergammaglobulinaemia[20,21]. However, the high incidence of anaemia at presentation of the disease (70–90% of the patients) has no relation to autoantibodies.

Thrombocytopenia, which occurs in 5–30% of infected individuals or AIDS patients, may be of autoimmune origin. Specific antiplatelet antibodies and platelet-bound immune complexes have been demonstrated in these cases[22,23]. Megakaryocytes may contain HIV-related RNA, which suggests direct involvement of progenitor cells in the development of thrombocytopenia[24]. According to Saba *et al.* anaemia, granulocytopenia and cytopenias in general are multifactorial, and among the factors that suppress haematopoiesis are antibodies specifically directed against the progenitor and haematopoietic cells in the bone marrow of HIV-infected individuals[25].

Other autoimmune phenomena in HIV-positive individuals include the presence of antinuclear antibodies but not anti-DNA in approximately 15% of patients, in a small percentage of whom the clinical symptoms mimic systemic lupus erythematosus (SLE)[26]. A few patients have symptoms that are compatible with Sjögren's syndrome and, because of the increasing incidence of HIV infection, patients with Sjögren's syndrome with atypical features should be checked for the presence of underlying HIV[27]. Via and

Shearer suggest that B-cell hyperactivity in HIV-positive individuals is multifactorial and that, despite the defects in T-cell-mediated immunity, T-cells may actively contribute to humoral autoimmunity[28]. It is also suggested, extrapolating from experiments in mice with SLE, that defective function of $CD4^+$ cells may reflect at least in part a compensatory immunosuppressive mechanism aimed at reducing further activation of $CD4^+$ cells.

TUMOURS ASSOCIATED WITH CONGENITAL IMMUNE DEFICIENCIES

The environment in which we live contains an immense number of viruses, bacteria, fungi and saprophytes that invade and colonize the body. Our defence mechanisms are usually efficient in coping with the invaders through our complex immune system, made up of a multitude of interdependent cellular and humoral components. When there is some type of breakdown of the immune system, various states of immune deficiency are identified and neoplasms may develop at a high incidence. According to Ioachim the tumours should be called opportunistic since they have the same mechanism of development as the opportunistic infections[29].

The immune deficiencies can be broadly divided into primary and secondary, congenital or acquired. The most important primary immunodeficiencies are the X-linked hyper-IgM syndrome, X-linked severe combined immunodeficiency (X-SCID), X-linked agammaglobulinaemia, SCID with absent $CD8^+$ T-cells, Wiskott–Aldrich syndrome and the bare lymphocyte syndrome. There are of course several other syndromes and subtypes, and their classification has become increasingly complex[30] and beyond the scope of this review.

Several groups of investigators have identified the genes responsible for classic immunodeficiencies. Mutations in the CD ligand, the CD4OL (cytokine gene locus Xq26), are responsible for the X-linked hyper-IgM syndrome[31]. The X-SCID syndrome is due to mutations in the γ-chain of the IL-2 receptor (IL-2Rγ), that transmits its downstream signal through the James family kinase, JAK3[32].

All primary immunodeficiency syndromes have a high incidence of neoplasms. Patients with SCID usually do not survive beyond the age of two years. Despite the short life-span of these patients 42 cases of neoplasms, 31 of which were non-Hodgkin lymphomas, were recorded up to 1987[35]. In patients with X-linked agammaglobulinaemia approximately 6% will develop neoplasms, usually leukaemias and lymphomas.

Patients with Wiskott–Aldrich syndrome have the highest incidence of neoplasms—around 10%—among the primary immunodeficiency syndromes. The majority are extranodal and brain lymphomas[36]. In ataxia–

telangiectasia, where the immune deficiencies are both cellular and humoral, with T-cell depletion and immunoglobulin abnormalities, a similar high incidence of leukaemias and lymphomas is found as in Wiskott–Aldrich syndrome. However, other solid tumours develop as well.

As is seen in most of these primary immune deficiencies the great majority of tumours are of haematological origin. An exception to this phenomenon appears to be the various dysgammaglobulinaemias in which defects of the B-lymphocytes result in marked decrease or absence of one or two of the three main classes of immunoglobulins. In IgA deficiency adenocarcinomas of the colon and stomach and carcinoma of the lungs and oesophagus are the main neoplasms developing, although cases of leukaemia and lymphoma are not few[36]. There is no doubt that qualitative and/or quantitative congenital abnormalities of the T- or B-lymphocytes, or both, after a period of time extending from a few to many years, may induce malignancies, mainly haematological, possibly with the help of other factors.

TUMOURS ASSOCIATED WITH ACQUIRED IMMUNE DEFICIENCIES

Neoplasms Associated with Autoimmune Disorders

In autoimmune diseases immune dysregulation initiates production of autoantibodies and autoreactive T-lymphocytes that play a pathogenetic role in the development of autoimmunity. This immune dysregulation associated with autoimmune disease may relate to a Th1–Th2 imbalance that involves mainly $CD4^+$ and possibly $CD8^+$ cells[37,38].

The close relationship between autoimmunity and cancer is manifested by the finding of increased incidence of malignancies among patients with autoimmune diseases and conversely an increased incidence of autoimmune conditions and autoantibodies in patients with neoplasms. Canoso and Cohen found eight patients from a series of 70 with SLE who were followed up for several years who developed lymphoma, myeloma, and carcinoma of the uterine cervix.

Autoimmune haemolytic anaemia is the most common autoimmune syndrome associated with cancer, usually with lymphomas and leukaemias and to a lesser extent with solid tumours. In one series of 175 patients malignant disease was found in 14%[39]. In autoimmune thrombocytopenia the incidence of neoplasms varies from 4% to 19%[40].

In a large series of patients with polymyositis cancer was diagnosed in 9% and in patients with dermatomyositis the incidence of neoplasms was 15%[41]. Further details of the incidence of cancer in autoimmune disorders can be found in the review by Sela and Shoenfeld[42].

Tumours Associated with Transplantation

Transplanted patients with allogenic organs are heavily immunosuppressed to prevent rejection. The most powerful immunosuppressant is cyclosporin A, which has a selective inhibitory activity on T-cell differentiation. As in the primary immunodeficiencies and the autoimmune diseases, lymphomas are commonly developed, having often increased anti-Epstein–Barr virus (anti-EBV) antibodies, especially against the viral capsid antigen. Lymphomas represent 26% of all tumours while in the general population they occur rarely. It should be stressed that brain lymphomas have also a high incidence[43]. Kaposi's sarcoma (KS) is also very common in transplanted patients, causing gastrointestinal bleeding and death in a substantial percentage of afflicted patients. In general, neoplasms are more aggressive when they develop in younger patients; the time of tumour diagnosis after transplantation varies from 23 months for Kaposi's sarcoma to 100 months for carcinomas of the vulva and the perineum[43].

Tumours Associated with Chemotherapy and Irradiation

There is no doubt that the incidence of second malignancies is significantly increased in patients treated with chemotherapy and/or radiotherapy if they live long enough. There is no need to reiterate the well-known facts regarding exposure to irradiation and radiotherapy as important factors in leukaemogenesis and the development of non-Hodgkin lymphomas and other solid tumours.

There is increasing evidence that alkylating agents and agents that inhibit the activity of topoisomerase II, such as the anthracyclines (dauno+doxo), the epipodophylotoxins (teniposide+etoposide) and actinomycin D are important leukaemogens[44,45]. The risk depends on the total administered dose and the schedule of administration. For example, the frequency of leukaemia is 2.6% in patients with germ cell tumours treated with <2000 mg/m^2 epipodophylotoxin, while it increases to 11.3% in those treated with >2000 mg/m^2 [46]. Patients treated with anthracyclines and irradiation have a significant increase in bone sarcoma and short time to diagnosis of the second malignancy. Second neoplasms—leukaemias, lymphomas, and solid tumours—developed after a mean of 7.5 years of observation in patients with Wilm's tumour treated with doxorubicin and irradiation[47]. Acute leukaemias, Hodgkin lymphomas and solid tumours are significantly increased in patients with rhabdomyosarcoma, non-Hodgkin lymphoma (NHL), breast cancer, ovarian cancer etc. The striking increase of second solid malignancies in patients with Hodgkin's disease who received combined modality treatment, and were followed up for almost 20 years, was recently reported by Doria[48]. At 20 years patients treated with chemotherapy and low-dose irradiation had an actuarial incidence of second malignancies of 12%, while in patients who were initially treated with radiotherapy only and on relapse with chemotherapy and radiotherapy the incidence was 41%[48].

The above findings stress the importance of repeated radiotherapy treatment over time and also the importance of combined modality treatment. They show in addition that the incidence of second malignancies is much higher in patients with Hodgkin's disease than in patients with other neoplasms, probably because of the additional well-known primary deficiency of cellular immunity in these patients.

HIV INFECTION AND CANCER

AIDS offers a new illustration of the relationship between immune deficiency and neoplasia. It also may illustrate the relationship between neoplasia and viral infection, but viral infection *per se* is rarely or ever sufficient to produce fully malignant change. Thus, if a virus is aetiologically involved in tumour development then it must form part of a complex multistep pathogenesis[49]. Although HIV is not believed to induce cell transformation directly, as already mentioned above, a recent report indicates that at least one type of T-cell lymphoma—the long terminal repeats (LTR) of an integrated HIV provirus—activates a cellular oncogene, fps, adjacent to its site of integration[50].

As in other states of primary and of acquired immune deficiencies, patients with a highly depressed number of T-helper lymphocytes have a high risk of developing tumours and NHL occurred in about 40% of all AIDS patients in the late 1970s and early 1980s[51]. Because patients are living longer in recent years, the incidence of neoplasms has increased and some other histological types and unusual locations have emerged and become prevalent.

Kaposi's Sarcoma (KS)

KS accounts for the highest percentage of malignancies occurring in AIDS patients. According to the population-based disease registries for AIDS and cancer, for San Francisco residents, during the time period 1980–1987, 83% of a total 1756 neoplasms were KS[52]. The difference in incidence of KS between homosexuals (50%) compared with non-homosexuals (8%), the absence of KS in women with HIV infection in upstate Yew York [53] and the presence of KS without HIV infection[54] show that the pathogenesis of HIV-related KS may be complex, as already mentioned, involving interrelated additional factors such as genetic predisposition, geographic cofactors and different ways of life and behaviour. KS shows an unexplained difference in incidence not only among the various groups of AIDS but also among the different types of immunodeficiency syndromes. It is rare in the congenital and acquired immunodeficiencies, with the exception of transplanted patients in whom the incidence is high but not approaching that of AIDS. KS develops in 5.5% of renal transplant patients, while in AIDS it is well over 35% of all patients. KS in recipients of renal transplants involving internal organs caused gastrointestinal bleeding and death on one-third of patients in one series. Recently, a substantial decrease of KS has been noted, possibly pathogenetically related to the decrease of some opportunistic infections due to prophylactic treatment with antibiotics[55].

Lymphomas

Non-Hodgkin Lymphomas (NHL)

The first cases of NHL in AIDs were described in 1982; 10 years later the projection was made that between 8% and 27% of all NHL in the USA would be attributable to HIV infection[56]. The ratio between Hodgkin's disease and NHL is changed because of the increase of NHL, especially in young adults. In one series of 72 cases of lymphoma in patients with HIV infection, 66 had NHL and 6 Hodgkin's disease[29]. Approximately 60–70% of patients have high-grade NHL and the rest intermediate or low grade. The low grade accounts for only 10% of cases[57]. These figures are quite different from those in the general population, in whom the incidence of high grade is 20% and of low grade 35%. In contrast to the general population there is also a reversal of nodal versus extranodal location ratio, with more tumours involving the viscera than the lymph nodes. The most commonly involved locations are the gastrointestinal tract, the brain and the bone marrow[58]. Unusual sites of NHL development include the heart, the sinuses, the soft tissues and the anus and rectum in homosexuals. Approximately 5–10% of HIV-infected patients will develop NHL. Because NHL is a relatively late complication of AIDS a cohort of patients on retroviral therapy have a risk of developing NHL of approximately 29% at 36 months, or three times more frequently at the time of death[59]. A large prospective study in patients with advanced HIV infection treated with zidovudine showed a projected incidence of NHL of 1.6% per year[60].

The pathogenesis of NHL in AIDS has not been elucidated but probably is complex and multifactorial and may be a step-by-step procedure. One very important factor is progressive immunological decline during HIV infection. The importance of this factor becomes evident from the fact that NHL in high incidence is seen in almost every immunodeficient disease—congenital or acquired. Another factor is the chronic antigenic stimulation by HIV that induces immune dysregulation and proliferation of B-lymphocytes resulting in persistent generalized lymphadenopathy and polyclonal hypergammaglobulinaemia[61.62].

IL-6 and IL-10, which act as strong B-cell autocrine growth factors, are elevated in AIDS patients who develop lymphoma[63,64].

Abnormal DNA rearrangements binding to chromosomal translocations (+8:14, +8:22, +8:2) result in the activation of c-myc, which has been shown to cause malignant transformation of B-lymphocytes. EBV may also be implicated in the pathogenesis of AIDS lymphoma because the EBV genome is found in 30–60% of patients with AIDS[65]. A recent report suggests an active pathogenetic role for HIV infection as viral genome has been found incorporated into the *fur* gene complex on chromosome 15 in non-B-lymphoma cells[66]. This is in contrast to our belief that generally HIV is not an oncogenic virus. In conclusion we suggest that immune deficiency induced by HIV infection results in reduced immunological surveillance which permits the abnormal B-lymphocytes produced by chronic viral antigenic stimulation to over-proliferate and become neoplastic. At some stage of proliferation the presence of the EBV genome together with the activation of c-myc enhance the neoplastic transformation. The AIDS-related lymphomas, in contrast to the general population, appear at a much younger age, are more aggressive, less sensitive to chemotherapy, with fewer and shorter complete remissions[58].

Another salient feature of AIDS-related NHL is the frequent involvement of the central nervous system (CNS). It occurs in 20–40% of patients with AIDS-related lymphoma, while in NHL of the general population it is less than 2%[61]. The incidence of CNS lymphoma in post-transplant lymphoproliferative disorders is approximately 20%, which is similar to that of AIDS patients. It is interesting that in two completely different disorders with immunodeficiency of different aetiology the incidence of CNS metastatic NHL is comparable.

The primary CNS lymphoma usually presents as a brain tumour but it may also involve the leptomininges, the eyes, the spinal cord or a combination of these sites. Systemic NHL is not present and only rarely does the lymphoma appear outside the CNS during the course of the disease. Approximately 6% of patients with HIV infection develop primary CNS lymphoma and it seems that its incidence continues to rise as HIV-infected individuals live longer[67,68]. The importance of the status of the immune system for the development of CNS lymphoma becomes obvious, since the peak of its incidence occurs when $CD4^+$ lymphocytes are less than 50/μl. On the contrary the incidence of systemic NHL has its peak incidence when $CD4^+$ lymphocytes are less than 200/μl[67].

The EBV genome, present in 30–60% of cases of systemic NHL, as already mentioned, is present in almost 100% of cases of CNS lymphoma, suggesting an important pathogenetic role of EBV infection[69,70]. The biological behaviour of CNS lymphoma is much more aggressive than systemic NHL of identical histology. Treatment with radiotherapy without or with chemotherapy gives significantly poorer results than in non-AIDS patients[71].

Hodgkin's Disease

Among the 1756 cases of malignancy diagnosed in patients with AIDS who were residents of San Francisco, 16 or 1% had Hodgkin's disease. The incidence is much higher than that of the general population. Similar findings were reported by Serraino *et al.*[72] and more recently by Lyter *et al.*[73], who reported the results of the study of the Pittsburg component of the multi-centre AIDS cohort study from 1984 to 1993. This study not only confirms the previous findings but it also shows the increasing incidence of the disease. In this study NHL had an incidence 83 times higher compared to the normal population and Hodgkin's disease 19.8 times. The disease in HIV-infected patients is more aggressive than in non-infected patients, the reponse to treatment less successful, the histology more unfavourable, the survival time shorter and the bone marrow is infiltrated in more than 50% of the cases.

Other Neoplasms

Cervical and Anal Neoplasia

It has been found recently that HIV-induced immunodeficiency may be responsible for the development of neoplasia of the cervical and anal mucosa. It is postulated that these cancers will become even more common in patients with AIDS in the future as they live much longer. In the San Francisco study the incidence of cervical and anal cancers, non-melanoma skin cancers and sinus cancers occurred more frequently than expected. The odds ratio for detection of anal cancer was 2.6 times compared to the pre-AIDS era[74]. The prolonged severe immunodeficiency provides the milieu for the emergence of diseases that develop after longer periods of latency such as anal and cervical cancers.

There is limited published experience regarding presentation and treatment outcome in HIV-infected persons with invasive anal cancer. However, there is general agreement that there is poor treatment outcome and short survival[75].

The incidence of cervical cancer is significantly higher than anal cancer. Maiman *et al.*[76] described the clinical features of invasive cervical cancer. They found no difference in histology or grade compared with non-HIV-infected women but a significant difference in the clinical and surgical stage. Only 6% of the HIV-infected women had limited stage disease, compared with 40% of non-infected women. In addition the disease is more aggressive, less likely to respond to standard therapy and consequently associated with poorer prognosis. The Centers for Disease Control have recently amended the AIDS surveillance case definition to include invasive cervical cancer among the conditions diagnostic of AIDS in HIV-infected women. For early diagnosis Papani colaov (PAP) smears and colposcopy every six months are indicated. Human papilloma virus (HPV) genotypes 16, 18 and 31 are detected in 90% of cervical intra-epithelial grade III lesions and invasive cervical cancers. The mechanisms by which HPV contributes to the development of cervical and anal neoplasia are not established. It seems that the E6 and E7 genes of HPV-16 are critical for the development of neoplasia[77]. E6 and E7 bind to p53 and the Rb protein respectively. These cellular protein products of the anti-oncogenes probably function as essential growth regulators in the normal cell. Loss of normal quantity or function of the above proteins is associated with the development of retinoblastoma, colorectal cancer and other tumours[78]. The HPV-16 E7 oncoprotein is able to bind the retinoblastoma gene product[78,79].

HIV-infected subjects are more likely to have detectable cervical or anal HPV-infection than non-HIV-infected controls. Also, detectable cervical and anal HPV infection is more common among HIV-infected subjects with low $CD4^+$ T-cell counts. It is therefore possible that the HIV infection causing immunodeficiency may be responsible for the propagation of HPV and the development of neoplasia.

Testicular Cancer

The incidence of testicular cancer is increased in HIV-infected subjects[73]. Lyter *et al.* found an eight-fold increase of testicular cancers but their conclusions on increased incidence are based on a very small number of patients. According to Gunthel *et al.*[80] there is no increased incidence of testicular cancers, the proportion of seminomas and non-seminomas is similar to the general population, and the clinical picture and response to treatment are also similar. However, the duration of response cannot be compared because AIDS patients die quite early from other complications of their disease.

Skin Cancers

Non-melanoma skin cancers are significantly increased according to various investigators[43,81–83]. These tumours include condyloma, carcinoma *in situ* or Bowen's disease, squamous cell carcinoma of the oral cavity and metastatic basal cell carcinoma. This is similar to the findings of the epidemiological study of San Francisco, in which increased incidence of cancer of the skin and lips was found. Conversely, others did not find any increase of the incidence in their HIV infected patients.

Other Cancers

In most large series lung cancer is not increased in HIV-infected subjects. Braun, however, found 6 cases among 500 HIV-seropositive individuals. If this is extrapolated then there is a 14-fold increased risk compared with that of white men. The patients present at a younger age than is typical for lung cancer in the general population, they have a more advanced disease at diagnosis and the histology shows increased incidence of adenocarcinomas.

There is some indication that gastrointestinal neoplasia may be increased in young patients, hepatobiliary cancer, soft tissue sarcomas and other solid tumours[43,84].

We believe that as patients with AIDS live longer because of proper prophylactic and disease treatment there will be a significant increase in the incidence of solid tumours and every other type of cancer.

CONCLUSIONS

This review deals with the abnormalities of the immune system caused by HIV infection and their gradual progression to profound immunodeficiency and development of AIDS. It also reviews the consequences of immune deficiency in AIDS patients with the development of autoimmune phenomena and of various neoplasms.

There is a variety of immunodeficiencies, unrelated to HIV infection, congenital and acquired, primary or induced by immunosuppressive drugs in transplanted patients, in chemotherapy patients or in patients with autoimmune disorders, all of which show an increased incidence of similar neoplasms as in AIDS patients. This phenomenon indicates that immunodeficiency of any origin and of almost any part of the complex immune system may be responsible for the development of malignancy. Only the triggering mechanism that initiates the immunodeficiency is different in these unrelated disorders.

The question as to whether HIV may be the sole cause of AIDS is still unanswered and the debate continues, with different theories each supported by experimental findings. It is probable that more than one factor plays a role in the development of the disease. A very important factor in HIV infection is autoimmunity. Patients may have abnormalities of B-cell function, autoreactive T-cells may be present, autoantibodies against lymphocytes are frequently detected, and increased synthesis with the production of unusual kinds of interferons are present that trigger autoimmune disease through disturbance of several immunological and interferon cascades[85].

All these events may suggest that, as in the chronic myeloproliferative disorders, there is overlap of the expression and consequences of HIV infection, of autoimmunity and of development of cancer. There are experiments and clinical data suggesting that autoimmunity plays a role in the development of cancer[86] and, conversely, that various types of cancers exhibit autoimmune phenomena considered as paraneoplastic. In the case of AIDS the initial triggering mechanism is HIV infection. During the incubation period there is immune disregulation favouring the development of autoimmune phenomena through the presence of viral particles mimicking parts of immune cell molecules leading to their destruction, so that in conjunction with the hyperproliferation of lymphocytes and induction of apoptosis, lymphomas and other neoplasms develop.

In other immune deficiency disorders the triggering mechanisms may be different, such as other types of viruses, bacteria, drugs or natural substances inducing mutations, but with similar end results as in HIV infection.

REFERENCES

1. Ho DD, Neumann AU, Perelson AS *et al.* Rapid turnover of plasma virions and CD4 lymphocytes in HIV-1 infection. *Nature* 1995; 373: 123–126.
2. Duesberg PH. The role of drugs in the origin of AIDS. *Biomed Pharmacother* 1992; 46: 3–15.
3. Schnittman SM, Psallidopoulos MC, Lane HC *et al.* The reservoir for HIV-1 in human peripheral blood is a T-cell that maintains expression of CD4. *Science* 1989; 245: 305–308.
4. Pantaleo G. HIV infection is active and progressive in lymphoid tissue during the clinically latent stage of disease. *Nature* 1993; 362: 355–358.
5. Embretson J, Zupancic M, Ribas JL *et al.* Massive covert infection of helper T lymphocytes and macrophages by HIV during the incubation period of AIDS. *Nature* 1993; 362: 359–362.
6. Ho DD, Moudgil T, Alam M. Quantitation of human immunodeficiency virus type 1 in the blood of infected persons. *N Engl J Med* 1989; 321: 1621–1625.
7. McLean AP. The balance of power between HIV and the immune system. *Trends Microbiol* 1993; 1: 9–13.
8. Clerici M, Stocks NT, Zaiac RA *et al.* Detection of three distinct patterns of T helper cell dysfunction in asymptomatic, human immunodeficiency virus-seropositive patients. *J Clin Invest* 1989; 84: 1892–1899.
9. Shearer GM, Clerici M. How human immunodeficiency virus ravages the immune system. *Curr Opinion Immunol* 1992; 4: 463–465.
10. Miedema F, Tersmette M, vanLier RAW. AIDS pathogenesis: a dynamic interaction between HIV and immune system. *Immunol Today* 1993; 14: 193–297.
11. Roberts JD, Bebenek K, Kunkel TA. The accuracy of reverse transcriptase from HIV-1. *Science* 1988; 242: 1171–1173.
12. Ameisen JC, Capron A. Cell dysfunction and depletion in AIDS: the programmed cell death hypothesis. *Immunol Today* 1991; 12: 102–105.
13. Shearer GM. Type 1 helper T-cell response: a leader in HIV control. *Clin Immunol Spectrum* 1994; 6(3): 1, 12–13.
14. Dalgleish AG. The immune response to HIV: potential for immunotherapy? *Immunol Today* 1995; 16: 356–358.
15. Fauci AS. The human immunodeficiency virus: infectivity and mechanisms of pathogenesis. *Science* 1988; 239: 617–622.
16. Mizuma H, Zolia-Pazner S, Litwin S *et al.* Serum IgD elevations as a marker of B cells activation during infection with the human immunodeficiency viruses. *Clin Exp Immunol* 1987; 68: 5–14.
17. Spivak JL, Selonick SE, Ruinn TC. Acquired immune deficiency syndrome and pancytopenia. *JAMA* 1983; 250: 3084–3087.

18. Golding H, Robey FA, Gates FT III *et al.* Identification of monologous regions in human immunodeficiency virus I gp 41 and human MHC class II β 1 domain. I. Monoclonal antibodies against gp41-derived peptide and patients' sera react with native HLA class II antigens suggesting a role for autoimmunity in the pathogenesis of acquired immune deficiency syndrome. *J Ex Med* 1988; 167: 914–923.
19. Klaassen RJL, Mulder JW, Viekk ABJ *et al.* Autoantibodies against peripheral blood cells appear early in HIV infection and their prevalence increases with disease progression. *Clin Exp Immunol* 1990; 81: 11–17.
20. Perkocha LA, Rodgers GM. Hematologic aspects of human immunodeficiency virus infection: laboratory and clinical considerations. *Am J Hematol* 1988; 29: 94–105.
21. Rapoport AP, Rowe JM, McMican A. Life-threatening autoimmune hemolytic anemia in a patient with the acquired immune deficiency syndrome. *Transfusion* 1988; 28: 190–191.
22. Battaib A, Oksenhendler E, Fromont P *et al.* Immunochemical analysis of platelet autoantibodies in HIV-related thrombocytopenic purpura: a study of 68 patients. *Br J Haematol* 1989; 73: 241–247.
23. Karpatkin S, Nardi M, Lennette ET *et al.* Antihuman immunodeficiency virus type I antibody complexes on platelets of seropositive thrombocytopenic homosexuals and narcotic addicts. *Proc Natl Acad Sci USA* 1988; 85: 9763–9767.
24. Zon LI, Groopman JE. Haematologic manifestations of the human immune deficiency virus (HIV). *Semin Hematol* 1988; 25: 208–218.
25. Saba HI, Spiers ASD, Greene JN, Alkan S. Hematologic effects of human immunodeficiency virus infection. *Cancer Control* 1995; 2: 104–112.
26. Kopelman RG, Zolia-Pazner S. Association of human immunodeficiency virus infection and autoimmune phenomena. *Am J Med* 1988; 48: 82–88.
27. Ulirsch RC, Jaffe ES. Sjögren's syndrome-like illness associated with the acquired immunodeficiency syndrome-related complex. *Hum Pathol* 1987; 18: 1063–1068.
28. Via CS, Shearer GM. T-cell interactions in autoimmunity: insights from a murine model of graft-versus-host disease. *Curr Opinion Immunol* 1989; 1: 753–756.
29. Ioachim HL. The opportunistic tumors of immune deficiency. *Adv Cancer Res* 1990; 54: 301–317.
30. Stiehm RE. In Stiehm RE, Fulginity VA (eds) *Immunologic Disorders in Infants and Children*. Philadelphia: Saunders, 1980; pp. 183–218.
31. Conley ME. X-linked immunodeficiencies. *Curr Opinion Genet Dev* 1994; 4: 401–406.
32. Conley ME. Primary immunodeficiencies: a flurry of new genes. *Immunol Today* 1995; 16: 313–315.
33. Derry JM, Ochs HD, Francke U. Isolation of a novel gene mutated in Wiskott–Aldrich syndrome. *Cell* 1994; 78: 635–644.
34. Kirchgessner CU, Patil CK, Evans JW *et al.* DNA-dependent kinase (p350) as a candidate gene for the murine SCID defect. *Science* 1995; 267: 1178–1183.
35. Filipovich AH, Heinitz KJ, Robison LL, Frizzera G. The Immunodeficiency Cancer Registry. A research resource. *Am J Pediatr Hematol Oncol* 1987; 9: 183–184.
36. Ammann AJ, Hong AR. In Stiehm RE, Fulginiti VA (eds) *Immunologic Disorders in Infants and Children*. Philadelphia: Saunders, 1980; pp. 291–297.
37. Sakaguchi S, Ermak TH, Toda M *et al.* Induction of autoimmune disease in mice by germline alteration of the T cell receptor gene expression. *J Immunol* 1994; 152: 1471–1484.
38. Wen L, Roberts SJ, Viney JL *et al.* Immunoglobulin synthesis and generalized autoimmunity in mice congenitally deficient in alpha beta (+) T cells. *Nature* 1994; 369: 654–658.

39. Dacie JV. *The Haemolytic Anaemias, Congenital and Acquired* (3rd ed, Part II), London: Churchill, 1962.
40. Doan C, Bouroncle BA, Wiseman BK. Idiopathic and secondary thrombocytopenic purpura: clinical study and evaluation of 381 cases over a period of 28 years. *Ann Intern Med* 1960; 53: 861–867.
41. Sigurgeirsson B, Lindelof B, Edhag O, Assander E. Risk of cancer in patients with dermatomyositis or polymyositis: a population-based study. *N Engl J Med* 1992; 326: 363–367.
42. Sela O, Shoenfeld V. Cancer in autoimmune diseases. *Semin Arthritis Rheum* 1988; 18: 77–87.
43. Penn J. Tumors of the immunocompromised patient. *Annu Rev Med* 1988; 39: 63–73.
44. Tervey KM, Rowe TC, Young L *et al.* Adriamycin-induced DNA damage mediated by mammalian DNA-topoisomerase II. *Science* 1984; 226: 466–468.
45. Long BH, Stringfellow DA. Inhibitors of topoisomerase II: structure–activity relationships and mechanism of action of podophyllin congeners. *Adv Enzyme Regul* 1988; 17: 223–256.
46. Smith MA, Rubenstein L, Ungerleider RS. Therapy related acute myeloid leukemia following treatment with epipodophyllotoxins: estimating the risks. *Med Pediatr Oncol* 1994; 23: 86–98.
47. Breslow NE, Takashima JR, Whitton JA *et al.* Second malignant neoplasms following treatment for Wilm's tumor: a report from the National Wilm's tumor study group. *J Clin Oncol* 1995; 13: 1851–1859.
48. Doria R, Hofford TH, Farber LR *et al.* Second solid malignancies after combined modality therapy for Hodgkin's disease. *J Clin Oncol* 1995; 13: 2016–2022.
49. Rickinson AB. Introduction: viruses and human cancer. *Cancer Biol* 1992; 3: 249–251.
50. McGrath MS, Herndier BG, Reyes G, Shiramizu BT. HIV-associated T-cell lymphoma: evidence that HIV may cause directly T-cell transformation. *J Cell Biochem* 1992; 53 (Suppl. 16E, Abstract Q) 335.
51. Friedman-Kien AE, Laubenstein LJ, Rubinstein P *et al.* Disseminated Kaposi's sarcoma in homosexual men. *Ann Intern Med* 1982; 96: 693–700.
52. Reynolds P, Saunders LD, Layefsky ME, Lemp GF. The spectrum of acquired immunodeficiency syndrome (AIDS)-associated malignancies in San Francisco, 1980–1987. *Am J Epidemiol* 1993; 137: 19–30.
53. Rabkin CS, Biggar RJ, Baptiste MS *et al.* Cancer incidence trends in women at high risk of human immunodeficiency virus (HIV) infection. *Intern J Cancer* 1993; 55: 208–212.
54. Levine AM. HIV related malignancies. *Proc AACR* 1992; 33: 590–591.
55. Selwyn PA. Prophylactic administration of antibiotics in patients with HIV infection. *Hosp Pract* 1986; 21: 149–153.
56. Gail MH, Pluda JM, Rabkin CS *et al.* Projections of the incidence of non-Hodgkin's lymphoma related to acquired immunodeficiency syndrome. *J Natl Cancer Inst* 1991; 83: 685–690.
57. Freter CE. Acquired immunodeficiency syndrome-associated lymphoma. *Monogr Nat Cancer Inst* 1990; 10: 45–54.
58. Remick SC. Acquired immunodeficiency syndrome-related non-Hodgkin's lymphoma. *Cancer Control* 1995; 2: 97–103.
59. Kaplan MH. Clinical insights in HIV related malignancies. *Proc AACR* 1992; 33: 591–592.
60. Moore RD, Kessler H, Richman DD *et al.* Non-Hodgkin's lymphoma in patients with advanced HIV infection treated with zidovudine. *JAMA* 1991; 265: 1208–1221.

61. Ziegler JL, Beckstead JA, Volberding PA *et al.* Non-Hodgkin's lymphoma in 90 homosexual men: relation to generalized lymphadenopathy and acquired immunodeficiency syndrome. *N Engl J Med* 1984; 311: 565–570.
62. Shiramizu B, McGrath MS. Molecular pathogenesis of AIDS-associated non-Hodgkin's lymphoma. *Hematol Oncol Clin North Am* 1991; 5: 323–330.
63. Birx DL, Redfield RR, Tencer K *et al.* Induction of interleukin-6 during human immunodeficiency virus infection. *Blood* 1990; 76: 2303–2310.
64. Masoon R, Zhang Y, Bond MW, Scadden DT *et al.* Interleukin-10 is an autocrine growth factor for acquired immunodeficiency syndrome-related B-cell lymphoma. *Blood* 1995; 85: 3423–3430.
65. Subar M, Neri A, Inghiranmi G *et al.* Frequent c-myc oncogene activation and infrequent presence of Epstein–Barr virus genome in AIDS-associated lymphoma. *Blood* 1988; 72: 667–671.
66. Shiramizu B, Herndier BG, McGrath MS. Identification of a common clonal human immunodeficiency virus integration site in human immunodeficiency virus-associated lymphoma. *Cancer Res* 1994; 54: 2069–2972.
67. Pluda JM, Yarhoan R, Jaffe ES *et al.* Development of non-Hodgkin's lymphoma in a cohort of patients with severe human immunodeficiency (HIV) infection on long-term anti-retroviral therapy. *Ann Intern Med* 1990; 113: 276–282.
68. Levine AM. AIDS-related malignancies: the emerging epidemic. *J Natl Cancer Inst* 1993; 85: 1382–1397.
69. Hanto DW, Frizzera G, Gail-Peczalska KJ *et al.* Epstein–Barr virus, immunodeficiency and B-cell lymphoproliferation. *Transplantation* 1985; 39: 461–472.
70. McMahon EM, Glass JD, Hayward SD *et al.* Epstein–Barr virus in AIDS-related primary central nervous system lymphoma. *Lancet* 1991; 338: 969–973.
71. DeAngelis L. Current management of primary central nervous system lymphoma. *Oncology* 1995; 9: 63–71.
72. Serraino M, Bellas C, Campo E *et al.* Hodgkin's disease in patients with antibodies to immunodeficiency virus: a study of 22 patients. *Cancer* 1990; 65: 2248–2254.
73. Lyter DW, Bryant J, Thackeray R *et al.* Incidence of human immunodeficiency virus-related and non-related malignancies in a large cohort of homosexual men. *J Clin Oncol* 1995; 15: 2540–2546.
74. Rabkin CS, Biggar RJ, Horn J. Cancer trends associated with increasing AIDS (abstract). *VIth International Conference on AIDS, San Francisco* 1990; 1: 295.
75. Lorenz HP, Wilson W, Leigh B *et al.* Squamous cell carcinoma of the anus and HIV infection. *Dis Colon Rectum* 1991; 34: 336–338.
76. Maiman M, Fruchter RG, Guy L *et al.* Human immunodeficiency virus infection and invasive cervical carcinoma. *Cancer* 1993; 71: 402–406.
77. Northfield DW. Cervical and anal neoplasia and HPV infection in persons with HIV infection. *Oncology* 1994; 4: 33–37.
78. Dyson N, Howley PM, Munger K *et al.* The human papilloma virus-16E7 oncoprotein is able to bind the retinoblastoma gene product. *Science* 1989; 243: 934–937.
79. Werness BA, Levine HJ, Howley PM. Association of human papilloma virus types 16 and 18E6 proteins with p53. *Science* 1990; 248: 76–79.
80. Gunthel CJ, Northfeld DW. Cancers not associated with immunodeficiency in HIV infected persons. *Oncology* 1994; 8: 59–64.
81. Ioachim HL. *Pathology of AIDS*. Philadelphia: Lippincott/Gower, 1988.
82. Ourcy WL, Jakubek DJ. Multiple squamous cell carcinomas and human immunodeficiency virus infection. *Ann Intern Med* 1987; 106: 334.
83. Sitz KV, Keppen M, Johnson DM. Metastatic basal cell carcinoma in acquired immunodeficiency syndrome-related complex. *JAMA* 1987; 257: 340–343.

84. Ravalli S, Chabon AB, Khan AA. Gastrointestinal neoplasia in young HIV antibody-positive patients. *Am J Clin Pathol* 1989; 91: 458–461.
85. Skurkovich S, Skurkovich B, Bellanti JA. A disturbance of interferon synthesis with the hyperproduction of unusual kinds of interferon can trigger autoimmune disease and play a pathogenetic role in AIDS: the removal of these interferons can be therapeutic. *Med Hypotheses* 1993; 41: 177–185.
86. Prehn RT, Prehn LM. The autoimmune nature of cancer. *Cancer Res* 1987; 47: 927–932.

7

AIDS and Lymphomas

Jill Lacy and Vincent T. DeVita Jr
Yale University School of Medicine, New Haven, Connecticut, USA

INTRODUCTION AND HISTORICAL PERSPECTIVE

An increased incidence of lymphoid neoplasms has been observed in a variety of conditions of impaired immunity. The role of immunodeficiency in predisposing individuals to the development of lymphoma was first appreciated in patients with congenital immunodeficiency syndromes, such as ataxia–telangiectasia and Wiskott–Aldrich syndrome, and then subsequently in allograft recipients receiving potent immunosuppressive drugs[1–3]. Not surprisingly, the profound impairment of the immune system that evolves in the setting of human immunodeficiency virus (HIV) infection is associated with a dramatic increase in the risk of developing lymphoma, and, indeed, acquired immunodeficiency syndrome (AIDS)-related lymphomas now represent the overwhelming majority of lymphoid neoplasms that are diagnosed in the setting of immunodeficiency. Although lymphomas that occur in the general population can be effectively treated and often cured, the development of lymphoma in the setting of HIV infection is associated with a poor prognosis. Despite recent advances in the therapy of AIDS-related lymphomas resulting from the incorporation of hematopoietic growth factors and antiretroviral agents into chemotherapeutic regimens, more than half of the patients with AIDS-related lymphoma will die within a year from diagnosis with progressive tumor or other complications of HIV infection. Clearly, long-term success in controlling this neoplastic complication of HIV infection will ultimately depend on the development of successful therapeutic strategies to reverse HIV-associated immunosuppression that can be integrated into effective antineoplastic therapies.

Although Kaposi's sarcoma (KS) was recognized early in the AIDS

AIDS and Malignancies: Current Concepts and Perspectives.
Edited by B.C. Golematis and V.T. DeVita Jr

pandemic as an AIDS-related neoplasm and became one of the initial criteria for diagnosis of AIDS in 1981 by the US Centers for Disease Control (CDC)[4], the recognition that HIV-infected patients were at increased risk of developing lymphoma emerged more slowly. This delayed recognition undoubtedly resulted from the propensity of AIDS-related lymphomas to emerge late in the course of HIV infection[5,6]. In 1982 the first cases of Burkitt's lymphoma in association with AIDS were reported in the literature[7–9], and it was appreciated that primary central nervous systems (CNS) lymphoma occurred with a dramatically increased incidence in AIDS patients, earning it the distinction of an AIDS-defining disease in 1982[10]. In 1985 the CDC revised its criteria for the diagnosis of AIDS to include HIV-infected individuals with systemic diffuse undifferentiated (Burkitt's and non-Burkitt's) high-grade non-Hodgkin lymphoma (NHL). Subsequently, several large clinico-pathological series of AIDS-related NHL were reported from New York[12–14], Houston[15], Los Angeles[16], and San Francisco[17], leading to the recognition that large cell and immunoblastic lymphomas, as well as high-grade diffuse undifferentiated NHLs, occurred as a neoplastic complication of AIDS. In 1987 the CDC expanded its criteria for the diagnosis of AIDS to include intermediate as well as high-grade NHLs in the setting of HIV infection[18]. Thus, primary CNS lymphoma (PCL) and systemic lymphoma of the intermediate-grade large cell and the high-grade diffuse undifferentiated and immunoblastic subtypes represent AIDS-defining illnesses. Although aggressive Hodgkin's disease (HD) has been linked to HIV infection, with over 200 cases reported in the literature[19–22], the incidence of HD is not consistently appreciated to be increased to a statistically significant degree in the HIV-infected population and thus is not a criterion for diagnosis of AIDS[23]. Nonetheless, epidemiological and pathogenetic evidence supports the association of HD with HIV infection[24–26].

Not surprisingly, lymphoid malignancies have emerged as a major clinical problem in HIV-infected patients. Since 1982 when the first cases of NHL were described in relationship to AIDS, there has been a dramatic increase in the incidence of AIDS-related lymphomas[27]. This increase is a result of not only the increased incidence of HIV-infected individuals in the general population, but also reflects the prolongation in survival of AIDS patients in recent years. The central role of impaired immunity in the genesis of AIDS-related NHL is exemplified by the recognition that the risk of developing NHL in AIDS increases dramatically as the CD4 count decreases, particularly below 50/mm^3. Based on this relationship, we can anticipate that the number of cases of AIDS-related NHL will continue to increase sharply as our successes with antiretroviral therapy and prophylaxis of opportunistic infections prolongs the survival of HIV-infected patients. Indeed, it has been suggested that 8–27% of new cases of NHL may be related to AIDS in the USA. Although much progress has been made in elucidating the complex pathobiology of AIDS-related NHL, major obstacles remain with respect to effective therapy for this neoplasm in the setting of HIV infection.

In this chapter we will discuss the epidemiology, pathogenesis, clinical features and therapy of the common lymphoid malignancies encountered in the setting of HIV infection, including systemic NHL, PCL, and HD.

SYSTEMIC NON-HODGKIN LYMPHOMA

Epidemiology

NHL is the second most common malignancy in persons with HIV infection, after KS, and represents the most common malignancy in all risk groups except the homosexual/bisexual risk group[29]. An analysis of AIDS cases reported to the CDC in the USA up to 1989 revealed that the risk of developing NHL is 60 times greater in HIV-infected patients than in the general population[30]. Based on patients diagnosed with AIDS in New York City between 1981 and 1986, other investigators have calculated the relative risk of developing NHL in the setting of AIDS to be over 500 times greater than for age- and sex-matched individuals without AIDS[31]. The exact incidence of NHL in the HIV-infected population is uncertain. Based on the number of cases of NHL reported to the CDC between 1981 and 1989, the incidence rate of NHL in AIDS patients was calculated to be 2.9%[30]. However, since immunoblastic/large cell lymphoma was reportable only after 1985, and since NHL occurring after another AIDS-defining illness is often not reported to the CDC, the actual incidence is undoubtedly substantially higher. In two large AIDS clinical trials of AZT (zidovudine) in asymptomatic HIV-seropositive individuals (ACTG 019 and the Concorde study), lymphoma represented 5% of clinical endpoints[32,33]. A large prospective study projected that 1.6% of patients with advanced HIV infection on AZT therapy will develop NHL each year[34]. Thus, it has been estimated that at least 5–10% of HIV-infected persons will develop NHL.

Recent studies have revealed that the risk of developing NHL in the AIDS population is not constant over time. Rather, the incidence appears to increase sharply in the later stages of HIV infection, confirming that the degree of immunodeficiency is a critical factor in the emergence of this neoplasia in HIV-seropositive individuals. Thus, Pluda *et al.* have shown that the incidence of NHL in AIDS patients increases sharply as the CD4 count falls below 50/mm^3 [5,6]. In an analysis of the cohort of patients undergoing long-term antiretroviral therapy with AZT at the National Cancer Institute (NCI) between 1985 and 1987, 8 of 55 patients (14.5%) developed NHL at a mean of two years after initiating antiretroviral therapy; the estimated actuarial probability of developing NHL rose to approximately 30% at 36 months of antiretroviral therapy[5]. The median CD4 count decreased from

74/mm^3 at the onset of antiretroviral therapy to 6/mm^3 at the time of diagnosis of NHL. In this cohort of patients, NHL developed exclusively in patients with CD4 counts of $<50/mm^3$ for greater than 12 months (median 18 months). A similar trend has been observed in a different cohort of patients receiving prolonged ddI (didanosine) antiretroviral therapy[6]. In both of these cohorts, the risk of developing NHL was significantly increased in patients with CD4 counts < 50 mm^3. Although AIDS-related NHL does occur in patients with CD4 counts $>50/mm^3$, and indeed, can occur in HIV-seropositive patients with normal CD4 counts, profound immunosuppression over an extended time period represents the major risk factor for the development of AIDS-related NHL. These studies suggest that the incidence of AIDS-related NHL is likely to increase further as patient survival continues to increase with advances in prophylaxis and therapy of opportunistic infections.

In contrast to KS, which occurs almost exclusively in homosexual males[35], AIDS-related NHL occurs in all groups at risk for HIV infection[30,36], including homosexual males[15,37], hemophiliacs[38], transfusion recipients[30], intravenous drug users[39], children with perinatally acquired infection[30], and heterosexual adults[30]. The incidence of NHL appears to be similar in all risk groups and in different geographic areas, suggesting that environmental cofactors have minimal impact on the development of AIDS-related NHL[33,34,40]. Furthermore, the clinical characteristics of NHL in each risk group are similar. However, clinicopathological differences may exist in different age groups and with different levels of immunodeficiency. Thus, Burkitt's lymphoma is reported more commonly in children and young adults with HIV infection and in individuals with high median CD4 counts, whereas immunoblastic and large cell NHL is encountered more frequently in older adults and in patients with more profound immunodeficiency as reflected in the CD4 count[30,41].

Pathology

The vast majority of AIDS-associated systemic NHLs are intermediate or high grade and fall into one of three diffuse, aggressive histologies in the NCI Working Formulation: small non-cleaved cell (SNCC), large cell immunoblastic plasmacytoid (LC-IBPL), or large cell cleaved or non-cleaved (LC). Based on several large series from the USA and Europe, these three subtypes are represented approximately equally in the HIV-infected population[12–17,41–43]. Thus, nearly 70% of NHLs in HIV-seropositive individuals are high-grade tumors (SNCC or LC-IBPL). In contrast, these high-grade lymphomas comprise only about 10% of all NHLs in the general population.

The diffuse, aggressive NHLs occurring in the setting of HIV infection share the same morphological features of non-AIDS-associated NHLs in the same histopathological category[44]. However, mitotic figures and necrosis occur more commonly, suggesting a higher rate of proliferation compared to non-AIDS NHLs[44]. The SNCC lymphomas in AIDS patients include both the classical Burkitt's lymphoma with a diffuse monomorphic population of medium-sized cells with distinct nucleoli, and the Burkitt-like lymphoma displaying a more variable population of cells with respect to size and shape. Both variants of SNCC are characterized by the 'starry sky' pattern of abundant macrophages, numerous mitotic figures, and necrosis, consistent with the high proliferative index of these tumors. The LC-IBPL lymphomas display a diffuse population of cells that are larger and more variable in size than the cells of SNCC. The eccentric nuclei are surrounded by abundant cytoplasm, and a plasmacytoid appearance is common. Like SNCC, LC-IBPL is a high-grade tumor with abundant mitotic figures, numerous macrophages, and necrosis. The LC lymphomas are characterized by a diffuse infiltrate of cells intermediate in size between SNCC and LC-IBPL lymphomas with abundant cytoplasm and round regular nuclei that may be non-cleaved, cleaved, or even multilobed. The features suggesting a high proliferative index (abundant macrophages and mitotic figures with necrosis) are less prominent in LC lymphomas compared to the high-grade tumors. There is considerable overlap in histopathological features of the LC-IBPL and LC lymphomas, rendering definitive distinctions difficult at times.

The majority of AIDS-related NHLs display an immunophenotype consistent with derivation from the B-cell lineage, expressing monoclonal surface immunoglobulin and B-cell-associated antigens (e.g. CD19, CD20, and CD22) and lacking T-cell-associated antigens[13,17,42,43,45,46]. The immunophenotypic profile of the three histopathological subtypes of AIDS NHL tends to mirror that of the same subtype encountered in the general population. Thus, the SNCC lymphomas are usually IgMκ/ CD10-positive and CD21-negative. As expected, the immunogenotype of the majority of AIDS-related NHLs is consistent with a monoclonal B-cell derivation[13,17,45]. Immunoglobulin gene rearrangement studies generally reveal one predominant immunoglobulin heavy chain gene rearrangement, indicating the monoclonal nature of these tumors. Although there have been reports of clinically aggressive polyclonal AIDS-related B-cell NHLs, this finding has not been widely confirmed, and precise incidence and clinical features of polyclonal B-cell NHLs remain uncertain[46,47].

In addition to the classical AIDS-related intermediate and high-grade B-cell NHLs, a variety of other non-Hodgkin lymphoid malignancies have been reported in the literature, including the B-cell low-grade lymphomas and plasma cell tumors and the full spectrum of T-cell lymphomas[13,48–51]. These tumors occur only sporadically in the AIDS population, and although there is no evidence that these tumors occur with increased frequency in HIV-seropositive individuals, their pathogenetic relationship to HIV infection remains unclear.

Recently, there have been several reports and series describing AIDS-associated NHLs that display the histological and immunophenotypic characteristics of CD30 (Ki-1)-positive anaplastic large cell lymphomas (ALC)[52–55]. In one large series a surprising 12% of AIDS-related NHLs were classified as ALC lymphomas[53]. Immunophenotyping of these anaplastic tumors revealed the consistent presence of CD30 (Ki-1) and epithelial membrane antigen; approximately half expressed T-cell antigens, whereas the remaining lacked both B- and T-cell antigens. The strong association of anaplastic NHL with Epstein–Barr virus in AIDS patients, in contrast to ALC occurring in the general population, supports a pathogenetic relationship to HIV infection and immunodeficiency[53,54].

Pathogenesis

During the past decade there have been dramatic advances in our understanding of the pathogenesis of AIDS-related lymphomas. We have learned that lymphoid tumorigenesis in the context of HIV infection is enormously complex and involves the interplay of diverse oncogenic factors. Some of these factors have been identified and extensively studied, including the role of (1) EBV, (2) aberrant expression or function of cellular oncogenes and tumor suppresser genes resulting from genetic mutations or chromosomal translocations, and (3) aberrant cytokine production that accompanies HIV infection. In this section, we will summarize our current understanding of the putative role of each of these three factors in the etiology of AIDS-related NHLs and postulate how they may interact in the pathogenesis of these tumors. Importantly, although we do not fully understand the genesis of AIDS-related lymphomas, we have learned that AIDS-related NHLs are pathogenetically heterogeneous. The molecular pathways that lead to the development of AIDS-related NHLs may diverge for different histopathological subtypes and for different sites of origin. Thus, we have begun to appreciate that novel therapeutic approaches may not necessarily be applicable to all types of AIDS-related NHLs.

There is no substantial evidence to date to implicate HIV directly in the pathogenesis of AIDS-related NHLs. HIV is not a transforming virus[56], and HIV DNA, RNA, or proteins are rarely identified in lymphoma specimens from AIDS patients[57]. There are no reports of the presence of HIV sequences in AIDS-related B-cell neoplasms, and only rare reports of integrated HIV provirus in T-cell neoplasias[58]. The significance of HIV proviral HIV DNA in T-cell NHLs remains uncertain. Thus, the pathogenetic role of HIV in the development of AIDS-related NHLs relates primarily to its suppressive effects on the immune system rather than any direct transforming functions.

Role of Epstein–Barr Virus

EBV is a ubiquitous human B-lymphotropic herpesvirus that has been causally linked to endemic Burkitt's lymphoma and transplant-associated lymphoproliferative diseases by virtue of the consistent presence of EBV DNA and proteins in these lymphoid tumors[59–64]. EBV has also been implicated causally in a significant percentage of lymphoid tumors arising in the setting of congenital immunodeficiency and in the AIDS population[59–63]. Although the precise role of EBV in the genesis of the EBV-associated lymphomas remains uncertain, there is compelling evidence that this virus is, in fact, a human transforming virus[65–70]. EBV is capable of transforming resting human B-cells to lymphoblastoid cells that will proliferate continuously *in vitro*, a phenomenon referred to as immortalization[59–68]. This highly efficient process of immortalization occurs *in vivo* as well, and in all likelihood, B-cell immortalization represents an early step in the multi-step process of EBV-associated lymphomagenesis[59]. In addition to its immortalizing properties, additional evidence supports a causal role for EBV in the EBV-associated lymphomas. Inoculation of infectious EBV into certain primate species leads to the development of lymphoid tumors that are EBV-positive[59,69]. In endemic Burkitt's lymphoma, viral titers predict the development of Burkitt's and, furthermore, correlate with remissions and relapses of the disease[70]. A consistent feature of all EBV-associated lymphoid tumors is the uniform presence of viral DNA and proteins in virtually 100% of cells; loss of viral DNA has not been documented, revealing the tight association with this virus with the transformed phenotype[59–64]. Although impaired immune function is a consistent factor in the development of EBV-associated lymphomas, the role of the virus in lymphomagenesis appears to vary in the different subtypes of EBV-associated tumors. Thus, a significant proportion of transplant-associated tumors are virus-driven proliferations that will regress when immune function is restored[64]. In contrast, in endemic Burkitt's lymphoma the virus most likely functions to promote or increase the likelihood of superimposed cellular oncogenic events, such as the c-myc oncogene translocation and mutations of the tumor suppresser gene, p53[59]. In the setting of AIDS, there is now evidence indicating that the role of EBV may also differ in different histopathological subtypes as discussed below.

There are conflicting reports in the literature regarding the overall proportion of AIDS-related NHLs that harbor EBV. Disparities undoubtedly result from the use of different techniques for detection as well as potential technical limitations with each technique. Based on the sensitive technique of *in situ* hybridization (ISH) for detection of the ubiquitous and abundant EBV-encoded small RNA transcripts (EBER-1) that are indicative of latent viral infection, it appears that approximately two-thirds of AIDS-related lymphoma are EBV-positive[41,53,71–75]. Several investigators have shown that the frequency of EBV positivity varies with the histological subtype or site of origin of disease, concluding that EBV is preferentially associated with the immunoblastic morphology (Table 7.1)[41,72,73]. In a representative series of 101 systemic NHLs, 11 Hodgkin's lymphomas, and 16 primary CNS lymphomas exam-

Table 7.1 Pathogenetic lesions of AIDS-related NHL[a]

Pathogenetic lesion	Total (%)	Histopathology (%)[b]			Specific sites (%)	
		SNCC	LC + LC-IBPL	ALC	1°CNS	Body cavity based
EBV	60–70	30–40	70–90	80	100	100
c-myc	70–80	100	30–40	–	0	–
N-*ras*	10–15	20	20	–	–	–
bcl-6	10–15	0	20	–	–	–
p53	40	60	0–15	–	–	–
KSHV[c]	–	0	0	0	–	100

[a] Data compiled from the following references: 41, 52–54, 71–77, 89, 90, 93, 96, 103, 115.
[b] SNCC, small non-cleaved cell; LC, diffuse large cell; LC-IBPL, large cell diffuse immunoblastic plasmacytoid; ALC, anaplastic large cell.
[c] KSHV, Kaposi's sarcoma herpesvirus.

ined by ISH, 77% of immunoblastic NHLs, 34% of SNCC NHLs, 100% of Hodgkin's lymphomas, and 94% of primary CNS lymphomas were positive for EBV[71]. It is now apparent that EBV is strongly associated with the immunoblastic morphology and, in particular, occurs consistently in primary CNS lymphomas where LC-IBPL morphology predominates. EBV is also identified in the majority of AIDS-related Hodgkin's lymphomas[71] and CD30 (Ki-1)-positive anaplastic large cell lymphomas[52–54,76]. Recently EBV has also been identified in all of the body cavity-based NHLs which display an indeterminate immunophenotype consistent with late stages of B-cell differentiation[77]. In contrast, the minority of SNCC AIDS-related NHLs harbor EBV[41,71].

A causal role for EBV in the genesis of the EBV-positive AIDS-related NHLs derives from recent molecular studies indicating that EBV infection occurs before clonal expansion of the malignant cell[78]. This conclusion derives from the finding that each cell of an EBV-positive AIDS-related NHL is infected with a single, clonal form of EBV DNA as determined by analysis of the molecular structure of the viral genome. The monoclonality of the EBV genome indicates that viral infection must have preceded clonal expansion rather than occurring at some point after expansion of the neoplastic cell population.

Based on these observations, it has been speculated that the development of the EBV-associated AIDS-related NHLs is a multi-step process that involves immortalizing events mediated by the virus and cellular genetic events that result in activation of oncogenes or inactivation of tumor suppresser genes. A favored hypothesis regarding the role of EBV in the genesis of AIDS-related NHLs is that in the context of HIV-associated severe immunodeficiency EBV-infected B-cells are able to proliferate unchecked as a result of an impaired T-cell response to virus-infected B-cells. The proliferation of EBV-infected B-cells leads to massive expansion of the polyclonal B-cell population. In this expanded pool of proliferating EBV-infected B-cells, secondary genetic events such as c-myc translocation or p53 mutations are more likely to occur, ultimately giving rise to a single fully transformed B-cell that clonally expands to overt NHL. Support for this hypothesis derives from several clinical observations. It has been shown that in patients with full-blown AIDS there is a dramatic increase in the number of circulating EBV-infected cells in the peripheral blood[79]. Furthermore, in HIV-infected patients with generalized lymphadenopathy, EBV is detectable by ISH in over one-third of specimens, in contrast to none of the lymph node specimens from HIV-negative individuals. Furthermore, the presence of EBV in lymph nodes is associated with a high risk of eventual development of lymphoma in comparison to HIV-seropositive patients with EBV-negative lymph nodes[80]. Additional support for the multi-step process of lymphomagenesis involving EBV-mediated immortalization and cellular genetic events derives from *in vitro* studies demonstrating that the introduction of activated c-myc genes by gene transfer technology into EBV-immortalized lymphoblastoid cells results in the acquisition of full-blown tumorigenic properties such as tumor formation in immunodeficient mice[81].

Although there is general agreement that EBV is involved in the genesis of the EBV-positive AIDS-related NHLs, the role of the virus in maintaining the transformed phenotype remains uncertain. Given our understanding of the function of the viral proteins expressed in latent infection, several recent studies revealing striking differences in patterns of EBV gene expression in different subtypes of AIDS-related lymphomas indicate that the role of the virus in the pathogenesis of different subtypes of AIDS-related NHL may vary[53,82,83]. Three patterns of latent viral gene expression have been described from *in vitro* and *in vivo* studies[82,84–87]. In the pattern known as Latency III there is broad expression of all nine latent viral proteins, including the EBV nuclear antigens EBNA-1 and EBNA-2 and the latent membrane protein, LMP-1; this form characterizes *in vitro* EBV-immortalized lymphoblastoid cell lines and the transplant-associated lymphoproliferative lesions. In contrast, in Burkitt's lymphoma there is restricted expression of viral proteins, known as Latency I, in which only EBNA-1 is expressed; other latent viral genes are downregulated and their protein products are undetectable. A third form of latency, designated Latency II, has recently been described for EBV-positive nasopharyngeal carcinoma, Hodgkin's disease, and T-cell NHLs. This form is characterized by protein expression restricted to EBNA-1 and the latent membrane proteins, LMP-1 and LMP-2.

In the AIDS-related NHLs all three forms of latent viral gene expression are encountered, but they are not distributed randomly among the different histopathological subtypes[53,82,83]. Thus, in the majority of EBV-positive SNCC NHLs, expression is restricted to EBNA-1, resembling the pattern observed in endemic Burkitt's lymphoma (Latency I). All three patterns of expression are encountered in the LC and LC-IBPL subtypes; interestingly, the broad pattern of expression, Latency III, is associated with extranodal tumors, whereas the intermediate pattern, Latency II, correlates with nodal disease[82]. AIDS-related Hodgkin's disease and anaplastic LC NHLs both display the pattern observed in non-HIV-infected patients with these tumors, that is, the intermediate pattern with expression of EBNA-1 and the LMP-1[53]. Since EBNA-1 functions to replicate and maintain latent viral DNA in progeny cells but does not exert direct transforming effects, whereas EBNA-2 and LMP-1 modulate cellular gene expression and alter cellular growth and adhesive properties[65,67], the role of the virus in maintaining the transformed state is likely to be different in the three forms of latency. Thus, it has been speculated that the LC and LC-IBPL subtypes that manifest broad expression of viral gene products are more likely to be virus-driven, analogous to the transplant-associated lymphoproliferative disorders[64], in contrast to the SNCC subtypes that express only EBNA-1. The full clinicopathological significance of the three forms of viral gene expression encountered in the AIDS-related lymphomas remains under active investigation.

In summary, although EBV has been causally implicated in the majority of AIDS-related lymphomas, the role of EBV in the pathogenesis of these tumors remains to be fully defined. There is substantial evidence to suggest that the EBV-positive AIDS-related NHLs are pathogenetically heterogeneous with respect to EBV, and, furthermore, there may be different mechanisms by which the virus contributes to lymphomagenesis. Finally, the pathogenetic relationship between EBV and the cellular genetic events encountered in the AIDS-related NHLs such as the c-myc oncogene translocation has not yet been established.

Role of Cellular Genetic Events: Oncogene Activation and Tumor Suppressor Gene Inactivation

Early in the AIDS epidemic it was recognized that specific reciprocal chromosomal translocations occurred frequently in the AIDS-related NHLs[88–90]. These translocations involved the c-myc oncogene on chromosome 8 and the immunoglobulin heavy chain, κ-light chain, or λ-light chain on chromosomes 14, 2, or 22 (t(8;14), t(2;8), and t(8;22), respectively) and proved to be similar to the characteristic translocations observed in endemic and sporadic Burkitt's NHL in HIV-seronegative individuals[91–94]. Thus, activation of the c-myc oncogene as a consequence of chromosomal translocation is recognized as an important pathogenetic event in the etiology of a majority of AIDS-related NHLs.

Since the initial reports of the c-myc translocation in AIDS-related NHL, molecular studies of large numbers of tumor specimens have revealed that approximately 75% of AIDS-related NHLs exhibit the chromosomal translocation involving c-myc[72,89,90,95,96]. The high frequency of this genetic lesion, however, is not uniform in each histopathological subtype (Table 7.1). In several large published series, nearly 100% of the AIDS-related NHLs displaying the SNCC morphology exhibit c-myc rearrangement, in contrast to only about 30% of the LC and LC-IBPL subtypes[72,95,96]. Interestingly, primary CNS lymphomas rarely display this genetic abnormality and retain germline c-myc alleles[46,47]. Importantly, this genetic lesion does not appear to be tightly linked to the presence of EBV, occurring in both EBV-positive and EBV-negative tumors[46,47,72,96]. Similarly, tumors in which c-myc remains in the germline configuration may be either EBV-positive or EBV-negative[46,47,72,96].

Given the frequent occurrence of c-*myc* rearrangement in AIDS-related NHL and its strong association with the SNCC subtype, it is widely held that activation of c-myc as a consequence of the translocation is an important molecular event in genesis of AIDS-related NHLs. Detailed molecular studies of the specific mutations and breakpoints that occur in endemic and sporadic Burkitt's lymphoma in HIV-seronegative patients have revealed the mechanisms by which the translocation may lead to deregulated transcription of the c-myc oncogene[92,93]. Thus, in the EBV-associated endemic Burkitt's, the breakpoint is usually well outside of the c-myc gene, often many kilobases upstream, and is associated with point mutations or small rearrangements within the transcriptional regulatory region of c-myc that lead to deregulated expression. In sporadic Burkitt's, which is generally EBV-negative, the breakpoint often occurs within the c-myc gene in the first exon or intron with truncation of the gene, or in the immediate 5' flanking regulatory sequences, thereby disrupting normal transcriptional regulatory mechanisms. In the sporadic variant of Burkitt's, c-myc generally recombines with the switch region of the heavy chain immunoglobulin locus, in contrast to the immunoglobulin joining region characteristic of translocation seen in endemic Burkitt's lymphoma. It appears that similar molecular mechanisms of deregulation of c-myc occur in the AIDS-related NHLs, where approximately 75% of breakpoints involve the 5' region of c-myc and the immunoglobulin switch region, as observed in sporadic Burkitt's, and the remainder are similar to the translocations encountered in endemic Burkitt's[72,90,96,97,98]. Clustered somatic mutations in the coding region of c-myc, specifically the critical transactivation domain of the protein, have been described in both HIV-negative Burkitt's and AIDS-related NHLs[96,99,100]. Thus, with respect to activation of c-myc, the AIDS-related NHLs share the same mutations and breakpoints as occur in Burkitt's lymphoma in HIV-seronegative patients, indicating overlapping pathogenetic pathways.

Other specific chromosomal translocations that have been associated with histopathologic subtypes of NHL that are not associated with HIV infection, such as t(14;18) in follicular lymphomas[101] and t(11;14) in mantle zone lymphomas[102], do not occur in the AIDS-related NHLs[90]. Thus activation of the bcl-2 gene arising from the t(14;18) translocation in follicular lymphomas does not appear to play a role in the genesis of AIDS-related NHLs. Likewise, the bcl-1 gene that is activated in mantle zone (centrocytic) NHLs as a result of the t(11;14) translocation is not involved in the AIDS-related NHLs. However, activation of the bcl-6 gene has recently been described in AIDS-related LC and LC-IBPL NHLs (Table 7.1)[103]. Bcl-6 is a putative oncogene with structural features of a transcription factor that is structurally altered by chromosomal translocations involving band 3q27 (e.g. t(3;22) and t(3;14)) that occur in about 45% of diffuse large cell lymphomas occurring in the general population[104–106]. Rearrangement of bcl-6 was observed in 20% of AIDS-related LC NHLs, did not correlate with the presence or absence of EBV, and was not associated with c-myc gene rearrangement or p53 mutations[103]. Furthermore, bcl-6 rearrangements were not encountered in any cases of SNCC. The frequent occurrence of bcl-6 rearrangements in diffuse large cell lymphomas occurring both in the general population and in the setting of HIV infection reveals common mutational events in the pathogenesis of this histopathological subtype.

Although activation of the ras family of oncogenes by point mutations has been causally associated with a variety of human cancers, including some hematological malignancies[107], this genetic lesion rarely occurs in the NHLs occurring in the general population[108]. However, it has recently been reported that point mutations involving ras genes (preferentially N-ras) were found in 4 of 27 (15%) AIDS-related NHLs[72]. Thus, this genetic lesion may represent a pathogenetic feature that is distinctive NHLs occurring in the setting of HIV infection.

In addition to the activation or deregulation of growth-promoting genes, or oncogenes, the inactivation of growth-inhibiting genes, or tumor suppresser genes, plays a significant pathogenetic role in the development of many human malignancies[109–111]. The tumor suppresser gene, p53, is a nuclear phosphoprotein that functions to inhibit progression from G1 to S phase of the cell cycle[109–111]. Mutations in p53 and/or its allelic loss due to loss of the short arm of chromosome 17 is a frequent finding in many solid human tumors and in specific histopathological subtypes of NHL, including Burkitt's lymphoma/leukemia and adult T-cell leukemia/lymphoma[112–114]. Several recent molecular studies of AIDS-related NHLs have revealed that p53 mutations are detectable in a significant proportion of AIDS-related NHLs (Table 7.1)[72,115]. Ballerini *et al.* demonstrated p53 mutations in 37% of AIDS-related NHLs, and, in addition, found that this genetic lesion occurred exclusively in lymphomas with the SNCC morphology. Furthermore, the location of the mutational 'hot spots' and the spectrum of mutations was similar to that encountered in other human tumors[72]. Nakamura *et al.* examined AIDS-related NHLs with immunoblastic features and found that approximately 15% harbored mutations in p53[115]. Thus, p53 mutations occur frequently in the AIDS-related NHLs and cluster in the SNCC subtype. Interestingly, the two genetic lesions, c-myc activation and p53 mutation, are associated with SNCC tumors encountered in both the AIDS population and in the general population. These findings support the concept that similar pathogenetic mechanisms may be operative in the development of specific histopathological subtypes of NHL in HIV-infected and -uninfected individuals.

Role of Aberrant Cytokine Production

HIV infection is characterized by enhanced production of a variety of cytokines in response to HIV infection, and there is considerable evidence implicating specific cytokine networks as playing a role in the development of AIDS-related NHLs. T-cells, monocytes, tissue macrophages, and cells of the reticuloendothelial system all produce a variety of cytokines in response to HIV infection, including interleukin 1 (IL-1), IL-4, IL-6, IL-10, and tumor necrosis factor (TNF)[116–118]. Based on several observations, IL-6 has been implicated as a candidate for promoting the development of lymphoma in the setting of AIDS. Among the many effects of IL-6, its critical role in promoting the growth and differentiation of B-cells implicates it in the genesis of B-cell tumors[119,120]. IL-6 production is induced early in the course of HIV infection, and increased serum levels of IL-6 are often detected in HIV-seropositive individuals[117,121,122]. Interestingly, in the cohort of patients entered onto the early AZT trials at the NCI, those who eventually developed NHL had elevated serum levels of IL-6 at the onset of the study which were persistent[6]. IL-6 has been shown to function as an autocrine growth factor for malignant plasma cells *in vitro*, and has been implicated in the pathogenesis of plasma cell dyscrasias[119,123,124]. High levels of IL-6 and IL-6 receptors have been detected in large cell lymphomas with immunoblastic features in both HIV-seronegative and -seropositive patients, suggesting an autocrine growth loop may be operative in this subtype of NHL. This finding was independent of the presence or absence of EBV[125]. Thus, IL-6 may play a role in the genesis of AIDS-related NHL by promoting B-cell proliferation and immunoglobulin synthesis in HIV-infected patients, thereby increasing the likelihood of oncogenic genetic events (e.g., c-myc rearrangement, p53 mutations) or, alternatively, by its involvement in maintaining autocrine growth of malignant immunoblasts.

In addition to IL-6, the cytokine synthesis inhibitory factor, or IL-10, has also been implicated in the pathogenesis of AIDS-related NHLs. B-cell lines derived from EBV-positive AIDS-related SNCC NHLs have been shown to secrete high levels of this cytokine constitutively and, furthermore, IL-10 can function as an autocrine growth factor for these B-cell lymphoma lines[126,127]. Since IL-10 suppresses helper T-cell function[128], it may also contribute to the development of AIDS-related NHLs by impairing immune surveillance mechanisms and, in particular, permitting the activation of EBV and expansion of the EBV-infected B-cell population.

In summary, the pathogenesis of AIDS-related NHLs involves several complex cellular and molecular processes, including impaired immune surveillance mechanisms, transforming events mediated by EBV, activation of cellular oncogenes, inactivation of tumor suppresser genes, and paracrine and autocrine growth stimulation mediated by the lymphohematopoietic growth factors that are produced in excess in response to HIV. Some of these pathogenetic events are particularly important to the development of lymphomas arising in the setting of HIV infection, e.g. impaired immune surveillance, excessive cytokine production, and EBV activation, whereas others represent more general mechanisms that occur in lymphomas of the same morphology in the general population, e.g. c-myc and bcl-6 rearrangements and p53 mutations. It has become clear that certain genetic lesions correlate with specific histopathological subtypes (Table 7.1). Thus, AIDS-related NHLs of the SNCC morphology usually exhibit c-myc rearrangement and p53 mutations, and EBV is often absent or its gene expression is restricted. Large cell lymphomas, particularly those with immunoblastic features, are generally EBV-positive with broad viral gene expression, and c-myc activation occurs inconsistently in this subtype. Furthermore, the bcl-6 rearrangement is restricted to the large cell subtypes.

CLINICAL FEATURES

The presenting clinical features of AIDS-related NHL from four representative series are summarized in Table 7.2. The majority of AIDS-related NHLs occur in adult males, reflecting the overall male/female ratio of HIV seropositivity. In the USA and Western Europe the median age at diagnosis is 38 and 28 years, respectively[12–17,42]. Approximately half of the patients diagnosed with AIDS-related NHL have prior AIDS-defining diagnoses such as KS (20%) or opportunistic infections (50%)[12–17,42]. The overwhelming majority of patients who develop AIDS-related NHL manifest immune dysfunction, as evidenced by depressed CD4 counts, depressed T4/T8 T-lymphocyte subset ratios, and polyclonal hypergammaglobulinemia[12–14,37]. The mean CD4 count in published series at the time of diagnosis of AIDS-related NHL ranges from 64 to 166/mm^3 [37,38].

The characteristic clinical hallmark of the AIDS-related NHL is advanced stage of disease at presentation with the frequent occurrence of extranodal involvement and systemic 'B' symptoms[12–17,36–38,42]. Approximately 70% of patients have stage III or IV disease at initial diagnosis, and an additional 20% have stage I or IIE disease reflecting extranodal sites of involvement. Indeed, stage I or II disease confined to nodal sites is rare. Based on several large clinical series from the USA and Europe[12–17,37,38,42], the majority of patients (68–98%) present with extranodal involvement. 'B' symptoms, i.e. unexplained fevers, night sweats, or weight loss in excess of 10% of body weight, are present in 80–90% of patients with AIDS-related NHL, in contrast to less than 30% of patients with NHL in the general population. Fever occurs with such frequency in AIDS-related NHL that its presence in an HIV-seropositive individual should always suggest the possibility of lymphoma as well as opportunistic infection.

The sites of extranodal involvement in AIDS-related NHL are diverse, and in many cases reflect not only widely disseminated disease but also the site of origin. In some large series, the most frequent site of extranodal site is the CNS, primarily because of the high incidence of PCL in the AIDS population[17]. If PCL is excluded, the most frequent sites of involvement in systemic AIDS-related NHL are the gastrointestinal tract (20–35%), bone marrow (20–35%), liver (10–25%), and leptomeninges (10–20%)[12–17,37,38,42,43]. The gastrointestinal tract is a frequent site of origin of AIDS-related NHL, and lymphoma can originate in or involve virtually any region of the gastro-

Table 7.2 Clinical features of AIDS-related NHL from representative series

	Kaplan[37]	Knowles[13]	Lowenthal[14]	Carbone[42]
Number of patients	84	89	43	35
Median age (years)	39 (mean)	38	38 (mean)	29
h/o OI[a] (%)	26	45	23	50
h/o KS[a] (%)	15	23	23	0
T4/T8 < 1 (%)	–	100	95	–
CD4 count/mm^3	166 (mean)	–	–	130 (median)
Stage				
I/II (%)	17	36	19	29
III/IV (%)	83	64	81	71
Extranodal disease (%)	76	87	65	85
Bone marrow (%)	31	21	30	21
GI tract (%)	11	24	28	32
Histopathology[a]				
SNCC (%)	34	40	37	40
LC + LC-IBPL (%)	63	59	53	38
Median survival (months)	4.3	5	10.5	22

[a] OI, opportunistic infections; KS, Kaposi's sarcoma; SNCC, small non-cleaved cell; LC, large cell; LC-IBPL, large cell immunoblastic plasmacytoid; GI, gastrointestinal.

intestinal tract, from the oropharynx to the anus. A recently recognized presentation of AIDS-related NHL is primary anorectal lymphoma in homosexual males[129]. These patients usually present with rectal bleeding and perianal pain, and although the disease is often localized at diagnosis, the prognosis remains poor with rapid dissemination of disease and median survival of seven months[129]. It is important to appreciate that virtually any anatomical site can be involved with AIDS-related NHL, including bizarre sites such as the myocardium, common bile duct, urethra, conjunctiva, and ear lobe. Indeed, the possibility of HIV infection should be considered when the diagnosis of a diffuse large cell or high-grade B-cell NHL involving an unusual extranodal site is made.

The diagnosis of AIDS-related NHL depends on an adequate biopsy, and in many cases will be made from biopsy of an extra nodal site[13]. The appropriate staging evaluation includes a careful history and physical examination, computed axial tomographic scanning of the chest, abdomen, and pelvis, and bone marrow biopsy. Gallium scanning may be useful for assessing response to therapy in patients with bulky tumors. In addition, since leptomeningeal involvement occurs in 5–20% of patients at presentation[16,17,37,43,130], a lumbar puncture for spinal fluid cytology should be obtained; intrathecal chemotherapy (cytosine arabinoside or methotrexate) can be instilled at the time of initial lumbar puncture. Since patients with systemic AIDS-related NHL rarely develop parenchymal brain involvement, in contrast to primary CNS lymphoma, routine brain imaging is not indicated in the absence of neurological symptoms. Finally, when the diagnosis of NHL is made in an AIDS patient who is experiencing fevers, it is important to vigorously pursue concurrent opportunistic infections and, if diagnosed, institute appropriate therapy.

PROGNOSTIC FACTORS

In aggressive systemic NHL that arises in the general population, prognosis is determined by extent of tumor burden as measured by stage, LDH, and involvement of extranodal sites[131]. In AIDS-related systemic lymphoma, the depth of immunodeficiency, as measured by CD4 counts and history of opportunistic infections, is a powerful predictor of survival, in addition to tumor burden. Thus, low CD4 counts, a history of a prior AIDS diagnosis, and poor performance status have been consistent adverse prognostic features in large published series from the USA and Europe (Table 7.3)[37,132,133]. In addition, some series have found the presence of extranodal disease, stage IV disease, or bone marrow involvement to represent adverse prognostic features[37,132]. Kaplan *et al.* reported that patients with AIDS-related NHL and a CD4 count $>100/mm^3$ had a median survival of 24 months, compared to a median survival of four months in patients with CD4 counts $<100/mm^3$ [37]. Patients with no prior AIDS-defining disease survived longer than patients with a prior AIDS diagnosis (8.3 versus 2.2 months), and the median survival of patients without extranodal involvement was 12.2 months versus 3.4 months for patients with an extranodal site of disease. Levine and colleagues also determined that low CD4 counts, history of prior opportunistic infection, poor performance status, and bone marrow involvement were all predictors of shortened survival[132]. In these two series, the pathological subtype of NHL, 'B' symptoms, elevated LDH, bulky disease, and specific site of disease (other than primary CNS lymphoma) were not predictors of survival. In a large series from Europe, multivariate analysis of 141 cases of AIDS-related NHL treated on a French–Italian Cooperative Group trial revealed that CD4 counts $<100/mm^3$, performance status >1, immunoblastic subtype, and prior AIDS diagnosis were strongly associated with shortened survival[133].

The importance of histopathological subtype as an independent predictor for survival remains uncertain. Although Kaplan *et al.* and Levine *et al.* failed

Table 7.3 Adverse prognostic features in AIDS-related NHL

CD4 count $<100/mm^3$
Prior AIDS diagnosis
Performance status <70% (Karnofsky)
Extranodal disease
Bone marrow involvement
Immunoblastic morphology

to identify statistically significant differences in survival among the three histological subtypes of NHL[37,132], Knowles *et al.* reported that patients with LC-IBPL has median survivals of only two months, in comparison to median survival of 7.5 and 5.5 months for patients with LC and SNCC lymphomas, respectively; these differences achieved statistical significance[13]. The French–Italian Cooperative Group identified immunoblastic histology as an adverse prognostic factor[133]. Additional large prospective series in which patients are treated uniformly and histological subtype is carefully confirmed are needed to resolve this issue.

CLINICOPATHOLOGICAL CORRELATES

Several molecular pathological correlates have now been identified in the AIDS-related NHLs, as described above and summarized in Table 7.1. In addition, several clinicopathological correlations have emerged with the analysis of large series of patients with AIDS-related NHL (Table 7.4). Two large series correlated sites of involvement with specific morphologies[13,43]. Thus, the SNCC subtypes display a greater propensity to involve the bone marrow (39% of patients) compared to the LC morphologies (16% of patients), whereas the LC subtypes display a greater propensity to involve the gastrointestinal tract (41% of patients) compared to the SNCC subtypes (8% of patients)[13]. Primary CNS lymphomas consistently display the large cell morphology, usually with immunoblastic features, and harbor EBV[15,43,73]. Recently, a distinct group of AIDS-related NHLs that exclusively or predominantly involve the body cavities (pleura, peritoneum, pericardium) have been described[134–136]. These tumors are nearly all of LC-IBPL morphology, display the immunophenotype of a B-cell in the late stages of differentiation, and, in addition, harbor both EBV and the recently described herpesvirus identified in KS lesions[135,136].

Table 7.4 Correlations between clinical features of AIDS-related NHL and histopathology[a]

Clinical feature	SNCC[b]	LC + LC-IBPL[b]
Age	Children Younger adults	Older adults
Prior AIDS	Uncommon	Frequent
Median CD4 count/mm^3	>200	<100
Disease sites	Bone marrow Lymph nodes Muscle	GI tract 1° CNS

[a] Derived from data published in the following references: 13, 30, 43, 137.
[b] SNCC, small cell non-cleaved; LC, large cell; LC-IBPL, large cell immunoblastic plasmocytoid; GI, gastrointestinal.

In addition to correlations with sites of involvement, the histopathological subtype also correlates with immune function (Table 7.4). Thus, the SNCC subtypes are encountered more frequently in patients with higher CD4 counts, representing an earlier manifestation of AIDS, in contrast with the LC subtypes which occur in patients who are more profoundly immunosuppressed with lower CD4 counts and a history of prior opportunistic infections[30,137]. The LC subtype of AIDS-related NHL that presents in the brain parenchyma, or primary CNS lymphoma, is seen almost exclusively in the late stages of HIV infection with profound immunodeficiency and CD4 counts that are invariably <50 mm^3, as described below[133].

TREATMENT AND SURVIVAL

The majority of patients with systemic AIDS-related NHL will experience symptoms attributable to their neoplasm and have a sufficient life expectancy that the institution of therapy is generally indicated. Given the histological grade and the disseminated nature of AIDS-related NHL, a multi-drug chemotherapeutic regimen is the standard therapy[138–148]. Radiation therapy as the initial and sole therapeutic modality is inadequate, even in the unusual patient with apparent localized disease. Although the majority of patients respond rapidly to chemotherapy and nearly 50% of patients treated will achieve a complete remission, there are major challenges in the treatment of AIDS-related NHL. Nearly 50% of patients who achieve a complete remission will relapse; remission durations tend to be short (less than 12 months), and approximately half of the patients die due to progressive lymphoma[12–14,17,140,141,148]. Survival times of patients diagnosed with AIDS-related NHL remain short, with a median survival of approximately seven months for treated patients in most series[38,133,139,140–142]. In addition, the use of chemotherapeutic agents in the setting of HIV infection poses unique problems, such as overlapping toxicities with antiretroviral agents or other drugs used to treat opportunistic infections and impaired marrow reserve resulting from HIV or antiretroviral drugs. Ultimately, the inevitable progression of the underlying HIV infection remains the greatest obstacle to successful long-term outcome for these patients.

The treatment of AIDS-related NHL has evolved substantially since the first cases emerged more than a decade ago. It has been appreciated that in the majority of patients dose-intensive chemotherapeutic regimens that are used in uninfected patients with high-grade NHL do not confer an overall survival advantage when compared to less intensive regimens. In addition, the introduction of growth factors in the 1990s has permitted the treatment of many patients who otherwise would not have had the marrow reserve to tolerate even modest myelosuppressive chemotherapy. Finally, more effective prophylaxis and treatment of opportunistic infections have enhanced our ability to deliver uninterrupted cycles of chemotherapy. Thus, it is now possible to treat the majority of patients with effective chemotherapeutic agents, and the identification of the optimum regimen for different prognostic subgroups of patients with AIDS-related NHL has become a major focus of clinical investigation.

The appreciation that dose-reduced chemotherapeutic regimens may be as effective as standard or dose-intensive regimens with less toxicity derives from the early experience in treating these malignancies from single institutions and has been substantiated in a recent multi-institution randomized prospective trial. In one of the earliest published experiences using an intensive chemotherapy regimen consisting of high-dose cyclophosphamide, cytosine arabinoside, and methotrexate for AIDS-related NHL, Gill *et al.* reported only a 33% complete remission rate, and 78% of patients developed intercurrent opportunistic infections that were associated with a high mortality rate[138]. Retrospective analysis of patients treated at San Francisco General Hospital indicated that patients who received higher doses of cyclophosphamide ($>1 g/m^2$) experienced significantly shorter median survivals than patients treated with less intensive regimens (4.6 months versus 12.2 months, respectively)[37]. The experience of these investigators and others prompted the AIDS Clinical Trial Group (ACTG) in the USA to test the efficacy and toxicity of a dose-reduced modification of the M-BACOD regimen, utilizing 50% reduction in the doses of cyclophosphamide and doxorubicin for four to six cycles[141]. A complete remission rate of 50% was achieved, and opportunistic infection occurred in only 20% of patients, thus substantiating the efficacy and acceptable morbidity of this approach.

With the introduction of hematopoietic growth factors, it became possible to administer standard chemotherapeutic regimens used to treat aggressive NHLs in the general population (e.g. CHOP or M-BACOD) to patients with HIV infection with acceptable toxicity[140,145]. To determine whether the greater dose intensity of the standard regimens plus hematopoietic growth factors yields superior outcomes compared to the low-dose regimens, in 1991 the ACTG embarked on an important randomized prospective trial to address the issue of dose intensity[148]. One hundred and eighty-eight patients were randomized to receive four to six cycles of standard M-BACOD with granulocyte–macrophage colony-stimulating factor (GM-CSF) or low-dose M-BACOD with GM-CSF only as needed. The two groups were similar with respect to major predictors of outcome such as the CD4 count (103 and $100/mm^3$, respectively) and stage of disease. There was no significant difference in complete response rates (50% versus 46%), median survival (31 versus 34 weeks), or time to progression (22 versus 28 weeks) between the two arms. However, 36% of cycles were complicated by grade 4 neutropenia with the standard dose regimen, in comparison to 22% of cycles with the low-dose regimen—a statistically significant difference. Thus, response rate and overall survival with low-dose chemotherapy appear equivalent to the standard dose regimen with substantially less toxicity. However, whether there are subsets of patients that derive benefit from more intensive regimens, such as those with favorable prognostic features, remains to be determined. This possibility is supported by a large series reported from the French–Italian Cooperative Group. In this prospective multi-institutional trial 141 patients with AIDS-related NHL were treated with the intensive LNH84 protocol[133]. Although the overall median survival was only nine months, the probability of survival at two years was 50% for those patients without adverse prognostic features (low CD4 counts, poor performance status, prior AIDS diagnosis, immunoblastic subtype).

Several single- and multi-institution trials of various combination chemotherapy regimes for the treatment of AIDS-related NHL have been published in recent years[133,140–148]. Representative studies are summarized in Tables 7.5 and 7.6. Complete response rates range from 39% to 67% and median survivals range from 5.6 months to 17.4 months. Sparano *et al.* have reported the best outcome to date in 12 patients treated with continuous infusion chemotherapy incorporating cyclophosphamide, doxorubicin, and etoposide plus hematopoietic growth factors[143]. Treatment-related toxicity was acceptable, and there was only one treatment-related death. Despite a median CD4 count of $<100/mm^3$ [87], the complete response rate was 67% and median survival 17.4 months. Whether these encouraging results can be reproduced by other institutions with large numbers of patients will be determined in an ongoing multi-institutional trial.

There are several special management issues that must be considered in the therapy of AIDS-related NHL. The myelosuppressive effects of chemotherapy are more pronounced in the setting of HIV infection, particularly in patients with depleted CD4 counts, and, indeed, patients with advanced HIV infection may be pancytopenic prior to the initiation of chemotherapy. The administration of a hematopoietic CSF has been shown to be associated with significantly higher granulocyte nadirs, shorter duration of granulocytopenia, fewer episodes of neutropenic fever with shorter hospital stays for treatment of this complication, and fewer delays and dose reductions in chemotherapy[140]. Thus, it can be recommended that the majority of patients receive CSF while undergoing chemotherapy. The use of GM-CSF has been associated with laboratory evidence of activation of HIV infection as measured by increases in serum HIV p24 antigen levels[140]. Although there is no evidence that this phenomenon is clinically significant, the use of granulocyte CSF (G-CSF) rather than GM-CSF seems prudent.

Regarding the management of the underlying HIV infection during treatment of AIDS-related NHL, no evidence exists to support or refute clinical benefit from the administration of antiretroviral agents concurrent with chemotherapy. Nonetheless, controlling the underlying HIV infection and slowing the decline in immune function is a factor in prolonging survival of these patients. Because of the myelosuppressive effects of AZT, its use in

Table 7.5 Chemotherapy trials for AIDS-related NHL

	CHOP[130]	Low-dose m-BACOD[148]	m-BACOD[148]	CDE[133]	Oral regimen[142]	Low-dose m-BACOD[131]
Number of patients	26	77	74	12	18	42
Median CD4 count/mm^3	240 (mean)	100	103	87	73	150
Extranodal disease (%)	81	–	–	83	28	66
Stage III/IV (%)	54	74	61	75	76	57
Median performance status (%)	84 (mean)	–	–	60	1(ECOG)	>80
Prior AIDS (%)	15	–	–	8	28	23
Complete response (%)	62	46	50	67	39	46
Median survival (months)	9.0	7.5	7.0	17.4	7	5.6

Table 7.6 Combination chemotherapy regimens effective in the treatment of systemic AIDS-related NHL

Regimen	Drugs	Dose and frequency
M-BACOD	Cyclophosphamide	600 mg/m^2 i.v. day 1
	Doxorubicin	45 mg/m^2 i.v. day 1
	Vincristine	1.4 mg/m^2 (not to exceed 2 mg) i.v. day 1
	Bleomycin	4 mg/m^2 i.v. day 1
	Dexamethasone	6 mg/m^2 i.v. p.o. days 1–5
	Methotrexate	200 mg/m^2 i.v. day 15 with leucovorin rescue
	4–6 cycles; each cycle every 21–28 days	
low-dose M-BACOD	Cyclophosphamide	300 mg/m^2 i.v. day 1
	Doxorubicin	25 mg/m^2 i.v. day 1
	Vincristine	1.4 mg/m^2 (not to exceed 2 mg) i.v. day 1
	Bleomycin	4 mg/m^2 i.v. day 1
	Dexamethasone	3 mg/m^2 p.o. days 1–5
	Methotrexate	200 mg/m^2 i.v. day 15 with leucovorin rescue
	4–6 cycles; each cycle every 21–28 days	
CHOP	Cyclophosphamide	750 mg/m^2 i.v. day 1
	Doxorubicin	50 mg/m^2 i.v. day 1
	Vincristine	1.4 mg/m^2 (not to exceed 2 mg) i.v. day 1
	Prednisone	100 mg p.o. days 1–5
	4–6 cycles; each cycle every 21–28 days	
CDE	Cyclophosphamide	187.5 mg/m^2 continuous infusion days 1–4
	Doxorubicin	12.5 mg/m^2 continuous infusion days 1–4
	Etoposide	60 mg/m^2 continuous infusion days 1–4
	4–6 cycles; each cycle every 28 days	
Oral	CCNU	100 mg/m^2 p.o. day 1 (cycles 1, 3, 5)
	Etoposide	200 mg/m^2 p.o. days 1–3
	Cyclophosphamide	100 mg/m^2 p.o. days 22–31
	Procarbazine	100 mg/m^2 p.o. days 22–31
	Each cycle 42 days	

conjunction with chemotherapy has proven difficult[144], and the concurrent administration of AZT with chemotherapy cannot be routinely recommended. However, ddI, ddC (zalcitabine), and D4T (stavudine) are acceptable alternatives that do not suppress the marrow and can be administered safely in conjunction with chemotherapy. The overlapping neurotoxicity of the latter drugs with the vinca alkaloids must be considered, although this has not proven to be a significant clinical problem[149,150]. Thus, in general ddI, ddC, or D4T should be substituted for AZT if antiretroviral therapy is to be continued during chemotherapy. In addition, *Pneumocystis carinii* prophylaxis should be administered to all patients, irrespective of their CD4 counts. If patients are receiving treatment or prophylaxis for other opportunistic infections when chemotherapy is initiated, this therapy should continue.

Given the high incidence of leptomeningeal involvement in AIDS-related NHL (up to 20% in some series)[14,17,37,43,130,133], CNS prophylaxis with intrathecal methotrexate or cytosine arabinoside has been incorporated into many treatment regimens. However, there is not unanimity regarding the routine use of CNS prophylaxis in systemic AIDS-related NHL. Although patients who eventually develop lymphomatous meningitis have a poor prognosis, with a median survival of only four months in one retrospective series[130], there is no published data demonstrating that CNS prophylaxis alters survival in the setting of AIDS. In some series, patients at greatest risk for leptomeningeal involvement appear to be those with SNCC histology or bone marrow involvement, and some investigators recommend limiting routine prophylaxis to these two groups[143]. The administration of intrathecal chemotherapy to other patients with systemic AIDS-related NHL must be individualized, given the paucity of data showing efficacy. The diagnosis of systemic and lymphomatous meningitis is made simultaneously in approximately 5% of patients with AIDS-related NHL[130]. Although the prognosis of these patients is generally poor, intrathecal chemotherapy and whole brain radiotherapy can often relieve symptoms and provide substantial palliation.

In summary, the optimum chemotherapy regimen and dose for different prognostic subsets of patients with systemic AIDS-related NHL remain to be clarified. Thus, all patients who develop AIDS-related NHL should be considered for enrollment in clinical trials. In the absence of an available clinical trial, the treatment of any given patient must be individualized, taking into consideration the patient's immunological status and overall clinical status. There is now substantial data showing the poor-prognosis subsets of patients tolerate the standard doses of chemotherapy used for aggressive NHL in the general population poorly and that reduced doses of chemotherapy are as effective with less toxicity. Thus reduced doses of a standard regimen such as CHOP or M-BACOD is a reasonable therapeutic choice for patients with low CD4 counts (e.g., $<100/mm^3$). It is uncertain whether patients without adverse prognostic features derive additional benefit from more intensive chemotherapeutic regimens, but these patients are better able to tolerate full doses of the standard regimens used for intermediate and high-grade NHLs in the general population. All patients with AIDS-related NHL undergoing chemotherapy should receive hematopoietic CSFs and *Pneumocystis carinii* prophylaxis, regardless of the CD4 count, and ddI, ddC, or D4T should be substituted for AZT while patients are receiving myelosuppressive drugs. The administration of CNS prophylaxis should be individualized; those patients who are responding to systemic therapy and otherwise have a reasonable life expectancy should be considered for CNS prophylaxis. For those patients who fail to respond to initial therapy or relapse, the prognosis has been uniformly dismal, and effective salvage regimens have not been identified.

PRIMARY CENTRAL NERVOUS SYSTEM LYMPHOMA

Approximately 20–30% of AIDS-associated NHLs present as brain parenchymal lesions limited to the CNS, i.e. primary CNS lymphomas (PCLs)[14,17,30]. This complication occurs in 2–3% of all patients with HIV infection, and in some autopsy series the incidence is as high as 5%[151,152]. The majority of AIDS-related PCLs occur in patients who are in the terminal stages of HIV infection with profound immunodeficiency. In a series reported by Levine *et al.* the median CD4 count of patients with PCL was only 30/mm^3, in contrast to 189/mm^3 in patients with systemic AIDS-related NHL[132]. Most patients diagnosed with PCL have documented AIDS as manifested by a history of opportunistic infections or KS[14,153–157].

AIDS-related PCL represents a distinct pathological entity based on histopathology and molecular features. The majority of AIDS-related PCLs display the morphology of LC or LC-IBPL subtypes; the SNCC NHLs identified in the CNS in AIDS patients usually represent secondary involvement in the setting of systemic lymphoma[13,43,153,154,156]. All of the AIDS-related PCLs are monoclonal B-cell tumors, exhibiting B-cell-specific antigens and clonal rearrangements of immunoglobulin genes[13,43,47,73,154,156]. EBV is consistently associated with AIDS-related PCL. EBV is detected in virtually all AIDS-related PCLs when the sensitive technique of ISH is used to detect the abundant latent transcripts of the EBV EBER-1 gene[73]. These tumors generally display the broad pattern of latent viral gene expression (Latency III) with expression of EBNA-1, EBNA-2, and LMP-1[158]. Thus, this neoplastic complication of AIDS is considered an EBV-associated tumor. In contrast, less than 10% of PCLs encountered in the general population harbor EBV[73,158]. The c-myc oncogene is virtually never rearranged in the AIDS-related PCLs, whereas the majority of systemic AIDS-related NHLs exhibit a chromosomal translocation involving c-*myc*[47].

Patients with HIV infection who develop PCL are usually profoundly immunocompromised, and the majority have experienced opportunistic infections or other complications of AIDS[14,153,154,156,157]. Although patients may present with dramatic focal neurological signs such as paresis, aphasia, or seizures, the most common presentation consists of subtle and non-focal signs and symptoms, such as confusion, lethargy, headache, memory loss, and behavioral or personality changes[153–157]. Since the presentation of PCL may be indistinguishable from AIDS-related dementia or progressive multifocal leukoencephalopathy, there may be a delay in considering the possibility of a mass lesion, and, indeed, PCL is often a postmortem diagnosis[13,14,152–154]. Radiographic findings on magnetic resonance or computed axial tomographic imaging consist of multiple parenchymal lesions in 50–70% of patients and solitary masses of the remainder[154,155,157]. In 5–10% of patients the radiographic findings reveal a diffuse infiltrative tumor involving the hemispheres[154]. The most common sites of involvement are the cerebrum and basal ganglia, although virtually any site can be involved[154,155,157]. The lesions usually show some degree of enhancement that may be homogeneous, heterogeneous, or ring-enhancing[154,155]. Thus, it is virtually impossible to radiographically distinguish AIDS-related PCL from toxoplasmosis or other less common CNS disease processes encountered in AIDS patients[154,159]. Spinal fluid analysis often reveals non-specific, non-diagnostic abnormalities, such as elevation of protein, mild hypoglycorrhachia, or mild pleocytosis[154]. However, only 10% of patients with PCL exhibit concurrent leptomeningeal involvement that can be definitively diagnosed by cytological examination[153,154]. Thus, definitive diagnosis requires a stereotactic brain biopsy in the majority of patients with AIDS-related PCL. A reasonable approach to the evaluation and treatment of brain parenchymal mass lesions in the setting of AIDS is to obtain serum toxoplasmosis titers and begin empirical antitoxoplasmosis therapy. A diagnostic stereotactic brain biopsy is indicated if the toxoplasmosis titers are negative, if the patient deteriorates neurologically at any time, or if the patient fails to improve clinically and radiographically after two weeks of antitoxoplasmosis therapy. The utility of an extensive evaluation for systemic lymphoma is low, since these patients rarely exhibit clinical evidence of systemic lymphoma, and at autopsy lymphoma will be identified outside of the CNS in less than 5% of patients[154].

The prognosis of AIDS-related PLC is extremely poor and substantially worse than that reported in the non-AIDS population. The median survival of patients with AIDS-related PCL is two to three months, in contrast to 19–20 months for HIV-seronegative patients with PCL[154,160–162]. Despite the poor prognosis of AIDS-related PCL, the majority of patients will benefit from therapy incorporating whole brain irradiation. In the absence of therapy for AIDS-related PCL, most patients will deteriorate rapidly and die within four to six weeks[154]. Several retrospective series suggest that radiation therapy of PCL in the setting of AIDS will improve radiographic findings, neurological function, quality of life, and perhaps survival[154–157,163]. In a series of 21 patients with AIDS-related PCL reported by Nisce *et al.*, patients were treated with 30–40 Gy of whole brain radiotherapy plus a 14 Gy boost in responding patients[163]. An improvement in neurological function was observed in 79% of patients, and 88% of patients who underwent repeat radiographic imaging exhibited marked tumor regression. The median survival in this series was 4.8 months. Although the use of systemic and intrathecal chemotherapy with radiotherapy has improved the outcome of PCL in patients without AIDS[160,161], the value of chemotherapy in the treatment of AIDS-related PCL remains largely unexplored and unknown. A report by Chamberlain revealed that the median survival of highly selected patients with AIDS-related PCL who received three cycles of procarbazine, lomustine, and vincristine following whole brain radiotherapy was 13.5 months[164]. Whether these excellent results can be extended to unselected patients with AIDS-related PCL is uncertain. The Eastern Cooperative Oncology Group (ECOG) in the USA is currently investigating the role of chemotherapy in AIDS-related PCL in an ongoing clinical trial that incorporates one cycle of chemotherapy (cyclophosphamide, doxorubicin, vincristine, and dexamethasone) prior to whole brain radiotherapy.

HODGKIN'S DISEASE

Epidemiology

Since the onset of the AIDS epidemic, Hodgkin's disease (HD) has been observed to occur frequently in AIDS patients, and over 200 cases of HIV-associated HD have now been reported in the literature[12,13,19,20–22,24–26,42,165–171]. HD has not consistently been shown to occur with a statistically significant increased frequency in HIV-seropositive individuals compared to the general population[23]. Thus it is not considered an AIDS-defining malignancy. However, because HD is not a criterion for the diagnosis of AIDS according to the CDC, it is not consistently reported, and the actual incidence and increased risk of HD in the HIV-infected population remain uncertain. Nonetheless, there is substantial evidence to support a relationship between HD and HIV infection that is more than coincidental. HIV-infected patients with HD are more likely to lie outside the typical age range of HD (15–34 years and >50 years), and one study concluded that there is a statistically significant increase in the number of cases of HD occurring in the HIV-infected population compared to the general population within the age bracket of 35–49 years[168]. Based on the incidence of HD among 6704 HIV-infected homosexual males in San Francisco between 1978 and 1989, Hessol *et al.* reported a statistically significant increase in HD compared to the general population, calculating an excess risk of 19.3 cases per 100 000 person-years[25]. Furthermore, several investigators have observed that HIV-

Table 7.7 Comparison of clinical and pathological features of HD in HIV-seropositive and -seronegative patients

	HIV-seropositive	HIV-seronegative
MC + LD subtypes[a] (%)	60–80	<25
EBV-positive (%)	90–100	30–50
Clinical stage III/IV (%)	90	40
Bone marrow involvement (%)	40–50	<10
Median survival (years)	<1.5	>10

[a] MC, mixed cellularity; LD, lymphocyte-depleted.

associated HD occurs predominantly in the intravenous drug user (IVDU) risk group. The ratio of HD to NHL is significantly higher in the IVDUs compared to homosexual males[14,167], and in a large series of 46 patients with HIV infection and HD reported from Spain, 85% of patients were IVDUs and only 9% were homosexuals[26]. These data suggest that there may be an increased risk of HD in HIV patients and that this risk is not equal among all groups at risk for AIDS.

Histopathology and Pathogenesis

There are no apparent morphological differences between HIV-associated HD and HD occurring in the general population. However, the distribution of the histopathological subtypes of HD in HIV-infected patients contrasts with the distribution in the HIV-seronegative population (Table 7.7). The high-grade variants of the disease (mixed cellularity and lymphocyte-depleted subtypes) comprise the majority of cases encountered in HIV-infected patients (mixed cellularity, 40–60%; lymphocyte-depleted, 10–20%[19–22, 24–26,42,168,170–172]) in contrast to HD in the general population, where the high-grade variants represent less than 25% of cases (mixed cellularity, 20–25%; lymphocyte-depleted, 1%)[173]. The immunophenotypic and immunogenotypic characteristics of HD occurring in HIV-infected and -uninfected patients are similar. The Reed–Sternberg cells are generally CD30 (Ki-1)-positive and CD15-positive and fail to demonstrate clonal rearrangements of immunoglobulin or T-cell receptor genes. However, HD occurring in HIV-infected patients may differ pathogenetically from HD occurring in uninfected individuals. Virtually 100% of HD tumors from HIV-infected patients are EBV-positive, in contrast to 30–50% of HD tumors from HIV-seronegative patients[71,174].

Clinical Characteristics and Treatment

The age at diagnosis of HD is similar to the age at diagnosis of NHL in HIV-infected patients. In the USA the median age is about 36 years and in

Western Europe about 26 years[13,26,169]. In the USA the majority of reported cases have occurred in homosexual males, whereas in Europe the majority occur in IVDUs[13,26,168,169]. Although many patients diagnosed with HD have a prior history of opportunistic infections or KS, in a large series reported from Spain HD was the first manifestation of HIV infection in more than 90% of patients[26]. Most patients exhibit immunological derangements consistent with HIV infection, including depressed CD4 counts and hypergammaglobulinemia[13,26,168,169,171].

The clinical hallmark of HIV-associated HD is advanced stage at presentation with a high frequency of disseminated disease to extranodal sites. This is in marked contrast to HD in the general population, which is clinical stage I or II in the majority of patients and uncommonly involves extranodal sites at presentation (Table 7.7)[173]. Approximately 90% of patients with HIV-associated HD present with stage III or IV disease, 40–50% of patients have frank bone marrow involvement at diagnosis, and other extranodal sites are involved in up to 30% of patients[12,13,19–22,166,168–171]. Liver, bone marrow, and lungs are the most common sites of extranodal involvement in HIV-associated HD[13,26,169,170]. In contrast to HD in the general population, a variety of unusual sites of involvement have been reported in the setting of HIV infection, including the oropharynx, gastrointestinal tract, skin, and brain[14,171,175–177]. Thus, the diagnosis of HD in HIV-infected patients is often established from a biopsy of an extranodal site[13,170,177]. Furthermore, HD in HIV-infected patients appears to spread in a non-contiguous manner. Thus, patients may exhibit dissemination to liver and bone marrow in the absence of splenic involvement, and the mediastinum may be uninvolved despite widespread disease[13,14,169,170].

The presenting symptoms of HD in the setting of HIV infection are diverse, reflecting the diversity of organ systems that can be involved. More than 80% of patients will experience 'B' symptoms at presentation[13,26,169,177], in contrast to about one-third of patients with HD in the general population[173]. The clinical presentation of HIV-associated HD and NHL are strikingly similar, with constitutional symptoms and diverse localizing symptoms characteristic of both types of lymphoma in the setting of HIV infection. Staging evaluation for HIV-associated HD should include computed axial tomographic scanning of the chest, abdomen, and pelvis and bone marrow biopsies. Gallium scanning may be useful to assess response to therapy. Exploratory laparotomy has no role to play in the staging evaluation, since HIV-associated HD is usually widely disseminated at presentation and not amenable to locoregional radiotherapy.

Since HD occurring in HIV-infected patients is advanced at presentation with dissemination to extranodal sites, patients generally have been treated with combination chemotherapy rather than radiotherapy. Response rates to chemotherapy have been high, with about 80% of patients achieving a partial or complete response[26,169,171,178]. Approximately 50% of patients treated will achieve a complete remission[26,171,178], and in one large series about one-third of complete responders will relapse[26]. The overall median survival from several series has ranged from 11 to 16 months[13,26,167,168,171,178], which is considerably better than the median survivals reported for AIDS-related NHL[38,133,139,140,142,148]. Patients die primarily from opportunistic infections or progressive HD[13,26,168–170], and adverse prognostic factors for survival have included the presence of 'B' symptoms, failure to respond to chemotherapy, and CD4 counts less than 200/mm^3 [26].

The optimum chemotherapeutic regimen for the treatment of HIV-associated HD has not yet been established, and, ideally, all patients should be enrolled in clinical trials. In lieu of an appropriate clinical trial, it is reasonable to avoid regimens that incorporate large amounts of steroids and alkylating agents due to the lympholytic effects of these agents. Thus, the ABVD regimen (doxorubicin, bleomycin, vinblastine, and dacarbazine)[173] or similar regimens such as EBV (epirubicin, bleomycin, vinblastine)[178] are reasonable choices for these patients. Errante *et al*. reported that the use of six cycles of EBV in HIV-infected HD patients was not associated with a decrease in the median CD4 counts (184/mm^3 and 203/mm^3 before and after therapy, respectively), and only 1 out of 17 treated patients developed an intercurrent opportunistic infection[178]. Since many of the patients with HIV-associated HD are cytopenic at presentation or experience severe hematological toxicity from marrow-suppressive chemotherapeutic regimens, the use of colony-stimulating factors should be considered for all patients. Extrapolating from the experience in treating AIDS-related NHL, the concurrent use of AZT with chemotherapy is to be avoided due to overlapping hematological toxicity, and all patients should receive *Pneumocystis carinii* prophylaxis. Ongoing clinical trials should yield important new information regarding the natural history, prognostic variables, and optimum management of HIV-associated HD. A prospective ACTG trial using the ABVD regimen with G-CSF is currently accruing patients in the USA, and this trial should generate useful data regarding the toxicity and efficacy of this regimen in HIV-associated HD.

REFERENCES

1. Gatti RA, Good RA. Occurrence of malignancy in immunodeficient disease: a literature review. *Cancer* 1971; 28: 89–98.
2. Frizzera G, Rosai J, Dehner LP *et al.* Lymphoreticular disorders in primary immunodeficiency: new findings based on an updated histologic classification of 35 cases. *Cancer* 1980; 46: 692–699.
3. Penn I. Cancers complicating organ transplantation. *N Engl J Med* 1990; 323: 1767–1769.
4. Centers for Disease Control. Kaposi's sarcoma and *Pneumocystis* pneumonia among homosexual men: New York City and California. *MMWR* 1981; 30: 305–308.

5. Pluda JM, Yarchoan R, Jaffe ES *et al.* Development of non-Hodgkin's lymphoma in a cohort of patients with severe immunodeficiency virus (HIV) infection on long-term antiretroviral therapy. *Ann Intern Med* 1990; 113: 276–282.
6. Pluda JM, Venzon DJ, Tosata G *et al.* Parameters affecting the development of non-Hodgkin's lymphoma in patients with severe human immunodeficiency virus infection receiving antiretrovial therapy. *J Clin Oncol* 1993; 11: 1099–1107.
7. Doll DC, List AF. Burkitt's lymphoma in a homosexual. *Lancet* 1982; i: 1026–1027.
8. Centers for Disease Control. Diffuse, undifferentiated non-Hodgkin's lymphoma among homosexual males: United States. *MMWR* 1982; 31: 277–279.
9. Ziegler JL, Miner RC, Rosenbaum E *et al.* Outbreak of Burkitt's-like lymphoma in homosexual men. *Lancet* 1982; ii: 631–633.
10. Centers for Disease Control. Update on acquired immune deficiency syndrome AIDS: United States. *MMWR* 1982; 31: 507–508.
11. Centers for Disease Control. Revision of the case definition of acquired immunodeficiency syndrome for national reporting: United States. *MMWR* 1985; 34: 373–375.
12. Iochim HL, Cooper MC, Hellman GC. Lymphomas in men at high risk for acquired immunodeficiency syndrome (AIDS). *Cancer* 1985; 56: 2831–2842.
13. Knowles DM, Chamulak GA, Subar M *et al.* Lymphoid neoplasia associated with the acquired immunodeficiency syndrome (AIDS): the New York University Medical Center Experience with 105 patients (1981–1986). *Ann Intern Med* 1988; 108: 744–753.
14. Lowenthal DA, Strauss DJ, Campbell SW *et al.* AIDS-related lymphoid neoplasia: the Memorial Hospital experience, *Cancer* 1987; 61: 2325–2337.
15. Kalter SP, Riggs SA, Cabanillas F *et al.* Aggressive non-Hodgkin's lymphomas in immunocompromised homosexual males. *Blood* 1985; 55: 655–659.
16. Levine AM, Gill PS, Meyer PR *et al.* Retrovirus and malignant lymphomas in homosexual men. *JAMA* 1985; 254: 1921–1925.
17. Ziegler JL, Beckstead JA, Volberding PA *et al.* Non-Hodgkin's lymphoma in 90 homosexual men: relation to generalized lymphadenopathy and the acquired immunodeficiency syndrome (AIDS). *N Engl J Med* 1984; 311: 565–570.
18. Centers for Disease Control. Revision of the CDC surveillance case definition for acquired immunodeficiency syndrome. *MMWR* 1987; 36 (Suppl.): 1S–15S.
19. Robert NJ, Schneiderman H. Hodgkin's disease and the acquired immunodeficiency syndrome. *Ann Intern Med* 1984; 101: 142–143.
20. Scheib RG, Siegel RS. Atypical Hodgkin's disease and the acquired immunodeficiency syndrome. *Ann Intern Med* 1985; 102: 554.
21. Prior E, Goldberg AF, Conjalka MS *et al.* Hodgkin's disease in homosexual men: an AIDS-related phenomenon? *Am J Med* 1986; 81: 1085–1088.
22. Temple JJ, Andes WA. AIDS and Hodgkin's disease. *Lancet* 1986; ii: 454–455.
23. Bernstein L, Levin D, Mench H, Ross RK. AIDS-related secular trends in cancer in Los Angeles county men: a comparison by martial status. *Cancer Res* 1989; 49: 466–470.
24. Roithman S, Tourani JM, Andrieu JM. Hodgkin's disease in HIV-infected intravenous drug abusers. *N Engl J Med* 1990; 323: 275–276.
25. Hessol NA, Katz MH, Liu JY *et al.* Increased incidence of Hodgkin disease in homosexual men with HIV infection. *Ann Intern Med* 1992; 117: 309–311.
26. Rubio R. Hodgkin's disease associated with human immunodeficiency virus infection: a clinical study of 46 cases. Cooperative Study Group of Malignancies Associated with HIV infection of Madrid. *Cancer* 1994; 73: 2400–2407.
27. Rabkin CS, Biggar RJ, Horm JS. Increasing incidence of cancers associated with the human immunodeficiency virus epidemic. *Int J Cancer* 1991; 47: 692–696.

28. Gail MH, Pluda JM, Rabkin CS *et al.* Projections of the incidence of non-Hodgkin's lymphoma related to acquired immunodeficiency syndrome. *J Natl Cancer Inst* 1991; 83: 695–700.
29. Safai B, Dias BM. Kaposi's sarcoma and cloacogenic carcinoma associated with AIDS. In Broder S, Merigan TC Jr, Bolognesi D (eds) *Textbook of AIDS Medicine*. Baltimore: Williams & Wilkins, 1994; pp. 410–414.
30. Beral V, Peterman T, Berkelman R, Jaffe H. AIDS-associated non-Hodgkin's lymphoma. *Lancet* 1991; 337: 805–809.
31. Beckhardt RN, Farley N, May M *et al.* Increased incidence of malignant lymphoma in AIDS: a comparison of risk groups and possible etiologic factors. *Mount Sinai J Med* 1988; 55: 383–389.
32. Volberding PA, Lagakos SW, Koch MA *et al.* Zidovudine in asymptomatic HIV infection: a controlled trial in persons with fewer than 500 CD4-positive cells per cubic millimeter. *N Engl J Med* 1990; 322: 941–949.
33. Concorde MRC/ANRS randomized double-blind controlled trial of immediate and deferred zidovudine in symptom-free HIV infection. Concorde Coordinating Committee. *Lancet* 1994; 343: 871–881.
34. Moore RD, Kessler H, Richman DD *et al.* Non-Hodgkin's lymphoma in patients with advanced HIV infection treated with zidovudine. *JAMA* 1991; 265: 2208–2211.
35. Beral V, Peterman TA, Berkelman RC, Jaffe HW. Kaposi's sarcoma among persons with AIDS: a sexually transmitted disease? *Lancet* 1990; 335: 123–128.
36. Levine AM. Acquired immunodeficiency syndrome-related lymphoma. *Blood* 1992; 80: 8–20.
37. Kaplan LD, Abrams DI, Feigal E *et al.* AIDS-associated non-Hodgkin's lymphoma in San Francisco. *JAMA* 1989; 261: 719–724.
38. Ragni MV, Belle SH, Jaffe RA *et al.* Acquired immunodeficiency syndrome-associated non-Hodgkin's lymphomas and other malignancies in patients with hemophilia. *Blood* 1993; 81: 1889–1997.
39. Monfardini S, Vaccher E, Tirelli U, and others for the Italian Cooperative Group on AIDS-related Tumors (GI-CAT). AIDS-associated non-Hodgkin's lymphoma in Italy: intravenous drug users versus homosexual men. *Ann Oncol* 1990; 1: 208–211.
40. Casabona J, Melbye M, Biggar RJ. Kaposi's sarcoma and non-Hodgkin's lymphoma in European AIDS cases: no excess risk of Kaposi's sarcoma in Mediterranean countries. *Int J Cancer* 1991; 47: 49–53.
41. Pedersen C, Gerstoft J, Lundgren JD *et al.* HIV-associated lymphoma: histopathology and association with Epstein–Barr virus genome related to clinical, immunological, and prognostic features. *Eur J Cancer* 1991; 27: 1416–1423.
42. Carbone A, Tirelli U, Vaccher E *et al.* A clinicopathologic study of lymphoid neoplasias associated with human immunodeficiency virus infection in Italy. *Cancer* 1991; 68: 842–852.
43. Raphael J, Gentihomme O, Tulliez M *et al.* Histopathologic features of high grade non-Hodgkin's lymphomas in acquired immunodeficiency syndrome. *Arch Pathol Lab Med* 1991; 115: 15–20.
44. Knowles DM, Chadburn A. Lymphadenopathy and the lymphoid neoplasms associated with the acquired immune deficiency syndrome (AIDS). In Knowles DM (ed.) *Neoplastic Hematopathology*. Baltimore: Williams & Wilkins, 1992; pp. 773–836.
45. Knowles DM, Chamulak GA, Subar M *et al.* Clinicopathologic, immunophenotypic, and molecular genetic analysis of AIDS-associated lymphoid neoplasia: clinical and biologic implications. *Pathol Annu* 1988; 23: 33–67.
46. McGrath MS, Shiramizu B, Meeker TC *et al.* AIDS-associated polyclonal lym-

phoma: identification of a new HIV-associated disease process. *J AIDS* 1991; 4: 408–415.
47. Shiramizu B, Herndier B, Meeker T *et al.* Molecular and immunophenotypic characterization of AIDS-associated, Epstein–Barr virus-negative, polyclonal lymphoma. *J Clin Oncol* 1992; 10: 383–389.
48. Voelkerding KV, Sandhaus LM, Kim HC *et al.* Plasma cell malignancy in the acquired immune deficiency syndrome. *Am J Clin Pathol* 1989; 92: 222–228.
49. Nasr SA, Byrnes RK, Garrison CP, Chan WC. Peripheral T-cell lymphoma in a patient with acquired immunodeficiency syndrome. *Cancer* 1988; 61: 947–951.
50. Herndier BG, Shiramizu BT, Jewett NE *et al.* Acquired immunodeficiency syndrome-associated T-cell lymphoma: evidence for human immunodeficiency virus type 1-associated T-cell transformation. *Blood* 1992; 79: 1768–1774.
51. Goldstein J, Becker N, DelRowe J, Davis L. Cutaneous T cell lymphoma in a patient infected with human immunodeficiency virus type 1: use of radiation therapy. *Cancer* 1990; 66: 1130–1132.
52. Tirelli U, Vaccher E, Zagonel V *et al.* CD30 (Ki-1)-positive anaplastic large-cell lymphomas in 13 patients with and 27 patients without human immunodeficiency virus infection: the first comparative clinicopathologic study from a single institution that also includes 80 patients with other human immunodeficiency virus-related systemic lymphomas. *J Clin Oncol* 1995; 13: 373–380.
53. Carbone A, Tirelli U, Gloghini A *et al.* Human immunodeficiency virus-associated systemic lymphomas may be subdivided into two main groups according to Epstein–Barr viral latent gene expression. *J Clin Oncol* 1993; 11: 1674–1681.
54. Carbone A, Gloghini A, Zanette I *et al.* Demonstration of Epstein–Barr viral genomes by in situ hybridization in acquired immune deficiency syndrome-related high grade and anaplastic large cell CD30+ lymphomas. *Am J Clin Pathol* 1993; 99: 289–297.
55. Chadburn A, Cesarman E, Jagidar J *et al.* CD30 (Ki-1) positive anaplastic large cell lymphomas in individuals infected with the human immunodeficiency virus. *Cancer* 1993; 72: 3078–3090.
56. Wong-Staal F, Gallo RC. Human T-lymphotropic retroviruses. *Nature* 1985; 317: 395–403.
57. Subar M, Neri A, Inghirami G *et al.* Frequent c-myc oncogene activation and infrequent presence of Epstein–Barr virus genome in AIDS-associated lymphoma. *Blood* 1988; 72: 667–671.
58. Shiramizu B, Herndier BG, McGrath MS. Identification of a common clonal human immunodeficiency virus integration site in human immunodeficiency virus-associated lymphoma. *Cancer* 1994; 54: 2069–2072.
59. Miller G. Epstein–Barr virus-biology, pathogenesis, and medical aspects. In Fields BN, Knipe DM, Chanock RM (eds.) *Virology*. New York: Raven Press, 1990; pp. 1921–1958.
60. Sullivan JL. Epstein–Barr virus and lymphoproliferative disorders. *Semin Hematol* 1988; 25: 269–279.
61. List AF, Greco A, Vogler LB. Lymphoproliferative diseases in immunocompromised hosts: the role of Epstein–Barr virus. *J Clin Oncol* 1987; 5: 1673–1689.
62. Penn I. Why do immunosuppressed patients develop cancer? *Crit Rev Oncog* 1989; 1: 27–52.
63. Purtilo DT, Strobach RS, Okano M, Davis JR. Epstein–Barr virus-associated lymphoproliferative disorders. *Lab Invest* 1992; 67: 5–23.
64. Nalesnik MA, Jaffe R, Starzl TE *et al.* The pathology of post-transplant lymphoproliferative disorders occurring in the setting of cyclosporine A–prednisone immunosuppression. *Am J Pathol* 1988; 133: 173–192.

65. Kieff E, Liebowitz D. Epstein–Barr virus and its replication. In Fields BN, Knipe DM, Chanock RM (eds) *Virology*. New York: Raven Press, 1990; pp. 1889–1920.
66. Klein G. Epstein–Barr virus strategy in normal and neoplastic B cells. *Cell* 1994; 77: 791–793.
67. Sugden B. An intricate route to immortality. *Cell* 1989; 57: 5–7.
68. Pope JH. Transformation by the virus in vitro. In Epstein MA, Achong BG (eds) *The Epstein–Barr Virus*. New York: Springer-Verlag, 1979; pp. 205–223.
69. Miller G. Experimental carcinogenicity by the virus in vivo. In Epstein MA, Achong BG (eds) *The Epstein–Barr Virus*. New York: Springer-Verlag, 1979; pp. 351–372.
70. Henle W, Henle G. Seroepidemiology of the virus. In Epstein MA, Achong, BG (eds) *The Epstein–Barr Virus*. New York: Springer-Verlag, 1979; pp. 61–78.
71. Hamilton-Dutoit SJ, Raphael M, Audouin J *et al.* In situ demonstration of Epstein–Barr virus small RNAs (EBER 1) in acquired immunodeficiency syndrome-related lymphomas: correlation with tumor morphology and primary site. *Blood* 1993; 82: 619–624.
72. Ballerini P, Gaidano G, Gong JZ *et al.* Multiple genetic lesions in acquired immunodeficiency syndrome-related non-Hodgkin's lymphoma. *Blood* 1993; 81: 166–167.
73. MacMahon EM, Glass JD, Hayward SD *et al.* Epstein–Barr virus in AIDS-related primary central nervous system lymphoma. *Lancet* 1991; 338: 969–973.
74. Shibata D, Weiss LM, Hernandez AM *et al.* Epstein–Barr virus-associated non-Hodgkin's lymphoma in patients infected with the human immunodeficiency virus. *Blood* 1993; 81: 2102–2109.
75. Raphael MM, Audouin J, Lamine M *et al.* Immunophenotypic and genotypic analysis of acquired immunodeficiency syndrome-related non-Hodgkin's lymphomas: correlation with histologic features in 36 cases. French Study Group of Pathology for HIV-associated Tumors. *Am J Clin Pathol* 1994; 101: 773–782.
76. Carbone A, Golghini A, Volpe R *et al.* High frequency of Epstein–Barr virus latent membrane protein-1 expression in acquired immunodeficiency syndrome-related Ki-1 (CD30)-positive anaplastic large-cell lymphomas. Italian Cooperative Group of AIDS and Tumors. *Am J Clin Pathol* 1994; 101: 768–772.
77. Cesarman E, Chang Y, Moore PS *et al.* Kaposi's sarcoma-associated herpesvirus-like DNA sequences in AIDS-related body-cavity-based lymphomas. *N Engl J Med* 1995; 332: 1186–1191.
78. Neri A, Barriga F, Knowles DM *et al.* Epstein–Barr virus infection precedes clonal expansion in Burkitt's and AIDS-associated lymphoma. *Blood* 1991; 77: 1092–1095.
79. Birx DL, Redfield RR, Tosata G. Defective regulation of Epstein–Barr virus infection in patients with acquired immunodeficiency syndrome (AIDS) or AIDS-related disorders. *N Engl J Med* 1986; 314: 874–879.
80. Shibata D, Weiss LM, Nathwani BN *et al.* Epstein–Barr virus in benign lymph node biopsies from individuals infected with the human immunodeficiency virus is associated with concurrent or subsequent development of non-Hodgkin's lymphoma. *Blood* 1991; 77: 1527–1533.
81. Lombardi L, Newcomb EW, Dalla-Favera R. Expression of an activated c-myc oncogene causes the tumorigenic conversion of EBV-infected human B lymphoblasts. *Cell* 1987; 49: 161–170.
82. Hamilton-Dutoit SJ, Rea D, Raphael M *et al.* Epstein–Barr virus-latent gene expression and tumor cell phenotype in acquired immunodeficiency syndrome-related non-Hodgkin's lymphoma: correlation of lymphoma phenotype with three distinct patterns of viral latency. *Am J Pathol* 1993; 143: 1072–1085.
83. Rea D, Delecluse HJ, Hamilton-Dutoit SJ *et al.* Epstein–Barr virus latent and

replicative gene expression in post-transplant lymphoproliferative disorders and AIDS-related non-Hodgkin's lymphomas. French Study Group of Pathology for HIV-associated Tumors. *Ann Oncol* 1994; 5 (Suppl. 1): S113–116.
84. Speck SH, Strominger JL. Transcription of Epstein–Barr virus in latently infected growth transformation lymphocytes. In Klein G (ed.) *Advances in Viral Oncology.* New York: Raven Press, 1989; pp. 133–150.
85. Sample J, Brooks L, Sample C *et al.* Restricted Epstein–Barr virus protein expression in Burkitt lymphoma is due to different Epstein–Barr virus nuclear antigen 1 transcriptional initiation site. *Proc Natl Acad Sci USA* 1991; 88: 6343–6347.
86. Deacon EM, Pallesen G, Niedobitek G *et al.* Epstein–Barr virus latent gene transcription in Hodgkin's disease. *J Exp Med* 1993; 177: 339–349.
87. Brooks L, Yao QY, Rickinson AB, Young LS. Epstein–Barr virus latent gene transcription in nasopharyngeal carcinoma cells: coexpression of EBNA 1, LMPI, and LMP2 transcripts. *J Virol* 1992; 66: 2689–2697.
88. Chaganti RSK, Jhanawar SC, Kozener B *et al.* Specific translocations characterize Burkitt's-like lymphoma of homosexual men with acquired immunodeficiency syndrome. *Blood* 1993; 61: 1265–1268.
89. Pelicci P-G, Knowles DM, Arlin ZA *et al.* Multiple monoclonal B cell expansions and c-myc oncogene rearrangements in acquired immune deficiency syndrome-related lymphoproliferative disorders: implications for lymphomagenesis. *J Exp Med* 1986; 164: 2049–2076.
90. Subar M, Neri A, Inghirami G *et al.* Frequent c-myc oncogene activation and infrequent presence of Epstein–Barr virus genome in AIDS-associated lymphoma. *Blood* 1988; 72: 667–761.
91. Croce CM, Nowell PC. Molecular basis of human B cell neoplasia. *Blood* 1985; 65: 1–7.
92. Shiramizu B, Barriga F, Neequaye J *et al.* Patterns of chromosomal breakpoint locations in Burkitt's lymphoma: relevance to geography and Epstein–Barr virus association. *Blood* 77: 1516–1526.
93. Pellici PG, Knowles DM, MaGrath I, Dalla-Favera R. Chromosomal breakpoints and structural alterations of the c-myc locus differ in endemic and sporadic forms of Burkitt lymphoma. *Proc Natl Acad Sci USA* 1986; 83: 2984–2988.
94. Magrath I. The pathogenesis of Burkitt's lymphoma. *Adv Cancer Res* 1990; 53: 133–270.
95. Delecluse HJ, Raphael M, Magaud JP *et al.* Variable morphology of human immunodeficiency virus-associated lymphomas with c-myc rearrangements. The French Study Group of Pathology for Human Immunodeficiency Virus-associated Tumors, I. *Blood* 1993; 82: 552–563.
96. Bhatia K, Spangler G, Gaidano G *et al.* Mutations in the coding region of c-myc occur frequently in acquired immunodeficiency syndrome-associated lymphomas. *Blood* 1994; 84: 883–888.
97. Lanfrancone L, Pelicci PG, Dalla-Favera R. Structure and expression of translocated c-myc oncogenes: specific differences in endemic, sporadic, and AIDS-associated forms of Burkitt's lymphomas. *Curr Top Microbiol Immunol* 1986; 132: 257–265.
98. Ladanyi M, Offitt K, Jhanwar SC *et al.* MYC rearrangement and translocations involving band 8q24 in diffuse large cell lymphomas. *Blood* 1991; 77: 1057–1063.
99. Clark HM, Yano T, Otsuki T *et al.* Mutations in the coding region of c-myc in AIDS-associated and other aggressive lymphomas. *Cancer Res* 1994; 54: 3383–3386.
100. Bhatia K, Huppi K, Spangler G *et al.* Point mutation in the c-Myc transactivation

domain are common in Burkitt's lymphoma and mouse plasmacytoma. *Nature Genet* 1993; 5: 56–61.
101. Weiss LM, Warnke RA, Sklar J, Cleary ML. Molecular analysis of the t(14;18) chromosomal translocation in malignant lymphomas. *N Engl J Med* 1987; 317: 1185–1189.
102. Raffield M, Jaffe ES. bcl-1, (t(11;14), and mantle cell-derived lymphomas. *Blood* 1991; 78: 259–263.
103. Gaidano G, Lo Coco R, Ye BH *et al*. Rearrangements of the Bc1-6 gene in acquired immunodeficiency syndrome-associated non-Hodgkin's lymphoma: association with diffuse large-cell subtype. *Blood* 1994; 84: 397–402.
104. Kerckaert J-P, Deweindt C, Tilly H *et al*. LAZ3, a novel zinc-finger encoding gene, is disrupted by recurring chromosome 3q27 translocations in human lymphomas. *Nature Genet* 1993; 5: 66–70.
105. Ye BH, Lista F, Lo Coco R *et al*. Alterations of a zinc-finger encoding gene, BCL6, in diffuse large-cell lymphoma. *Science* 1993; 262: 747–750.
106. Lo Coco F, Ye BH, Lista F *et al*. Rearrangements of the BCL6 gene in diffuse large cell non-Hodgkin's lymphoma. *Blood* 1994; 83: 1757–1759.
107. Bos JL. Ras oncogenes in human cancer: a review. *Cancer Res* 1989; 49: 4682–4689.
108. Neri A, Knowles DM, McCormick F, Dalla-Favera R. Analysis of ras oncogene mutations in human lymphoid malignancies. *Proc Natl Acad Sci USA* 1988; 85: 9268–9272.
109. Stanbridge EJ, Nowell PC. Origins of human cancer revisited. *Cell* 1990; 63: 867–874.
110. Stanbridge EJ. Human tumor suppressor genes. *Annu Rev Genet* 1990; 24: 615–657.
111. Hollingsworth RE, Lee W-T. Tumor suppressor genes: new prospects for cancer research. *J Natl Cancer Inst* 1991; 83: 91–96.
112. Nigro JM, Baker SJ, Preisinger AC *et al*. Mutations in the p53 gene occur in diverse human tumor types. *Nature* 1989; 342: 705–708.
113. Gaidano G, Ballerini P, Gong JZ *et al*. p53 mutations in human lymphoid malignancies: association with Burkitt's lymphoma and chronic lymphocytic leukemia. *Proc Natl Acad Sci USA* 1991; 88: 5413–5417.
114 Cesarman E, Chadburn A, Inghirami G *et al*. Structural and functional analysis of oncogenes and tumor suppressor genes in adult T cell leukemia/lymphoma (ATLL) reveals frequent p53 mutations. *Blood* 1992; 80: 3205–3216.
115. Nakamura H, Said JW, Miller CW, Koeffler HP. Mutation and protein expression of p53 in acquired immunodeficiency syndrome-related lymphomas. *Blood* 1993; 82: 920–926.
116. Doweiko JP, Groopman JE. Hematological consequences of HIV infection. In Broder S, Merigan TC Jr, Bolognesi D (eds) *Textbook of AIDS Medicine*. Baltimore: William & Wilkins, 1994; pp. 617–628.
117. Birx DL, Redfield RR, Tencer K *et al*. Induction of interleukin-6 during human immunodeficiency virus infection. *Blood* 1990; 76: 2303–2310.
118. Scadden DT, Zeira M, Woon A *et al*. Human immunodeficiency virus infection of human bone marrow stromal fibroblasts. *Blood* 1990; 76: 317–322.
119. Hirano T. Interleukin-6 (IL-6) and its receptor: their role in plasma cell neoplasias. *Int J Cloning* 1991; 9: 166–184.
120. Kishimoto T. The biology of interleukin-6. *Blood* 1989; 74: 1–10.
121. Berberian L, Valles-Ayoub Y, Sun N *et al*. A VH clonal deficit in human immunodeficiency virus-positive individuals reflects a B-cell maturational arrest. *Blood* 1991; 78: 175–179.
122. Breen EC, Rezai AR, Nakajima K *et al*. Infection with HIV is associated with elevated IL-6 levels and production. *J Immunol* 1990; 144: 480–484.

123. Schwab G, Siegall CB, Aarden LA *et al.* Characterization of an interleukin-6 mediated autocrine growth loop in the human multiple myeloma cell lines U266. *Blood* 1991; 77: 587–593.
124. Zhang XG, Klein B, Bataille R. Interleukin-6 is a potent myeloma-cell growth factor in patients with aggressive multiple myeloma. *Blood* 1989; 74: 11–13.
125. Emilie D, Coumbaras J, Raphael M *et al.* Interleukin-6 production in high grade B lymphomas: correlation with the presence of malignant immunoblasts in acquired immunodeficiency syndrome and in human immunodeficiency syndrome virus-negative patients. *Blood* 1992; 80: 498–504.
126. Benjamin D, Knoblach TJ, Dayton MA. Human B-cell IL-10: B cell lines derived from patients with acquired immunodeficiency syndrome and Burkitt's lymphoma constitutively secrete large quantities of interleukin-10. *Blood* 1992; 80: 1289–1298.
127. Masood R, Zhang Y, Bond M *et al.* Interleukin-10 is an autocrine B-cell growth factor for acquired immunodeficiency syndrome-related B-cell lymphoma. *Blood* 1995; 85: 3423–3430.
128. Go NF, Castle BE, Barrett R *et al.* Interleukin-10, a novel B cell stimulatory factor: unresponsiveness of X chromosome-linked immunodeficiency B cells. *J Exp Med* 1990; 172: 1625–1631.
129. Iochim HL, Weinstein MA, Robbins RD *et al.* Primary anorectal lymphoma: a new manifestation of the acquired immunodeficiency syndrome (AIDS). *Cancer* 1987; 60: 1449–1453.
130. Enting RH, Esselink RA, Portegies P. Lymphomatous meningitis in AIDS-related systemic non-Hodgkin's lymphoma: a report of eight cases. *J Neurol Neurosurg Psychiatry* 1994; 57: 150–153.
131. International Non-Hodgkin's Lymphoma Prognostic Factors Group. A predictive model for aggressive non-Hodgkin's lymphoma. *N Engl J Med* 1993; 329: 987–994.
132. Levine AM, Sullivan-Halley J, Pikem MC *et al.* HIV-related lymphoma: prognostic factors predictive of survival. *Cancer* 1991; 68: 2466–2472.
133. Gisselbrecht C, Oksenhendler E, Tirelli U *et al.* Human immunodeficiency virus-related lymphoma treatment with intensive combination chemotherapy. French–Italian Cooperative Group. *Am J Med* 1995; 95: 188–196.
134. Walts AE, Shintaku IP, Said JW. Diagnosis of malignant lymphoma in effusions from patients with AIDS by gene rearrangement. *Am J Clin Pathol* 1990; 94: 170–175.
135. Green I, Espiritu E, Ladanyi M *et al.* Primary lymphomatous effusions in AIDS: a morphological, immunophenotypic, and molecular study. *Mod Pathol* 1995; 8: 39–45.
136. Cesarman E, Chang Y, Moore PS *et al.* Kaposi's sarcoma-associated herpesvirus-like DNA sequences in AIDS-related body-cavity-based lymphomas. *N Engl J Med* 1995; 332: 1186–1191.
137. Roithmann R, Tourani JM, Andrieu JM. AIDS associated non-Hodgkin's lymphoma. *Lancet* 1991; 338: 884–885.
138. Gill P, Levine A, Krailo M *et al.* AIDS-related malignant lymphoma: results of prospective treatment trials. *J Clin Oncol* 1987; 5: 1322–1328.
139. Bermudez MA, Grant KM, Rodvien R, Mendes R. Non-Hodgkin's lymphoma in a population with or at risk for acquired immunodeficiency syndrome: indications for intensive chemotherapy. *JAMA* 1989; 86: 71–76.
140. Kaplan L, Kahn J, Crowe S *et al.* Clinical and virologic effects of recombinant human granulocyte–macrophage colony-stimulating factor in patients receiving chemotherapy for human immunodeficiency virus-associated non-Hodgkin's lymphoma: results of a randomized trial. *J Clin Oncol* 1991; 9: 929–940.

141. Levine AM, Wernz JC, Kaplan L *et al.* Low-dose chemotherapy with central nervous system prophylaxis and zidovudine maintenance in AIDS-related lymphoma: a prospective multi-institutional trial. *JAMA* 1991; 266: 84–88.
142. Remick SC, McSharry JJ, Wolf BC *et al.* Novel oral combination chemotherapy in the treatment of intermediate-grade and high-grade AIDS-related non-Hodgkin's lymphoma. *J Clin Oncol* 1993; 11: 1691–1702.
143. Sparano JA, Wiernik PH, Strack M *et al.* Infusional cyclophosphamide doxorubicin, and etoposide in human immunodeficiency virus- and human T-cell leukemia virus type 1-related non-Hodgkin's lymphoma: a highly active regimen. *Blood* 1993; 81: 2810–2815.
144. Tirelli U, Errante D, Oksenhendler E. Prospective study with combined low-dose chemotherapy and zidovudine in 37 patients with poor-prognosis AIDS-related non-Hodgkin's lymphoma. French–Italian Cooperative Study Group. *Ann Oncol* 1992; 3: 843–847.
145. Walsh C, Wernz JC, Levine A *et al.* Phase I trial of m-BACOD and granulocyte–macrophage colony stimulating factor in HIV-associated non-Hodgkin's lymphoma. *J AIDS* 1993; 6: 265–271.
146. Taillan B, Garnier G, Ferrari E. MACOP-B chemotherapy for the treatment of high-grade lymphomas in patients with HIV-1 infection. *Acta Haematol* 1993; 89: 10–12.
147. Sawka CA, Shepherd FA, Brandwein J *et al.* Treatment of AIDS-related non-Hodgkin's lymphoma with a twelve week chemotherapy program. *Leuk Lymph* 1992; 8: 213–220.
148. Kaplan L, Straus D, Testa M, Levine AM, for the NIAID AIDS Clinical Trial Group (ACTG). Randomized trial of standard mBACOD with GM-CSF vs. reduced dose mBACOD for systemic HIV-associated lymphoma: ACTG 142. *Proc Am Soc Clin Oncol* 1995; 14: 288.
149. Mitsuyasu R, Gill P, Paredes J *et al.* Combination chemotherapy. Adriamycin, Bleomycim, and Vincristine (ABV) with dideoxyinosine (ddI) or dideoxycytidine (ddC) in advanced AIDS-related Kaposi's sarcoma. *Proc Am Soc Clin Oncol* 1995; 14: 289.
150. Levine AM, Katz-Willson E, Espina B *et al.* Low dose m-BACOD with concomitant dideoxycytidine (ddC) in AIDS-related lymphoma. *Blood* 1992; 80: 328a.
151. Levy RM, Janssen RS, Bush TJ *et al.* Neuroepidemiology of acquired immunodeficiency syndrome. In Rosenblum ML, Levy RM, Bredesen DE (eds) *AIDS and the Nervous System*. New York: Raven Press, 1988; pp. 13–27.
152. Wilkes MS, Fortin AH, Felix JC *et al.* Value of necropsy in acquired immunodeficiency syndrome. *Lancet* 1988; ii: 85–88.
153. Gill PS, Levine AM, Meyer PR *et al.* Primary central nervous system lymphoma in homosexual men: clinical, immunologic, and pathologic features. *Am J Med* 1985; 78: 742–748.
154. So YT, Beckstead JH, Davis RL. Primary central nervous system lymphoma in acquired immune deficiency syndrome: a clinical and pathological study. *Ann Neurol* 1986; 20: 566–572.
155. Goldstein JD, Dickson DW, Moser FG *et al.* Primary central nervous system lymphoma in acquired immunodeficiency syndrome: a clinical and pathologic study with results of treatment with radiation. *Cancer* 1991; 67: 2756–2765.
156. Formenti SC, Gill PS, Lean E *et al.* Primary central nervous system lymphoma in AIDS: results of radiation therapy. *Cancer* 1989; 63: 1101–1107.
157. Baumgartner JE, Rachlin JR, Beckstead JH *et al.* Primary central nervous system lymphomas: natural history and response to radiation therapy in 55 patients with acquired immunodeficiency syndrome. *J Neurosurg* 1990; 73: 206–211.

158. Bashir R, Luka J, Cheloha K *et al.* Expression of Epstein–Barr virus proteins in primary CNS lymphoma in AIDS patients. *Neurology* 1993; 43: 2358–2362.
159. Lee YY, Bruner JM, Van Tassle P, Libshitz H. Primary central nervous system lymphoma: CT and pathologic correlation. *AJNR* 1986; 7: 599–604.
160. Fine HA, Mayer RJ. Primary central nervous system lymphoma. *Ann Intern Med* 1993; 119: 1093–1004.
161. De Angelis LM, Yahalom J, Heinemann MH *et al.* Primary CNS lymphoma: combined treatment with chemotherapy and radiotherapy. *Neurology* 1990; 40: 80–86.
162. Ling SM, Roach M III, Larson DA, Wara WM. Radiotherapy of primary central nervous system lymphoma in patients with and without human immunodeficiency virus: ten years of treatment experience at the University of California San Francisco. *Cancer* 1994; 73: 2570–2582.
163. Nisce LZ, Kaufmann T, Metroka C. Radiation therapy in patients with AIDS-related central nervous system lymphoma. *JAMA* 1992; 267: 1921–1922.
164. Chamberlain MC. Long survival in patients with acquired immune deficiency syndrome-related primary central nervous system lymphoma. *Cancer* 1994; 73: 1728–1730.
165. Baer DM, Anderson ET, Wilkinson LS. Acquired immune deficiency syndrome in homosexual men with Hodgkin's disease. *Am J Med* 1986; 80: 738–740.
166. Cid JA, Cid JL, Sanudo EF *et al.* AIDS and Hodgkin's disease. *Lancet* 1986; ii: 1104–1105.
167. Tirelli U, Vaccher E, Rezza G *et al.* Hodgkin disease and infection with the human immunodeficiency virus (HIV) in Italy. *Ann Intern Med* 1988; 108: 309–310.
168. Gold JE, Altarac D, Ree HJ *et al.* HIV-associated Hodgkin's disease: a clinical study of 18 cases and review of the literature. *Am J Hematol* 1991; 36: 93–99.
169. Serrano M, Bellas C, Camp E *et al.* Hodgkin's disease in patients with antibodies to human immunodeficiency virus: a study of 22 patients. *Cancer* 1991; 65: 2248–2254.
170. Ree HJ, Strauchen JA, Khan AA *et al.* HIV-associated Hodgkin's disease: clinicopathologic studies of 24 cases: preponderance of mixed cellularity type characterized by the occurrence of fibro-histiocytoid stromal cells. *Cancer* 1991; 67: 1614–1621.
171. Monfardini S, Tirrelli U, Vaccher E *et al.* Hodgkin's disease in 63 intravenous drug users infected with human immunodeficiency virus. *Ann Oncol* 1991; 2 (Suppl. 2): 201–205.
172. Serraino D, Carbone A, Francheszchi S, Tirelli U. Increased frequency of lymphocyte depletion and mixed cellularity subtypes of Hodgkin's disease in HIV-infected patients. The Italian Cooperative Group of AIDS and Tumors. *Eur J Cancer* 1993; 29: 1948–1950.
173. DeVita VT, Hellman S, Jaffe ES. Hodgkin's disease. In DeVita VT, Hellman S, Rosenberg SA (eds) *Cancer Principles and Practice of Oncology*. Philadelphia: Lippincott, 1993; pp. 1819–1858.
174. Herbst H, Steinbrecher E, Niedobitek G *et al.* Distribution and phenotype of Epstein–Barr virus-harboring cells in Hodgkin's disease. *Blood* 1992; 80: 484–491.
175. Coonley CJ, Straus DJ, Filippa D, Watson R. Hodgkin's disease presenting with rectal symptoms in a homosexual male: a case report and review of the literature. *Cancer Invest* 1984; 2: 279–284.
176. Hair LS, Rogers JD, Chadburn A *et al.* Intracerebral Hodgkin's disease in a human immunodeficiency virus-seropositive patient. *Cancer* 1991; 67: 2931–2934.

177. Ames ED, Conjalka MS, Goldberg AF *et al.* Hodgkin's disease and AIDS: twenty three new cases and a review of the literature. *Hematol Oncol Clin N Am* 1991; 5: 343–356.
178. Errante D, Tirelli U, Gastaldi R *et al.* Combined antineoplastic and antiretroviral therapy for patients with Hodgkin's disease and human immunodeficiency virus infection: a prospective study of 17 patients. The Italian Cooperative Group on AIDS and Tumors (GICAT). *Cancer* 1994; 73: 437–444.

8

AIDS-related Kaposi's Sarcoma

Kevin J. Harrington and Konstantinos N. Syrigos
Royal Postgraduate Medical School, Hammersmith Hospital, London, UK

INTRODUCTION

In 1872 Moritz Kaposi described multiple, pigmented tumour masses in elderly men as 'sarcoma idiopathicum multiple haemorrhagicum'[1]. This clinical entity has come to be known as classical, or European, Kaposi's sarcoma (KS), an indolent condition which afflicts elderly men of Mediterranean or Eastern European Jewish descent. Another manifestation of the same disease process was described in the 1950s in an endemic form, occurring in sub-Saharan Africa. The clinical features of endemic KS are more heterogeneous, varying from a benign process in elderly patients to a fulminant, fatal lymphadenopathic disorder in infants and children. Recently, patients receiving chronic immunosuppressive therapy following renal transplantation have been found to have an increased incidence of KS and these lesions have been reported to resolve spontaneously upon withdrawal of immunosuppression[2,3]. However, in 1979–1980 what had previously been a rare disease assumed enormous importance as an epidemic of cases was reported from San Francisco, USA, in young homosexual or bisexual men[4,5].

EPIDEMIOLOGY

It soon became apparent that the epidemic of cases of KS was occurring as part of a syndrome involving a breakdown of the patient's immune system, since a number of patients also presented with opportunistic infections, such

AIDS and Malignancies: Current Concepts and Perspectives.
Edited by B.C. Golematis and V.T. DeVita Jr

as *Pneumocystis carinii* pneumonia and cerebral toxoplasmosis[6]. The occurrence of this acquired immunodeficiency syndrome (AIDS) in intravenous drug users and haemophiliacs receiving factor VIII indicated that a blood-borne transmissible factor was responsible. However, despite these indications of an infective aetiology of AIDS, the incidence of KS in patients infected through contaminated blood products was found to be significantly lower than in patients infected through sexual contact. Therefore, 1% of haemophiliacs and 21% of homosexuals with AIDS developed KS[7]. This data provides strong evidence that HIV infection *per se* is not the cause of AIDS-related KS.

The apparent incidence of KS has declined steeply since the early years of the epidemic[7–9], but, since fewer patients are succumbing to early infective complications of the disease, the overall prevalence of this condition has increased[10]. A recent survey from St Mary's Hospital, London, showed that KS represented the AIDS-defining diagnosis in 21% of patients[11]. AIDS-related KS, therefore, represents a significant health care problem, both in terms of the morbidity and mortality experienced by the patient, and the need for resources to provide therapy.

AETIOLOGY AND PATHOGENESIS

The specific aetiology of AIDS-related KS remains obscure. In the last decade several models have been proposed to explain the epidemiological and clinical features of this disease. Although an infective aetiology seems most likely, as supported by recent evidence, a number of different aetiological events may interact in a multifactorial process.

The role of immunosuppression in the development of KS was first documented in the setting of organ transplantation, where recipients were found to have a 400–500-fold increased risk. Furthermore, regression of lesions in 50% of cases was reported on withdrawal of immunosuppressive agents[3]. However, immunosuppression in itself is not the only factor, since neither bone marrow transplant recipients nor children with congenital immunodeficiency disorders have an increased risk of developing KS. It seems most likely that the immunosuppressed state provides a suitable milieu in which one or more other factors can exert an effect.

The fact that AIDS-related KS is more common in homosexual or bisexual men than in other human immunodeficiency virus (HIV)-infected groups, such as intravenous drug users or haemophiliacs[12], has led some investigators to presume the existence of a sexually transmitted factor, independent of HIV[7]. The development of KS has been shown to be strongly associated with sexual practices involving faeco-oral contact[7,13]. Furthermore, in Africa, where HIV is predominantly spread by the heterosexual route, there is no difference in prevalence between the sexes. There are also reports of cases of epidemic KS occurring in HIV-negative homosexual men in the USA[14,15].

Such evidence supports the notion of an independent transmissible agent which does not show the same propensity for blood-borne passage as HIV. An extensive search has been undertaken in an attempt to isolate the putative infective agent. Cytomegalovirus (CMV) was thought to be implicated in classical KS, but CMV DNA sequences were not detected in AIDS-related KS lesions[16]. Using polymerase chain reaction techniques, the presence of HPV-16 DNA sequences has been demonstrated in both KS tissue specimens and cell lines[17]. In addition, anti-HPV antibodies were shown to localize to KS tissues by means of immunohistochemical analysis[18]. However, the significance of this finding is uncertain since it has not been confirmed by other researchers[19]. More recently, the detection of DNA sequences from a previously undescribed herpes virus (HHV-8) in 10 of 11 cases of AIDS-related KS, six of six cases of classical KS and four of four cases of KS in HIV-negative homosexuals has lent strong support to suggestions of an infective aetiology[20,21]. This so-called Kaposi's sarcoma herpesvirus (KSHV) was also detected in some AIDS-related B-cell lymphomas[22]. However, the detection of HHV-8 viral DNA sequences in KS lesions is not conclusive proof of a direct aetiological role and this matter needs further research.

The growth of KS cells in long-term tissue cultures has facilitated investigation of the role of cytokines in the pathogenesis of AIDS-related KS[23]. KS cells express high-affinity receptors for many cytokines, including interleukin 1 (IL-1), IL-6, basic fibroblast growth factor (bFGF), tumour necrosis factor (TNF), platelet derived growth factor (PDGF) and oncostatin M. These growth factors, which are produced by activated T-cells and macrophages and also by KS cells themselves[24–27], promote KS cell proliferation by both paracrine and autocrine effects. The observation that TNF-α and IL-1 are increased by opportunistic infections may explain exacerbation of KS during such episodes[28,29]. On the other hand, normal mesenchymal cells fail to proliferate when exposed to these cytokines[30,31]. In addition, *in vitro* studies have shown a mitogenic effect of oncostatin M on KS cells in culture, transforming their histological appearance towards a more malignant phenotype[32]. A final strand of evidence linking cytokines to the pathogenesis of AIDS-related KS is provided by the observation that antibodies raised against IL-1, IL-6, bFGF and PDGF inhibit the growth of KS cells in culture[33,34].

The transactivating protein of HIV, HIV-tat may also act as a mitogenic signal for KS. Transgenic mice bearing the tat gene develop multifocal lesions of variable size composed of spindle-shaped cells[35]. These KS-like lesions are more common in male mice. Although the tat gene product promotes the growth of AIDS KS cells *in vitro* and anti-tat antibodies specifically inhibit this growth[36], tat is not expressed by KS cells *in vitro* or *in vivo*. This suggests that tat exerts its effects indirectly, perhaps by inducing the production of growth factors by tat-expressing HIV-infected T cells.

The striking preponderance of male KS sufferers has led to investigation of the possible aetiological role of male steroid hormones. HIV-positive patients with KS have higher levels of dehydroepiandrosterone and testosterone than seropositive males without KS[37]. In addition, glucocorticoid receptors have been detected in biopsy specimens from KS lesions and in AIDS-related spindle cell isolates. Such receptors are upregulated by cytokines, such as IL-6 and oncostatin M, providing circumstantial evidence that they are linked to positive growth signals. Glucocorticoids have also been shown to promote spindle cell proliferation[38]. Recent evidence of tumor responses to high-dose intramuscular human chorionic gonadotrophin[39] lends further weight to the hypothesis that KS is a hormonally responsive disease. Further work is required to define the repertoire of positive and negative hormonal signals to which KS cells are responsive.

A genetic component to the development of AIDS-related KS has been suggested in light of evidence of a correlation between KS and certain HLA types (mainly DR5 and DQ1)[40,41]. However, cytogenetic abnormalities in these tumours are rather rare and tend to be unstable[42].

The use of nitrite inhalants during homosexual sex is associated with an increased risk of developing KS. However, it is not clear if this is a direct effect of the nitrite or a consequence of enhanced transmission of an infective agent through the effects of vasodilation and loss of sexual inhibition[43,44].

CLINICAL FEATURES

The clinical manifestations of AIDS-related KS may be extremely variable, representing a continuous spectrum from asymptomatic, quiescent cutaneous lesions to rapidly progressing visceral disease. In general, epidemic KS tends to pursue a more aggressive course than its classical or endemic counterparts.

KS frequently represented the AIDS-defining diagnosis in the early years of the epidemic, but this phenomenon has decreased in recent years[45], most probably as a result of public health measures leading to a change in sexual practices amongst high-risk groups. Typically, the first lesions appear on the skin as maculopapular areas, ranging in size from a few millimetres to several centimetres. This phase of the disease may persist for prolonged periods, such that the patient succumbs to another AIDS-related condition before symptomatic KS intervenes. If progression occurs, it is to tumour plaques or nodules which may lead to diffuse skin thickening and eventual ulceration. The size and shape of the lesions may vary and their colour ranges from pink, through brown to deep purple. Lesions can occur on any area of the skin, but have a propensity to involve the upper half of the body, the head and neck area and the shins and feet. Cosmetically sensitive areas, such as the tip of the nose, the eyelids and conjunctiva, are, unfortunately, commonly involved[10,46]. There is some suggestion that patients in whom the first lesions develop on the lower extremities have a better prognosis[47]. The distribution of lesions may follow skin creases (Langer's lines) and the condition demonstrates the Koebner phenomenon of occurring in sites of trauma[10]. The development of extensive oedema of the face, extremities and scrotum, as a result of extensive infiltration of the subdermal lymphatics, may cause considerable cosmetic morbidity, in addition to predisposing to cellulitis and ulceration.

Oral mucosal involvement is common and can be the cause of distressing symptoms including pain, bleeding, difficulty eating and swallowing and dental instability. Gastrointestinal involvement is seen in up to 50% of patients with cutaneous KS[48] and should especially be suspected in patients presenting with oral disease. Although usually asymptomatic, gut involvement may cause obstructive lesions, diarrhoea, perforation, intussusception, protein-losing enteropathy and malabsorptive states. Bleeding is a relatively unusual occurrence by virtue of the submucosal distribution of the lesions. The gut is frequently affected by the infective complications of AIDS and so it is important to exclude infective causes of gastrointestinal symptoms before concluding that the likely cause is KS. On occasions a trial of chemotherapy may be required to resolve the diagnostic dilemma[10]. The response rate of gastrointestinal KS is equivalent to that of cutaneous disease[49].

Bronchopulmonary KS may involve the lung parenchyma, the tracheobronchial tree and the pleura. The true incidence of such lesions is not known, but clinical studies have reported an incidence of 6–32% in patients with KS involving the skin[50–52]. A postmortem study has demonstrated a higher incidence, with lesions in 47% of cases[53]. The presenting symptoms of bronchopulmonary involvement are non-specific, with shortness of breath, fever and cough, occasionally productive of blood, predominant. Indeed, only 8–10% of patients with AIDS and respiratory symptoms are found to have bronchopulmonary KS on investigation[54–56]. The chest radiograph is frequently normal[56,57], but may demonstrate the presence of diffuse, reticulonodular shadowing, mediastinal adenopathy and, on occasions, a pleural effusion. None of these features is pathognomonic of bronchopulmonary KS. The diagnosis may be extremely difficult by virtue of the non-specific symptomatology and lack of definitive non-invasive investigations. Flexible bronchoscopy may fail to yield a tissue diagnosis since the lesions are found in a patchy, submucosal distribution and biopsy carries a risk of inducing haemorrhage[58]. Often a transbronchial or open lung biopsy is required to provide a firm diagnosis, if there is sufficient clinical doubt of the diagnosis. However, on occasions, response to cytotoxic chemotherapy may provide the clearest evidence that the radiographic changes were due to bronchopulmonary KS.

Other organ systems are involved infrequently, but KS should be considered in any patient with AIDS presenting with symptoms, signs and investigational features of a mass lesion. Interestingly, KS involving the central nervous system (CNS) has not been described.

Table 8.1 TIS staging system for AIDS-related Kaposi's sarcoma

Tumour (T)	
T_0	Confined to the skin and/or lymph nodes and/or minimal oral disease
T_1	Tumour-associated oedema or ulceration
	Extensive oral disease
	Visceral involvement (other than lymph nodes)
Immune system (I)	
I_0	CD4 T cells $\geq$ 200/mm^3
I_1	CD4 T cells $\leq$ 200/mm^3
Systemic disease (S)	
S_0	No previous opportunistic infection or candidiasis
	No 'B' symptoms
	Karnofsky performance status $\geq$ 70
S_1	Previous opportunistic infection
	'B' symptoms (unexplained fever, night sweats, $\geq$ 10% weight loss)
	Karnofsky performance status $\leq$ 70

The clinical course of AIDS-related KS is unpredictable. In general terms, cutaneous disease usually pursues a relatively indolent course until the immune suppression is severe. At that time rapid progression is possible, with crops of new lesions appearing suddenly. Exacerbation of cutaneous KS has been reported in association with episodes of opportunistic infection, perhaps as a consequence of alterations in the levels of circulating inflammatory cytokines[28,29]. Gastrointestinal disease is often asymptomatic and rarely poses life-threatening problems. Respiratory KS tends to behave more aggressively and has a measurable associated mortality. Patients with bronchopulmonary KS have a median survival of approximately four to seven months[56,57].

The clearest indication of the likely progress of the disease is given by the patients' immune status. Patients who have well-maintained CD4 cell counts, above 200/mm^3, are more likely to have indolent disease. As the CD4 cell count falls the lesions may increase in size, number and sites of involvement. The AIDS Clinical Trials Group (ACTG) has devised a staging system for KS which derives information not only from the extent of the tumours, but also from the patients' general condition, immune status and concomitant illnesses[59] (Table 8.1). This system will be of benefit in guiding the selection of treatment modalities for different patient groups.

TREATMENT

The aim of treatment for patients with AIDS-related KS is palliative, since the underlying HIV infection and resulting immune suppression, which predispose to the development of these lesions, are incurable at present. In the early stages of the disease, small, asymptomatic cutaneous lesions may be present in unexposed areas and may remain clinically quiescent for prolonged periods. For such lesions, a watch-and-wait policy is most appropriate, reserving active treatment for such time as disease progression occurs or symptoms develop. Usually, active treatment is first required for cutaneous disease causing cosmetic disfigurement or local symptoms. Despite the fact that KS in incurable, once the decision to offer therapy is taken the objective should be to secure durable local control of each individual lesion with optimal cosmetic outcome at the cost of minimal toxicity. In the setting of generalized cutaneous or visceral disease, complete remissions are uncommon and the aim must be to control symptoms without producing excessive treatment-related toxicity.

Patients may receive a number of different treatment modalities throughout the course of their illness, reflecting the progressive nature of the immune suppression and extension of both orocutaneous and visceral disease. Treatment approaches may be either local or systemic, with many patients initially receiving local therapy to troublesome cutaneous lesions and later requiring systemic cytotoxic chemotherapy for progressive disease.

Local Treatment

Radiotherapy

Based on the experience gained from treating classical KS with moderate doses of external beam radiotherapy, this form of treatment was applied to patients with AIDS-related KS early in the epidemic. Considerable experience has been gained by a number of centres in the treatment of AIDS-related KS, resulting in rapid progress in understanding the response of this disease to palliative radiotherapy. It is generally accepted that radiotherapy is an effective local treatment for KS lesions which are causing symptoms such as pain, cosmetic disfigurement, mass lesions, ulceration or bleeding and oedema[60,61]. However, a number of important controversies persist which remain to be fully resolved.

The initial reports of the effect of radiotherapy in AIDS-related KS appeared within a few years of the description of the epidemic[62–64]. It was rapidly appreciated that, like endemic KS, the lesions responded to relatively modest doses of radiotherapy. Variations in the radioresponsiveness and local control rates of lesions in different areas of the body were noted, with evidence that lesions on the face, eyelids, conjunctivae, hands and feet, and genitalia are particularly well controlled[65–68]. Cosmetic outcome is also better in these areas, a fact that has been attributed to the patient presenting early for treatment because of cosmetic disfigurement. Early lesions are less likely to contain excessive haemosiderin deposits and, therefore, are less likely to leave residual pigmentation after treatment[10].

The contentious issues of the optimal total radiation dose and fractionation schedule were initially addressed by means of retrospective reviews and, more recently, by randomized trials. Berson *et al.*[69] treated 375 fields in 187 patients in a non-randomized fashion with doses ranging from 8 Gy in a single fraction to 15–40 Gy in 5–10 fractions. Response was documented in more than 90% of lesions with a median time to progression of 21 months and an actuarial freedom from relapse at six months of 69%. There was no evidence of improved outcome with higher total doses or fractionation of treatment. Severe radiation-induced reactions were significantly less common in the group of patients receiving single-fraction therapy. This view was supported by de Wit *et al.*[70], who reported subjective palliation in 90% of treated fields in 31 patients after an 8 Gy single fraction. However, the objective response rate was only 33%. The authors concluded that a single fraction of 8 Gy provided effective palliation for patients with a predicted survival of only a few months, but patients with a good performance status might gain more benefit from prolonged, fractionated treatment. In a large series, Cooper *et al.*[60] treated 226 lesions in 129 patients, again with non-randomly selected doses ranging from 8 Gy as a single fraction to 30 Gy in 10 fractions. The complete response rate was 68%, although residual pigmentation persisted in 20% of cases. The response of oedema to single-fraction radiotherapy was generally poor. These authors concluded that epidemic KS should not be regarded as a homogeneous disease process. Therefore, different dose and fractionation regimens might be required depending on the clinical circumstances. Geara *et al.*[61] reached a similar conclusion in their report on 149 patients treated with either local or extended field irradiation. They drew attention to the higher non-response (17% versus 3%) and local recurrence rates (67% versus 33%) for 20 Gy and 30 Gy, respectively. Stein *et al.*[71] treated a group of 56 patients with classical, African endemic or epidemic KS and found no evidence of dose or fractionation dependence of the response.

In a randomized, prospective trial Stelzer *et al.*[72] treated 71 cutaneous lesions with one of three regimens: 8 Gy/1 fraction; 20 Gy/10 fractions; 40 Gy/20 fractions. The complete response rate was significantly higher with 40 Gy (83%) and 20 Gy (79%) compared with 8 Gy (50%). The local control and cosmetic outcome was also significantly better for the fractionated regimens. Harrison *et al.*[68] reported on 172 lesions in 27 patients treated randomly with either 8 Gy/1 fraction or 16 Gy/4 fractions, with no difference in response rates, local control or cosmesis. Despite these findings, it was proposed that fractionated radiotherapy should be considered for lesions on sites other than the face and for mature lesions, in view of the modest performance of radiotherapy under these circumstances. From this brief survey of the literature, it can be seen that, as yet, conflicting evidence exists which makes it difficult to derive recommendations regarding the optimal dose and fraction schedule that should be employed. It would seem that single-fraction radiotherapy is generally acceptable, except for the treatment of larger, symptomatic lesions in patients with good performance status who are likely to live long enough to develop troublesome local recurrences. In these patients, fractionated therapy should be considered.

In addition to localized treatment of small lesions, wide-field radiotherapy may be useful in palliating certain specific problems. Extended field irradiation has been employed for the treatment of more extensive cutaneous disease, especially when associated with oedema[61]. Its use is limited by acute skin toxicity, which may be circumvented by careful fractionation of treatment[10]. Whole lung irradiation may play a role in patients with end-stage disease and symptomatic pulmonary involvement. Meyer[73] treated 25 patients with extensive pulmonary disease with a dose of 10.5–15 Gy in 7–10 fractions, treating four times a week. There was no acute toxicity and 89% of patients completing therapy reported an improvement in dyspnoea.

Patients receiving radiotherapy for AIDS-related KS are prone to develop severe acute reactions to treatment at doses which would be tolerated by patients without HIV infection. The basis of this increased radiosensitivity is not fully understood but it has been suggested that reduced systemic and intracellular glutathione levels are responsible[74]. There is some evidence that radiosensitivity increases with disease progression[75], which may be due to progressive reductions in systemic glutathione levels. The increased radiosensitivity of patients with AIDS-related KS must be taken into account when planning treatment, especially when it involves the oral mucosa, and if necessary treatment may be given as a split course[10].

In addition, radiation recall phenomena have been documented in patients receiving cytotoxic chemotherapy. Nemechek *et al.*[76] reported vinblastine-association radiation recall in a patient who received 27 Gy in 15 fractions to the foot. Stelzer *et al.*[77] reported a similar reaction in a patient treated with bleomycin chemotherapy. Interestingly, in this case, the reaction only developed in an area which had been treated to a dose of 40 Gy in 20 fractions, and not in other skin areas which had received either 20 Gy or 8 Gy. This suggests that there may be some radiation dose dependence in the development of radiation recall phenomena.

Intralesional Chemotherapy

This form of treatment is effective and easily performed for accessible lesions. Newman[78] treated 190 lesions, injecting 0.01–0.02 mg of vinblastine in 0.1 ml of saline every two weeks to a maximum of three injections per lesion. The response rate was 92% with a mean duration of response of 4.5 months. Treatment was associated with transient local pain and numbness at the site of injection. Scarring and alopecia in hair-bearing skin may preclude the use of intralesional chemotherapy in exposed areas[10]. Intralesional vinblastine is considered to be the treatment of choice for small oral lesions[79,80]. Epstein[79] treated 42 patients with 0.1 ml of vinblastine in a 0.2 mg/ml solution per 0.5 cm^2 of lesion. A response rate of 74% was documented with a mean duration of response of 3.5 months. This result is similar to the palliative effect of radiotherapy, but with considerably less mucosal toxicity.

Other Local Modalities

Simple camouflage of unsightly lesions with cosmetics may be effective and is particularly useful for lesions at the hairline, where radiotherapy or intralesional chemotherapy would be likely to cause alopecia[10]. Surgical removal of small troublesome lesions may also provide palliation with good cosmesis for selected sites[81]. Otherwise cryotherapy, laser or photodynamic therapy may have a role to play in certain selected situations[82,83]. However, at present, radiotherapy represents the most effective local therapy against which other new treatment modalities should be judged.

Systemic Therapy

Chemotherapy

The development of progressive or extensive skin disease, with or without visceral involvement, heralds the need to switch from local to systemic therapy. The important issue here is that toxicity, which was previously confined to the area of the lesion, may now be systemic and may, in particular, include myelosuppression with resulting immune depression. This can predispose the patient to life-threatening infective episodes. Therefore an optimal chemotherapeutic regimen should ideally have minimum myelotoxicity and maximal antitumour activity. In addition to concerns surrounding the acute toxicity of treatment, attention must be paid to the possible chronic effects of chemotherapy, since patients may require prolonged, repeated courses of treatment.

There exists an extensive literature on the use of cytotoxic chemotherapy in the treatment of AIDS-related KS, both in terms of single-agent and combination regimen therapy. There has been some difficulty in interpreting some of this data due to the fact that different response criteria have been used in some of the studies. Certain authors have included stable disease in the category of clinical response. The vinca alkaloids, the anthracyclines and bleomycin are the most widely used agents in this condition, although other agents such as etoposide have been used. These agents have important dose-limiting toxicities, such as lung, cardiac and neurological damage. Furthermore, patients with AIDS-related KS are also likely to develop non-KS-associated disorders in the major organ systems, potentially lowering the threshold at which chemotherapy-induced toxicity may become manifest. It is advisable that patients receiving cytotoxic chemotherapy for AIDS-related KS should be closely supervised, preferably in a joint HIV–Oncology clinic.

Single-agent chemotherapy A number of drugs have been shown to have useful single-agent activity. Volberding *et al.*[84] used weekly vinblastine in 38 patients at a median dose of 6 mg for a median duration of 72 weeks. Ten of the patients had a clinical response and a further 19 showed stable disease. Mintzer *et al.*[85] treated 23 patients with vincristine 2 mg, initially on a weekly basis for up to five weeks and thereafter fortnightly. There were 11 responses in 18 evaluable patients (61%), with a median duration of response in excess of four months. The response rates of the anthracyclines have been reported in small studies, varying from 0% for mitoxantrone and idarubicin, 14% for doxorubicin and 42% for epirubicin[86–89]. Bleomycin 5 mg intramuscularly every two weeks has been reported to have a response rate of 50% as a single agent in 38 patients[90]. Infusional bleomycin at a dose of 20 mg/m^2 per day for three days yielded a response rate of 65% with minimal toxicity[91]. Etoposide was investigated as an intravenous infusion of 150 mg/m^2 on days 1–3 of a four-week cycle for a median of seven cycles in 41 patients. The response rate was high (76%) but this was achieved at the expense of considerable treatment-related toxicity[92]. Tenoposide was evaluated in 25 patients treated with 350 mg/m^2 every three weeks, yielding a 40% response rate, achieved at the price of severe toxicity[93]. Most recently, a 3 h infusion of single-agent paclitaxel in a dose of 135 mg/m^2 (escalating to 175 mg/m^2) was administered to 20 patients[94]. A partial response rate of 65% was reported, with neutropenia as the most frequent dose-limiting side effect. The modest response rates of single-agent therapy have precluded their large-scale use and has fuelled the search for more active treatment.

Combination chemotherapy The drugs with documented single-agent activity have been combined in an attempt to increase the response rates in a number of studies. The greatest potential problem with such combinations is the potential for overlapping toxicity to the bone marrow, resulting in severe immune suppression. This matter may be further compounded by the continued use of zidovudine as an antiretroviral therapy.

Alternating doses of vincristine 2 mg and vinblastine 0.1 mg/kg were employed by Kaplan *et al.*[95] in an attempt to circumvent the neurotoxicity of the former and reduce the myelotoxicity of the latter. Despite this approach, peripheral neurotoxicity was the major dose-limiting problem. The response rate was only 43%, with a further seven patients achieving a state of stable disease. The median duration of response was greater than nine months. The combination of adriamycin 40 mg/m^2 day 1, vinblastine 6 mg/m^2 day 1 and bleomycin 15 U days 1 and 15, has been investigated by Laubenstein *et al.*[92] in 31 patients who received a median of six cycles. The response rate of 84% was a considerable improvement on the single-agent data but was only achieved at the expense of considerable toxicity, necessitating dose reductions due to myelotoxicity in more than half of the patients. In an attempt to ameliorate the bone marrow toxicity, vincristine 2 mg was substituted for vinblastine and the bleomycin and doxorubicin doses were reduced to 10 mg/m^2 and 20 mg/m^2, respectively, by Gill *et al.*[96] A response rate of 8/10 patients was obtained but there was still considerable immune suppression as evidenced by the occurrence of bacterial infections in five patients. Further experience with this regimen was reported by the same authors, with a response rate of 79% in 33 patients[97]. There seemed to be no obvious survival benefit from using higher doses of adriamycin.

The trend in Europe has been to omit anthracyclines from the first-line combination regimen. Most patients receive a combination of a vinca alkaloid and bleomycin as initial systemic therapy. Gompels *et al.*[98] reported a partial response rate of 56% in 46 patients treated every three to four weeks with vincristine 2 mg and bleomycin 30 U, with manageable toxicity. Lipman *et al.*[99] used the same regimen but in a more intensive two-weekly schedule. The response rate was 84%, with a median survival of six months. Neutropenia occurred in 21% of patients, but there were only three episodes of opportunistic infection during the study.

In one of the few prospective randomized trials which has been performed, Gill *et al.*[96] treated 61 patients every two weeks with either low-dose ABV (doxorubicin 20 mg/m^2, bleomycin 10 mg/m^2, vincristine 1.4 mg/m^2) or single-agent doxorubicin 20 mg/m^2. There was a significantly improved response rate for the combination chemotherapy (88% versus 48%). The disease-free survival, but not the median survival, was significantly better for ABV. One-quarter of the evaluable patients developed an opportunistic infection, although there was no significant difference in the rates between the two regimens.

Attempts have been made to deliver anthracycline-based combination chemotherapy and zidovudine on schedule by using haematopoietic growth factors to limit myelotoxicity. It has been shown that recombinant human granulocyte–monocyte colony-stimulating factor (rhGM-CSF) does not up-regulate HIV replication[100]. Recent studies have demonstrated that it is possible to deliver ABV chemotherapy in full doses with zidovudine 100 mg every 4 h with the aid of rhGM-CSF[101–103]. However, this did not seem to have a noticeable effect on the response rates that were achieved. Randomized trials will be required before growth factor support can be recommended as routine for patients receiving combination chemotherapy.

Liposomal chemotherapy Liposomes are synthetic structures comprised of single or multiple lipid bilayers, enclosing an aqueous phase in which various agents can be entrapped. Liposomes have been shown to accumulate preferentially at the site of tumours by means of histopathological studies in model mouse KS tumour systems[104], and in imaging studies with ^{111}In-labelled liposomes[105]. They are thought to extravasate from abnormal tumour vasculature and release their contents at the site of disease. Various liposomal formulations have been developed in an attempt to increase their circulation time and area under the curve. Stealth® liposomes have been derivatized with polyethylene glycol, which confers on them the ability to evade the reticuloendothelial system[106–108]. There is also evidence that liposomal drug delivery may circumvent the multiple drug-resistant phenotype. This offers the possibility of patients unresponsive to conventional anthracycline therapy responding to liposomal preparations of the same drug.

Liposomal doxorubicin has been shown to exert a considerable advantage in terms of *in vitro* cytotoxicity assays in KS-derived cell lines[109]. Its use in clinical situations has also been explored. Simpson *et al.*[110] reported a partial response rate of 87% in 16 patients treated with liposomal doxorubicin 20 mg/m^2 every three weeks. The use of Stealth® liposomes containing doxorubicin at a dose of 20 mg/m^2 every two weeks was reported in 21 patients by Hengge *et al.*[111], with response rates in excess of 90%. Harrison *et al.*[112] reported their results with this treatment modality in 34 patients with advanced cutaneous and systemic disease who were treated at a dose of 20 mg/m^2 every three weeks. The overall response rate was 73.5% (complete response (CR) 5.8%, partial response (PR) 67.7%), with a median time to response of six weeks.

Liposomal daunorubicin has also been investigated by a number of authors[113–115]. Money-Kyrle *et al.*[113] treated 11 patients with a dose of 40 mg/m^2 every two weeks, achieving a modest response rate of 36%. Presant *et al.*[114] documented a response rate of 62.5% (CR 8.3%, PR 54.2%) in 24 evaluable patients treated at a dose of 40 mg/m^2 every two weeks. In a recent phase I/II evaluation[115], liposomal daunorubicin was shown to display a favourable pharmacokinetic profile compared to free drug, in terms of the area under the plasma concentration curve (AUC), clearance, volume of distribution and terminal half-life. The drug was well tolerated, with no significant alopecia, mucositis or emesis. Importantly, myelosuppression was mild and no significant impact on cardiac function was demonstrated, even with cumulative doses in excess of 1000 mg/m^2. The favourable toxicity profile of liposomal anthracycline chemotherapy and the high response rates have led to randomized trials comparing liposomal and conventional chemotherapy.

A randomized trial of liposomal daunorubicin 40 mg/m^2 versus combination therapy with adriamycin 10 mg/m^2, bleomycin 15 U and vincristine 1 mg in 115 patients was recently reported in abstract form. There was no difference in response rates between the two arms of the study, but the liposomal therapy was significantly better tolerated in terms of alopecia and peripheral neuropathy[116]. The results of a multi-centre European trial of liposomal doxorubicin versus vincristine and bleomycin are awaited with interest.

Cytokines

Evidence that AIDS-related KS is associated with profound immune suppression led to early trials of cytokine therapy. The interferons with their wide range of antiviral, antineoplastic and immunomodulatory effects were amongst the first agents to be employed[117]. Such trials were supported by *in vitro* evidence of reduced interferon α (IFN-α) and IFN-γ production from HIV-infected patients and IFN-α- and IFN-β-mediated suppression of HIV replication[118,119].

Most clinical studies have focused on the use of α interferons, either as single recombinant species (IFN-α2a or -2b), or as a multi-species product from human lymphoblastoid cells (IFN-αn1)[117]. Many authors use an escalating dose induction regimen over 7–10 days, in order to minimize acute toxicity. Thereafter, treatment is given by subcutaneous injection daily or thrice weekly for two months and the response is assessed. Those patients demonstrating a clinical response continue treatment, usually thrice weekly. Acute toxicity usually takes the form of a flu-like illness with fever, rigors, myalgia and malaise. Myelosuppression, neutropenia, thrombocytopenia, elevated liver function tests, peripheral and central neurotoxicity and exacerbations of psoriasis have all been reported as later complications of treatment.

Small-scale studies employing a wide range of different doses, schedules and routes of administration have hampered comparison of data from the various trials[120–123]. The overall response rate for high-dose therapy is approximately 30–40%, and in up to 50% of these patients is a pathological complete response. The median duration of response has been reported as 11.5 months for partial and 24 months for complete responders[120]. Responses are generally seen within the first four to six weeks, but may take six months to evolve to their maximal extent. It is unknown if maintenance therapy prolongs the response duration but, since most patients who stop treatment relapse within six to eight months[117], it is usual to continue treatment until disease progression or toxicity intervenes. Low-dose therapy (<10 MU/m^2) has been investigated but reduced toxicity is counterbalanced by response rates of only 10%[124,125]. The use of intermediate-dose therapy has yielded mixed results, with some reports suggesting no responses and others showing moderate activity[125,126].

There is evidence that patients who respond to interferon therapy have a better prognosis than non-responders. It is not clear if this is a direct effect of the interferon on the tumour, the virus or the immune system, or if it is a manifestation of the fact that responding patients have better prognosis disease from the outset[117]. Patients with a history of opportunistic infections, 'B' symptoms and low CD4 counts are less likely to respond[59]. Factors positively correlated with response include preserved delayed-type hypersensitivity skin response, relatively high lymphoproliferative responses to mitogens, the absence of acid-labile IFN-α and low levels of inteferon-inducible products in the serum[124,127–130].

In addition to being used as single agent therapy, interferons have combined with anti-HIV agents, such as the reverse transcriptase inhibitor, zidovudine[127,131,132], and conventional chemotherapy[122,133,134]. Despite its lack of direct anti-KS activity[135], zidovudine affects the immune system of AIDS patients, leading to improved CD4 counts and skin reactivity, factors associated with interferon responsiveness[136]. *In vitro* and *in vivo* data suggests that IFN-α and zidovudine act synergistically to prevent HIV replication and viraemia[137]. Unfortunately each agent causes dose-limiting haematological toxicity which has impeded attempts to use them in combination. However, there is preliminary data suggesting that, with this combination, response rates of approximately 40% can be achieved[117]. Combinations of IFN-α and cytotoxic chemotherapy have been generally disappointing. There was little evidence of enhanced response rates with vinblastine or etoposide, but toxicity was severe[133,134].

At present there is little experience with other cytokines in this setting. IFN-βser has shown activity *in vitro* and *in vivo* in combination with zidovudine,with little evidence of haematological toxicity. A response rate of 16% to IFN-βser was reported by Miles *et al.*[138] in 39 patients, with a further 16 patients showing stable disease. IFN-γ has shown little antitumour activity in KS[139]. Tumour necrosis factor (TNF) has been used by intralesional injection, with high response rates[140]. However, the responses were only local despite frequent systemic toxicity. IL-2 has also been investigated, but the results were not promising[141].

Therefore, at present, it seems that the role of cytokines in the treatment of AIDS-related KS is limited. There may be a group of patients with relatively well-preserved immune function for whom local therapies alone are unsuitable. These patients may benefit from treatment with cytokines, with or without zidovudine, deferring the need for systemic chemotherapy to a later date. Further efforts are required to identify such patients.

Novel Therapies

Although radiotherapy is highly effective at controlling local disease with good cosmesis, it is associated with appreciable toxicity. An effective topical anti-KS treatment would be a welcome development. There is evidence of *in vitro* growth inhibition of KS cells with all-*trans*-retinoic acid and 13-*cis*-retinoic acid[142]. Preliminary data from eight patients treated with topical all-*trans*-retinoic acid showed a greater than 50% reduction in all lesions, suggesting that this may be a useful therapy[143]. However, oral all-*trans*-retinoic acid was associated with disease progression when given to six patients by von Roenn[144] at a dose of 175 mg/m^2. A recent evaluation of intermittent all-*trans*-retinoic acid alone or in combination with IFN-α2a failed to demonstrate any antitumour activity[145]. Further evaluation of this treatment will be required before its use can be widely recommended. Analogues of vitamin D are also under study at present.

The toxicity of cytotoxic chemotherapy and lack of efficacy of antiviral and cytokine treatment in patients who require systemic therapy fuels the search for effective new approaches in this setting. A number of exploratory studies are under way, seeking to apply advances in the understanding of the pathogenesis of AIDS-related KS to the clinic. New cytokine therapies, such as IL-4 and recombinant platelet factor 4 (rPF-4), have been shown to have potential activity *in vitro*. IL-4 downregulates IL-6 and oncostatin M expression, and inhibits AIDS-related KS spindle cell growth[38]. The results of preliminary clinical studies are awaited. Recombinant PF-4 possesses angiostatic activity[146] and has been used in early phase I/II studies[147]. It has been found to be relatively non-toxic by the intravenous route, although there is little evidence of efficacy at present. There is also considerable interest in developing inhibitors of trophic cytokines and it has been suggested that agents such as pentoxifylline or anti-sense oligonucleotides may fulfil this function[38].

Other inhibitors of angiogenesis have been investigated. SP-PG is a bacterial cell wall component which has been shown to inhibit endothelial cell and AIDS-related KS cell proliferation *in vitro*[148]. TNP-470 is an analogue of fumagillin and possesses similar properties to SP-PG *in vitro*[38].

CONCLUSION

Since the recognition of epidemic KS as part of the acquired immunodeficiency syndrome, there has been an enormous expansion in the understanding of this disease process. The epidemiology of KS in patients with HIV infection has been well characterized. Research into the biology of the disease has yielded important insights in the aetiological and pathogenetic mechanisms as well as providing useful clues for future therapeutic intervention. Within a very short space of time effective treatment strategies have been derived for both local and systemic disease based on known predictive factors, and further advances may be expected from refinements of these modalities. However, despite these potential therapeutic improvements, AIDS-related KS will remain incurable until the underlying immunosuppression can be addressed. In the meantime the search for novel agents should continue with the aim of achieving better response rates with reduced local and systemic toxicity.

Table 8.2 Response criteria for AIDS-related Kaposi's sarcoma

Complete response (CR)
Complete resolution of all existing lesions for a period of at least 4 weeks with no new lesions appearing in that time. Flat pigmented lesions must be biopsied to confirm the absence of residual disease. Endoscopic confirmation of complete response of previously detected visceral lesions must be obtained

Clinical complete response (CCR)
Absence of clinically detectable residual disease for at least 4 weeks, but without biopsy or endoscopic confirmation

Partial response (PR)
One or more of the following in the absence of: (a) new skin lesions, (b) new oral/visceral lesions, (c) progressive disease-associated oedema, (d) ≥ 25% increase in the product of the bidimensional diameters of any index lesion:

(1) ≥ 50% decrease in the number of measurable cutaneous, or visceral lesions
(2) ≥ 50% decrease in the size of the lesions, defined by one of the following criteria:
  (a) ≥ 50% decrease in the sum of the products of the largest bidimensional diameters of the index lesion
  (b) Complete flattening of ≥ 50% of the lesions
  (c) ≥ 75% of nodular lesions become indurated plaques

Stable disease
Any response which fails to meet the above conditions

Progressive disease
Any of the following:

(1) ≥ 25% increase in the product of the bidimensional diameter of any index lesion
(2) The appearance of new lesions
(3) ≥ 25% of previously flat lesions become raised
(4) The appearance of new or increased disease-associated oedema

REFERENCES

1. Kaposi M. Idiopathisches multiples Pigmentsarkom der haut. *Arch Dermatol Syphilis* 1872; 4: 265–273. (English translation: Idiopathic multiple pigmented sarcoma of the skin. *CA* 1982; 32: 342–347.)
2. Harwood AR, Osoba D, Hofstader SL *et al*. Kaposi's sarcoma in recipients of renal transplants. *Am J Med* 1979; 67: 759–765.
3. Penn I. The changing pattern of posttransplant malignancies. *Transplant Proc* 1991; 23: 1101–1103.
4. Centres for Disease Control. Epidemiologic aspects of the current outbreak of Kaposi's sarcoma and opportunistic infections. *N Engl J Med* 1982; 306: 248–252.
5. Reynolds P, Saunders LD, Layefsky ME, Lemp GF. The spectrum of acquired

immune deficiency syndrome (AIDS)-associated malignancies in San Francisco, 1980–1987. *Am J Epidemiol* 1993; 137: 19–30.
6. Friedman-Kein A, Laubenstein L, Marmor M *et al.* Kaposi's sarcoma and pneumocystis pneumonia among homosexual men: New York City and California. *MMWR* 1981; 30: 305–308.
7. Beral V, Perterman AT, Berkelman RL, Jaffe HW. Kaposi's sarcoma among persons with AIDS: a sexually transmitted infection? *Lancet* 1990; 335: 123–128.
8. Serraino D, Zaccarelli M, Franceschi S, Grego D. The epidemiology of AIDS-associated Kaposi's sarcoma in Italy. *AIDS* 1992; 6: 1015–1019.
9. Casabona J, Melbye M, Biggar R, AIDS Registry Contributors. Kaposi's sarcoma and non-Hodgkin's lymphoma in European AIDS cases. No excess risk of Kaposi's sarcoma in Mediterranean countries. *Int J Cancer* 1991; 47: 49–53.
10. Stewart S. AIDS-related cancer. In Price P, Sikora K (eds) *Treatment of Cancer*, 3rd edn. London: Chapman & Hall, 1995.
11. Poznansky MC, Coker R, Skinner C *et al.* HIV positive patients first presenting with an AIDS defining illness: characteristics and survival. *Br Med J* 1995; 311: 156–158.
12. Tirelli U, Franceschi S, Carbone A. Malignant tumors in patients with HIV infection. *Br Med J* 1994; 308: 1148–1153.
13. Beral V, Bull D, Darby S *et al.* Risk of Kaposi's sarcoma and sexual practices associated with faecal contact in homosexual or bisexual men with AIDS. *Lancet* 1992; 339: 632–635.
14. Friedman-Kein AE, Saltzmann BR, Cao YZ *et al.* Kaposi's sarcoma in HIV-negative homosexual men. *Lancet* 1990; 335: 168–169.
15. Garcia Muret MP, Pujol RM, Puig I *et al.* Disseminated Kaposi's sarcoma not associated with HIV infection in a bisexual man. *J Am Acad Dermatol* 1990; 23: 1035–1038.
16. Drew WL, Conant MA, Miner RC. Cytomegalovirus and Kaposi's sarcoma in young homosexual men. *Lancet* 1982; ii: 125–127.
17. Hyang YQ, Li JJ, Rush MG *et al.* HPV-16 related DNA sequences in Kaposi's sarcoma. *Lancet* 1992; 339: 515–518.
18. Nickoloff BJ, Hyang YQ, Li JJ *et al.* Immunohistochemical detection of papillomavirus antigens in KS. *Lancet* 1992; 339: 548–549.
19. Biggar RJ, Dunsmore N, Kurman RJ *et al.* Failure to detect human papillomavirus in Kaposi's sarcoma. *Lancet* 1992; 339: 1604–1605.
20. Moore PS, Chang Y. Detection of herpesvirus-like DNA sequences in Kaposi's sarcoma in patients with and those without HIV infection. *N Engl J Med* 1995; 332: 1181–1185.
21. Chang Y, Cesarman E, Pessin MS *et al.* Identification of herpesvirus-like DNA sequences in AIDS-associated Kaposi's sarcoma. *Science* 1994; 266: 1865–1869.
22. Cesarman E, Chang Y, Moore PS *et al.* Kaposi's sarcoma associated herpesvirus-like DNA sequences in AIDS-related body-cavity-based lymphomas. *N Engl J Med* 1995; 332: 1186–1191.
23. Nakamura S, Salahuddin SZ, Biberfeld P *et al.* Kaposi's sarcoma cells: long-term culture with growth factor from retrovirus-infected CD4+ T-cells. *Science* 1988; 242: 426–340.
24. Barillari G, Buonaguro L, Fiorelli V *et al.* Effects of cytokines from activated immune cells on vascular cell growth and HIV-1 gene expression. *J Immunol* 1992; 149: 3727–3734.
25. Strunzl M, Roth WK, Brockmeyer NH *et al.* Expression of platelet-derived growth factor and its receptor in AIDS-related Kaposi sarcoma in vivo suggests paracrine and autocrine mechanisms of tumour maintenance. *Proc Natl Acad Sci USA* 1992; 89: 7046–7052.

26. Nair BC, DeVico AL, Nakamura S *et al.* Identification of a major growth factor for AIDS–Kaposi's sarcoma cells as oncostatin M. *Science* 1992; 255: 1430–1432.
27. Samaniego F, Markham PD, Gallo RC, Ensoli B. Inflammatory cytokines induce AIDS-Kaposi's sarcoma-derived spindle cells to produce and release basic fibroblast growth factor and enhance Kaposi's sarcoma-like lesions in nude mice. *J Immunol* 1995; 154: 3582–3592.
28. Ammann AJ, Palladino MA, Volberding P *et al.* Tumour necrosis factor alpha and beta in acquired immunodeficiency syndrome (AIDS) and AIDS-related complex. *J Clin Immunol* 1987; 7: 481–485.
29. Berman MA, Sandborg CI, Calabia BS *et al.* Interleukin-1 inhibitor masks high interleukin-1 production in acquired immunodeficiency syndrome (AIDS). *Clin Immunol Immunopathol* 1987; 42: 133–140.
30. Roth WK, Werner S, Schirren CG, Hofschneider PH. Depletion of PDGF from serum inhibits growth of AIDS-related and sporadic Kaposi's sarcoma cells in culture. *Oncogene* 1989; 4: 483–487.
31. Mitsuyasu R. Clinical aspects of AIDS-related Kaposi's sarcoma. *Curr Opinion Oncol* 1993; 5: 835–844.
32. Miles SA, Martinez-Maza O, Rezai A *et al.* Oncostatin M as a potent mitogen for AIDS–Kaposi's sarcoma derived cells. *Science* 1992; 255: 1432–1434.
33. Ensoli B, Nakamura S, Salahuddin SZ *et al.* AIDS–Kaposi's sarcoma-derived cells express cytokines with autocrine and paracrine growth effects. *Science* 1989; 243: 223–226.
34. Miles SA, Rezai AR, Salazar-Gonzales JF *et al.* AIDS–Kaposi's sarcoma derived cells produce and respond to interleukin. *Proc Natl Acad Sci USA* 1990; 87: 4068–4072.
35. Vogel J, Hinrichs SH, Reynolds RK *et al.* The HIV tat gene induces dermal lesions resembling Kaposi's sarcoma in transgenic mice. *Nature* 1990; 345: 84–86.
36. Ensoli B, Barillari G, Salahuddin SZ *et al.* Tat protein of HIV-1 stimulates growth of cells derived from Kaposi's sarcoma lesions of AIDS patients. *Nature* 1990; 345: 84–86.
37. Christeff N, Thubie N, Nunez AE *et al.* Differences in the androgens of HIV positive patients with or without Kaposi's sarcoma. *IX International Conference on AIDS* 1993; Abstr. PO-B12-1588.
38. Masood R, Cai J, Law R, Gill P. AIDS-associated Kaposi's sarcoma pathogenesis, clinical features, and treatment. *Curr Opinion Oncol* 1993; 5: 831–834.
39. Harris PJ. Treatment of Kaposi's sarcoma and other manifestations of AIDS with human chorionic gonadotrophon. *Lancet* 1995; 346: 118–119.
40. Brunson ME, Balakrishnan K, Penn I. HLA and Kaposi's sarcoma in solid organ transplantation. *Human Immunol* 1990; 29: 56–63.
41. Man DI, Murray C, O'Donnell M *et al.* HLA antigen frequencies in HIV-1 related Kaposi's sarcoma. *J AIDS* 1990; 3: 51–55.
42. Delli Bovi P, Donti E, Knoeles DM *et al.* Presence of chromosomal abnormalities and lack of AIDS–retrovirus DNA sequence in AIDS-associated Kaposi's sarcoma. *Cancer Res* 1986; 46: 6333–6338.
43. Archibald CP, Schechter MT, Le TN *et al.* Evidence for a sexually transmitted co-factor for AIDS-related Kaposi's sarcoma in a cohort of homosexual men. *Epidemiology* 1992; 3: 203–209.
44. Bernstein L, Hamilton AS. The epidemiology of AIDS-related malignancies. *Curr Opinion Oncol* 1993; 5: 822–830.
45. Drew WL, Mills J, Haner LB *et al.* Declining prevalence of Kaposi's sarcoma in homosexual AIDS patients paralleled by fall in cytomegalovirus transmission. *Lancet* 1988; i: 66.

46. Shuler JD, Holland GN, Miles SA *et al.* Kaposi's sarcoma of the conjunctiva and eyelids associated with the acquired immune deficiency syndrome. *Arch Opthalmol* 1989; 107: 858–862.
47. Myskowski PL, Niedzwiecki D, Shurgot BA *et al.* AIDS-associated Kaposi's sarcoma: variables associated with survival. *J Am Acad Dermatol* 1988; 18: 1299–1306.
48. Friedman SL, Wright JL, Altman DF. Gastrointestinal Kaposi's sarcoma in patients with acquired immunodeficiency syndrome: endoscopic and autopsy findings. *Gastroenterology* 1985; 89: 102–108.
49. Laine L, Amerian J, Rarick M *et al.* The response of symptomatic gastrointestinal Kaposi's sarcoma to chemotherapy: a prospective evaluation using an endoscopic method of disease quantification. *Am J Gastroenterol* 1990; 85: 959–961.
50. Zibrak JD, Silvestri RC, Costello P *et al.* Bronchoscopic and radiographic features of Kaposi's sarcoma involving the respiratory tract. *Chest* 1986; 90: 476–479.
51. Garay SM, Belenko M, Fazzini E, Schinella R. Pulmonary manifestations of Kaposi's sarcoma. *Chest* 1987; 91: 39–43.
52. Gill PS, Akil B, Colletti P *et al.* Pulmonary Kaposi's sarcoma: clinical findings and results of therapy. *Am J Med* 1989; 87: 57–63.
53. Meduri GU, Stover DE, Lee M *et al.* Pulmonary Kaposi's sarcoma in the acquired immunodeficiency syndrome. *Am J Med* 1986; 81: 11–18.
54. Report of the National Heart, Lung and Blood workshop. Pulmonary complications of the acquired immunodeficiency syndrome. *N Engl J Med* 1984; 310: 1682–1688.
55. Fouret PJ, Touboul JL, Maynaud CD *et al.* Pulmonary Kaposi's sarcoma in patients with acquired immune deficiency syndrome: a clinicopathological study. *Thorax* 1987; 42: 262–268.
56. Miller RF, Tomlinson MC, Cottrill CP *et al.* Bronchopulmonary Kaposi's sarcoma in patients with AIDS. *Thorax* 1992; 47: 721–725.
57. Mitchell DH, McCarty M, Fleming J, Moss FH. Bronchopulmonary Kaposi's sarcoma in patients with AIDS. *Thorax* 1992; 47: 726–729.
58. Pitchenick AE, Fischl MA, Saldana MJ. Kaposi's sarcoma of the tracheobronchial tree: clinical, bronchoscopic and pathological features. *Chest* 1985; 87: 122–124.
59. Krown SE, Metroka C, Wernz JC. Kaposi's sarcoma in the acquired immunodeficiency syndrome: a proposal for uniform evaluation, response and staging criteria. *J Clin Oncol* 1989; 7: 1201–1207.
60. Cooper JS, Steinfeld AD, Lerch I. Intentions and outcomes in the radiotherapeutic management of epidemic Kaposi's sarcoma. *Int J Radiat Oncol Biol Phys* 1991; 20: 419–422.
61. Geara F, Le Bourgeois JP, Piedbois P *et al.* Radiotherapy in the management of cutaneous epidemic Kaposi's sarcoma. *Int J Radiat Oncol Biol Phys* 1991; 21: 1517–1522.
62. Cooper JS, Fried PR, Laubenstein LJ. Initial observations of the effect of radiotherapy of epidemic Kaposi's sarcoma. *JAMA* 1984; 252: 934–935.
63. Harris JW, Reed TA. Kaposi's sarcoma in AIDS: the role of radiation therapy. *Front Radiat Ther Oncol* 1985; 19: 126–132.
64. Nisce L, Safai B. Radiation therapy of Kaposi's sarcoma in AIDS. *Front Radiat Ther Oncol* 1985; 19: 133–137.
65. Vapnek JM, Quivey JM, Carroll PR. Acquired immunodeficiency syndrome-related Kaposi's sarcoma of the male genitalia: management with radiation therapy. *J Urol* 1991; 146: 333–336.
66. Ghabrial R, Quivey JM, Dunn JP, Char DH. Radiation therapy of acquired immunodeficiency syndrome-related Kaposi's sarcoma of the eyelids and con-

junctiva. *Arch Opthalmol* 1992; 110: 1423–1426.
67. Le Bourgeois JP, Frikha H, Piedbois P *et al.* Radiotherapy in the management of epidemic Kaposi's sarcoma of the oral cavity, the eyelid and the genitals. *Radiother Oncol* 1994; 30: 263–266.
68. Harrison M, Harrington K, Tomlinson D, Stewart S. Response and cosmetic outcome of two fractionation regimes for AIDS-related Kaposi's sarcoma. *Int J Radiat Oncol Biol Phys.*
69. Berson AM, Quivey JM, Harris JW, Wara WM. Radiation therapy for AIDS-related Kaposi's sarcoma. *Int J Radiat Oncol Biol Phys* 1990; 19: 569–575.
70. de Wit R, Smit WGJM, Veenhof KHN, Bakker PJM *et al.* Palliative radiation therapy for AIDS-associated Kaposi's sarcoma by using a single fraction of 800 cGY. *Radiother Oncol* 1990; 19: 131–136.
71. Stein ME, Lakier R, Spencer D *et al.* Radiation therapy for non-AIDS associated (classic and endemic African) and epidemic Kaposi's sarcoma. *Int J Radiat Oncol Biol Phys* 1994; 28: 613–619.
72. Stelzer KJ, Griffin TW. A randomized prospective trial of radiation therapy for AIDS-associated Kaposi's sarcoma. *Int J Radiat Oncol Biol Phys* 1993; 27: 1057–1061.
73. Meyer JL. Whole lung irradiation for Kaposi's sarcoma. *Am J Clin Oncol* 1993; 16: 372–376.
74. Vallis KA. Glutathione deficiency and radiosensitivity in AIDS patients. *Lancet* 1991; 337: 918–919.
75. Hughes-Davies L, Young T, Spittle M. Radiosensitivity in AIDS patients. *Lancet* 1991; 337: 1616.
76. Nemechek PM, Corder MC. Radiation recall associated with vinblastine in a patient treated for Kaposi sarcoma related to acquired immune deficiency syndrome. *Cancer* 1992; 70: 1605–1606.
77. Stelzer KJ, Griffin TW, Koh W-J. Radiation skin toxicity with bleomycin in a patient with Kaposi sarcoma related to acquired immune deficiency syndrome. *Cancer* 1993; 71: 1322–1325.
78. Newman S. Treatment of epidemic Kaposi's sarcoma with intralesional vinblastine injection. *Proc Am Soc Clin Oncol* 1988; 7: 19.
79. Epstein JB. Treatment of oral Kaposi sarcoma with intralesional vinblastine. *Cancer* 1993; 71: 1722–1725.
80. Moyle G, Youle M, Barton S. Intralesional vinblastine in the treatment of oral Kaposi's sarcoma. *Br J Clin Prac* 1993; 47: 79–80.
81. Northfelt D, Volberding P. AIDS-related Kaposi's sarcoma: clinical presentation, biology and therapy. *Adv Oncol* 1991; 7: 9–17.
82. Langtry JA, Bottomley DM, Phillips RH, Staughton RC. The infra-red coagulator in the treatment of AIDS-related Kaposi's sarcoma and a comparison with radiotherapy. *Clin Exp Dermatol* 1994; 19: 23–25.
83. Bernstein ZP, Wilson D, Summers K *et al.* Pilot/Phase I study of photodynamic therapy (PDT) for treatment of AIDS-associated Kaposi's sarcoma (AIDS/KS). *Proc Am Soc Clin Oncol* 1995; 14: 289 (abstract 285).
84. Volberding PA, Abrams DI, Conant M *et al.* Vinblastine therapy for Kaposi's sarcoma in the acquired immune deficiency syndrome. *Ann Intern Med* 1985; 103: 335–338.
85. Mintzer DM, Real FX, Jovino L *et al.* Treatment of Kaposi's sarcoma and thrombocytopenia with vincristine in patients with acquired immunodeficiency syndrome. *Ann Intern Med* 1985; 102: 200–202.
86. Chachoua A, Green M, Laubenstine L *et al.* Phase II study of oral idarubicin in patients with AIDS-associated Kaposi's sarcoma. *Cancer Treat Rep* 1987; 71: 775–776.

87. Kaplan L, Volberding PA. Failure (and danger) of mitoxantrone in AIDS-related Kaposi's sarcoma. *Lancet* 1985; ii: 396.
88. Goss PE, Shepherd FA, Burkes R *et al.* Phase II study of epirubicin in the treatment of Kaposi's sarcoma and AIDS. *Proc Am Soc Clin Oncol* 1989; 8: 2.
89. Gill PS, Akil B, Colletti P *et al.* Pulmonary Kaposi's sarcoma: clinical findings and results of therapy. *Am J Med* 1989; 87: 57–61.
90. Guermonprez G, Katlama C, Caumes E *et al.* Bleomycin in treatment of AIDS-related Kaposi's sarcoma. *Abstracts: VI International Conference on AIDS* San Francisco, 1990; 3: 213 (poster SB511).
91. Remick S, Reddy M, Herrman D *et al* Continuous infusion bleomycin in AIDS-related Kaposi's sarcoma. *J Clin Oncol* 1994; 12: 1130–1136.
92. Laubenstein LJ, Krigel RL, Odajnyk CM *et al.* Treatment of epidemic Kaposi's sarcoma with etoposide or a combination of doxorubicin, bleomycin and vinglastine. *J Clin Oncol* 1984; 2: 1115–1120.
93. Schwartzsmann G, Sprinz E, Kronfeld M *et al.* Phase II study of tenoposide in patients with AIDS-related Kaposi's sarcoma. *Eur J Cancer* 1991; 27: 1637–1639.
94. Saville MW, Lietzau J, Pluda JM *et al.* Treatment of HIV-associated Kaposi's sarcoma with paclitaxel. *Lancet* 1995; 346: 26–28.
95. Kaplan L, Abrams D, Volberding P. Treatment of Kaposi's sarcoma in acquired immunodeficiency syndrome with an alternating vincristine–vinblastine regimen. *Cancer Treat Rep* 1986; 70: 1121–1122.
96. Gill PS, Rarick M, McCutchan JA *et al.* Systemic treatment of AIDS-related Kaposi's sarcoma: results of a randomised trial. *Am J Med* 1991; 90: 427–434.
97. Gill PS, Rarick MU, Espina B *et al.* Advanced acquired immune deficiency syndrome-related Kaposi's sarcoma: results of pilot studies using combination chemotherapy. *Cancer* 1990; 65: 1074–1078.
98. Gompels MM, Hill A, Jenkins P *et al.* Kaposi's sarcoma in HIV infection treated with vincristine and bleomycin. *AIDS* 1992; 6: 1175–1180.
99. Lipman MCI, Swaden LS, Sabin CA *et al.* Kaposi's sarcoma in HIV infection treated with vincristine and bleomycin. *AIDS* 1993; 7: 592–593.
100. Groopman JE, Mitsuyasu RT, DeLeo MJ *et al.* Effect of recombinant human granulocyte–macrophage colony stimulating factor on myelopoiesis in the acquired immunodeficiency syndrome. *N Eng J Med* 1987; 317: 593–598.
101. Gill PS, Bernstein-Singer M, Espina BM *et al.* Adriamycin, bleomycin, and vincristine chemotherapy with recombinant granulocyte macrophage colony-stimulating factor in the treatment of AIDS-related Kaposi's sarcoma. *AIDS* 1992; 6: 1477–1481.
102. Gill PS, Miles SA, Mitsuyasu RT *et al.* Phase I AIDS Clinical Trial Group (075) study of adriamycin, bleomycin and vincristine chemotherapy with zidovudine in the treatment of AIDS-related Kaposi's sarcoma. *AIDS* 1994; 8: 1695–1699.
103. Bakker PJM, Danner SA, ten Napel CHH *et al.* Treatment of poor prognosis epidemic Kaposi's sarcoma with doxorubicin, bleomycin, vindesine and recombinant human granulocyte–monocyte colony stimulating factor (rhGM-CSF). *Eur J Cancer* 1995; 31A: 188–192.
104. Huang SK, Lee K-D, Hong K *et al.* Microscopic localisation of sterically stabilised liposomes in colon carcinoma-bearing mice. *Cancer Res* 1992; 52: 5135–5143.
105. Presant CA, Blayney D, Proffitt RT *et al.* Preliminary report: imaging of Kaposi sarcoma and lymphoma in AIDS with indium-111-labeled liposomes. *Lancet* 1990: 335: 1307–1309.
106. Gabizon AA. Selective tumor localization and improved therapeutic index of anthracyclines encapsulated in long-circulating liposomes. *Cancer Res* 1992; 52: 891–896.

107. Huang SK, Lee K-D, Hong K *et al.* Microscopic localisation of sterically stabilised liposomes in colon carcinoma-bearing mice. *Cancer Res* 1992; 52: 5135–5143.
108. Mayhew EG, Lasic D, Babbar S, Martin FJ. Pharmacokinetics and antitumour activity of epirubicin encapsulated in long-circulating liposomes incorporating a polyethylene glycol-derivatized phospholipid. *Int J Cancer* 1992; 51: 302–309.
109. Masood R, Husain SR, Rahman A, Gill P. Potentiation of cytotoxicity of Kaposi's sarcoma related to immunodeficiency syndrome (AIDS) by liposome-encapsulated doxorubicin. *AIDS Res Hum Retrovir* 1993; 9: 741–746.
110. Simpson JK, Miller RF, Spittle MF. Liposomal doxorubicin for the treatment of AIDS-related Kaposi's sarcoma. *Clin Oncol* 1993; 5: 372–377.
111. Hengge UR, Brockmeyer NH, Baumann M *et al.* Liposomal doxorubicin in AIDS-related Kaposi's sarcoma. *Lancet* 1993; 342: 497.
112. Harrison M, Tomlinson D, Stewart S. Liposomal-entrapped doxorubicin: an active agent in AIDS-related Kaposi's sarcoma. *J Clin Oncol* 1995; 13: 914–920.
113. Money-Kyrle JF, Bates F, Ready J *et al.* Liposomal daunorubicin in advanced Kaposi's sarcoma: a phase II study. *Clin Oncol* 1993; 5: 367–371.
114. Presant CA, Scolaro M, Kennedy P *et al.* Liposomal daunorubicin treatment of HIV-associated Kaposi's sarcoma. *Lancet* 1993; 341: 1242–1243.
115. Gill PS, Espina BM, Muggia F *et al.* Phase I/II clinical and pharmacokinetic evaluation of liposomal daunorubicin. *J Clin Oncol* 1995; 13: 996–1003.
116. Gill PS, Wernz J, Scadden DT *et al.* A randomized trial of liposomal daunorubicin (DaunoXome) versus adriamycin, bleomycin and vincristine (ABV) in 232 patients with advanced AIDS-related Kaposi's sarcoma. *Proc Am Soc Clin Oncol* 1995; 14: 291 (abstract 830).
117. Krown SE. Interferon and other biologic agents for the treatment of Kaposi's sarcoma. *Hematol Oncon Clin North Am* 1991; 5: 311–322.
118. Hersh EM, Gutterman JU, Spector S *et al.* Impaired in vitro interferon, blastogenic, and natural killer cell responses to viral stimulation in acquired immune deficiency syndrome. *Cancer* 1985; 45: 406–410.
119. Ho DD, Hartshorn KL, Rota TR *et al.* Recombinant human interferon alpha-A suppresses HTLV-III replication in vitro. *Lancet* 1985; i: 602–604.
120. Real FX, Krown SE, Oettgen HF. Kaposi's sarcoma and the acquired immune deficiency syndrome: treatment with high and low doses of recombinant leukocyte A interferon. *J Clin Oncol* 1986; 4: 544–551.
121. Volberding PA, Mitsuyasu RT, Golando JP *et al.* Treatment of Kaposi's sarcoma with interferon alpha-2b (Intron® A). *Cancer* 1987; 59: 620–625.
122. Rios A, Mansell PWA, Newell GR *et al.* Treatment of acquired immunodeficiency syndrome-related Kaposi's sarcoma with lymphoblastoid interferon. *J Clin Oncol* 1985; 3: 506–512.
123. Lane HC, Kovacs JA, Feinberg J *et al.* Anti-retroviral effects of interferon alpha in AIDS-associated Kaposi's sarcoma. *Lancet* 1988; ii: 1218–1222.
124. Gelmann EP, Preble OT, Steis R *et al.* Human lymphoblastoid interferon treatment of Kaposi's sarcoma in the acquired immunodeficiency syndrome. *Am J Med* 1985; 78: 737–741.
125. Groopman JE, Gottlieb MS, Goodman J *et al.* Recombinant alpha-2 interferon therapy for Kaposi's sarcoma associated with the acquired immunodeficiency syndrome. *Ann Intern Med* 1984; 100: 671–676.
126. Kern P, Meigel W, Racz P *et al.* Interferon alpha in the treatment of AIDS-associated Kaposi's sarcoma. *Onkologie* 1987; 10: 50–52.
127. Krown SE, Gold JWM, Niedwiecki D *et al.* Interferon alpha with zidovudine:

safety, tolerance, and clinical and virological effects in patients with Kaposi sarcoma associated with the acquired immunodeficiency syndrome. *Ann Intern Med* 1990; 112: 812–821.
128. Mitsuyasu RT, Taylor JMG, Glaspy J *et al.* Heterogeneity of epidemic Kaposi's sarcoma: implications for therapy. *Cancer* 1986; 57: 1657–1661.
129. Raskokat H, Haussermann L, Minnemann M. Response of AIDS-related Kaposi's sarcoma to treatment with recombinant interferon alpha depends on the stage of underlying immunodeficiency. *J Invest Dermatol* 1987; 89: 444–445.
130. Vadhan-Raj S, Wong G, Gnecco C *et al.* Immunological variables as predictors of prognosis in patients with Kaposi's sarcoma and the acquired immunodeficiency syndrome. *Cancer Res* 1986; 46: 417–425.
131. Kovacs JA, Deyton L, Davey R *et al.* Combined zidovudine and interferon alpha therapy in patients with Kaposi's sarcoma and the acquired immunodeficiency syndrome (AIDS). *Ann Intern Med* 1989; 111: 280–287.
132. Gill PS. Phase I/II trials of alpha interferon alone or in combination with zidovudine as maintenance therapy following induction chemotherapy in the treatment of acquired immunodeficiency syndrome-related Kaposi's sarcoma. *Semin Oncol* 1991; 5 (Suppl. 7): 53–57.
133. Krown SE, Real FX, Lester T *et al.* Interferon alpha-2a ± vinblastine (VLB) in AIDS-related Kaposi's sarcoma (KS/AIDS): a prospective randomized trial. *Proc Am Soc Clin Oncol* 1986; 5: 6.
134. Krigel RL, Slywotsky CM, Lonberg M *et al.* Treatment of epidemic Kaposi's sarcoma with a combination of interferon alpha 2b and etoposide. *J Biol Response Modif* 1988; 7: 359–364.
135. de Wit R, Reiss P, Bakker PJ *et al.* Lack of activity of zidovudine in AIDS-related Kaposi's sarcoma. *AIDS* 1989; 3: 847–850.
136. Lane HC, Falloon J, Walker RE *et al.* Zidovudine in patients with human immunodeficiency virus (HIV) infection and Kaposi's sarcoma. *Ann Intern Med* 1989; 111: 41–50.
137. Ruprecht RM, Chou T, Chipty F *et al.* Interferon-alpha and 3′-azido-3′-deoxythymidine are highly synergistic in mice and prevent viremia after acute retrovirus exposure. *J AIDS* 1990; 3: 591–600.
138. Miles SA, Wang H, Cortes E *et al.* Beta-interferon therapy in patients with poor prognosis Kaposi's sarcoma related to the acquired immunodeficiency syndrome (AIDS). *Ann Intern Med* 1990; 112: 582–589.
139. Krigel RL, Odanjyk CM, Laubenstein LH *et al.* Therapeutic trial of interferon-gamma in patients with epidemic Kaposi's sarcoma. *J Biol Response Modif* 1985; 4: 358–364.
140. Kahn JO, Kaplan LD, Volberding PA *et al.* Intralesional recombinant tumour necrosis factor-alpha for AIDS-associated Kaposi's sarcoma: a randomised, double-blind trial. *J AIDS* 1989; 2: 217–223.
141. Volberding P, Moody DJ, Beardslee D *et al.* Therapy of acquired immune deficiency syndrome with recombinant interleukin-2. *AIDS Res Hum Retroviruses* 1987; 3: 115–124.
142. Guo W-X, Gill PS, Antakly T. Inhibition of AIDS–Kaposi's sarcoma cell proliferation following retinoic acid receptor activation. *Cancer Res* 1995; 55: 823–829.
143. Bonhomme L, Fredj G, Averous S *et al.* Topical treatment of epidemic Kaposi's sarcoma with all-trans retinoic acid. *Ann Oncol* 1991; 2: 234–235.
144. von Roenn J, von Gunter C, Mullane M *et al.* All-trans retinoic acid (TRA) in the treatment of AIDS-related Kaposi's sarcoma: a phase II Illinois Cancer Centre Study. *Proc. Am Soc Clin Oncol* 1993; 12: 51.
145. Bailey J, Pluda JM, Foli A *et al.* Phase I/II study of intermittent all-trans-retinoic

acid, alone and in combination with interferon alpha-2a, in patients with epidemic Kaposi's sarcoma. *J Clin Oncol* 1995; 13: 1966–1974.

146. Maione TE, Gray GS, Petro J *et al.* Inhibition of angiogenesis by recombinant human platelet factor 4 and related peptides. *Science* 1990; 247: 77–79.
147. Northfelt DW, Robles R, Lang W *et al.* Phase I/II study of intravenous (IV) recombinant platelet factor 4 (rPF-4) in AIDS-related Kaposi's sarcoma (AIDS-KS). *Proc Am Soc Clin Oncol* 1995; 14: 288 (abstract 820).
148. Tanaka NG, Sakamoto N, Inoue K *et al.* Anti-tumor effects of an antiangiogenic polysaccharide from an *Arthrobacter* species with or without a steroid. *Cancer Res* 1989; 49: 6727–6730.

9

Other AIDS-related Malignancies

Konstantinos N. Syrigos and Agamemnon A. Epenetos
Royal Postgraduate Medical School, Hammersmith Hospital, London, UK

Impairment of the function of the immune system and especially of cell-mediated defence was long ago recognized as a possible reason for the development of malignant disease. Both primary immunodeficiency disorders, such as Wiskott–Aldrich syndrome, and secondary deficiencies due to cytostatic or immunosuppressive treatment, have been associated with carcinogenic potential[1,2]. The above principle applies also to acquired immunodeficiency syndrome (AIDS) patients, of whom more than 40% will experience a neoplastic disease at some time during the course of their human immunodeficiency virus (HIV) infection[3]. These neoplasms are thought to contribute to morbidity and mortality of AIDS patients, while, as survival of patients with HIV disease improves, a steady increase in new cases of AIDS-related malignancies have been observed[4,5].

Of the malignant syndromes in AIDS patients only 5% involve tumours other than Kaposi's sarcomas and lymphomas. These mainly include cervical and anorectal neoplasias, squamous cell carcinomas of the head, neck and oral cavity as well as lung cancers[5,6]. The study of these HIV-associated malignancies is of particular interest mainly because they provide us with a fascinating model for the study of the role of viruses and other cofactors in oncogenesis, which may lead to a better understanding of tumour development.

AIDS-RELATED CERVICAL CANCER

Cervical cancer was originally reported to be increased in patients who had undergone renal transplantation[7,8]. The immunodeficient environment of

AIDS and Malignancies: Current Concepts and Perspectives.
Edited by B.C. Golematis and V.T. DeVita Jr

these patients is likely to predispose such individuals to human papillomavirus (HPV) infection, which has long been recognized as an important cause of cervical malignancy. Indeed, HPV types 16 and 18 are capable of transforming human keratinocytes *in vitro* into a malignant phenotype[9]. They encode the oncoproteins E6/E7, which target the product of the tumour suppressor gene p53 and form complexes. These two HPV types, although associated with approximately 80% of cervical carcinomas, do not appear capable of inducing cervical cancer on their own, mainly because most HPV infections regress spontaneously. Even when HPV infection is latent, an additional factor is needed for its reactivation. The mechanism is not fully understood, but it seems that a cofactor is needed for malignant transformation of the cervical epithelium[10,11].

Epidemiology

Almost immediately after the outset of the AIDS epidemic, several groups suggested that cervical malignancies (including cervical intraepithelial neoplasia (CIN) and invasive cervical cancer) are more frequent in HIV-seropositive than non-HIV-infected women[12]. Adachi *et al.* reported that 68% of the 25 HIV-positive women studied had cervical abnormalities as confirmed by Papanicolaou examination of the smear, compared with only 3% of the 13 seronegative women[13]. Feingnold *et al.* presented molecular evidence of HPV infection in women with HIV infection and showed that 49% of HIV-infected women had detectable HPV genomic material, compared with only 25% of non-infected women[14]. The odds ratio of detecting CIN and HPV DNA was significantly greater among HIV-infected individuals than HIV-negative women when prostitutes in Zaire were studied[15]. On the contrary, another group was not able to establish that discrepancy[16], making it difficult to establish an aetiological relationship between HIV infection and cervical cancer, mainly because both HPV and HIV may be sexually transmitted. Finally, Mandelblatt *et al.*, conducting a meta-analysis of previously published studies, provided supportive evidence for the prevalence of cervical cancer in HIV-infected women: the combined odds ratio was statistically significant[17]. Furthermore, it is now clear that HIV-seropositive women are more likely to be infected by the more aggressive HPV genotypes 16 and 18 than HIV-negative women. Indeed, infection with HPV-16 or -18 and cervical cancer were highly associated with the presence of antibodies to HIV-1. While HPV DNA of any type was found only 1.4-fold more often in the HIV-infected group than in the HIV-seronegative women, HPV-16 or -18 DNA was found 2.2-fold more often in the HIV-infected group[18].

Pathogenesis

The exact pathogenetic mechanism that leads HIV-seropositive women to enhanced cervical cancer is not understood. It seems that Langerhans cells in the cervix are important to the local immune response to HPV. In fact, Spinillo *et al.* studying cervical biopsy specimens were able to demonstrate lower Langerhans cells counts in HIV-infected women compared to non-HIV women matched with respect to stage of CIN, age and smoking habits. The number of Langerhans cells in HIV-seropositive women was correlated with the stage of HIV infection. Estimation of the degree of immunosuppression by CD4 and CD8 cell counts showed a direct relationship to the Langerhans cells counts[19]. In addition, the evaluation of 16 women with recurrent CIN showed that five immunosuppressed patients (including three with AIDS) had the same type of HPV, whereas the immunocompetent women had different strains[20]. The above findings provide enough evidence that immunocompetent women are able to develop HPV-specific immunity, whereas immunocompromised women are not.

Progress of the Disease

The development and prognosis of cervical disease are affected by the degree of immunosuppression. It has been demonstrated that there is a relationship between the degree of immunosuppression and the severity of the HIV-associated cervical dysplasia, as estimated with the Papanicolaou smear. In fact the presence of cytological abnormalities was related to low CD4 cell counts[21]. Furthermore, Maiman *et al.* studying the clinical course of 84 women with cervical cancer demonstrated that only 6% of HIV-infected patients had limited stage disease compared with 40% of HIV-seronegative patients. In addition, women with CIN II or III had significantly lower CD4 cell counts compared with patients with CIN I. The HIV-infected women were found to have significantly more advanced disease and poorer prognosis. It has also been demonstrated that within the group of seropositive patients, those with CD4 cell counts greater than 500/mm^3 showed a better response to treatment, with prolonged disease-free periods. Patients with a CD4 count less than 500/mm^3 have a 45% chance of developing recurrent CIN after local treatment, compared with only 18% of HIV-positive women with CD4 count higher than 500/mm^3 and 9% of seronegative women[22].

In general, the natural history of cervical disease is distinct in HIV-infected women, with more advanced disease on presentation, more aggressive clinical course, poorer response to therapy, increased risk of relapse and shorter survival.

Treatment

As there are not enough studies on the treatment of cervical cancer in HIV-seropositive women it is impossible to provide any guidelines. Patients should be treated according to conventional methods which include cone surgery, with or without chemotherapy. The additional therapy consists of cisplatin, bleomycin or vincristine, laser therapy and cryotherapy. One must always bear in mind that these patients are immunocompromised, and when radiotherapy is used there are increased reactions of normal tissues. Perilesional administration of interferon has also been given, with encouraging results. Its application may be useful for the prevention of relapse after initial treatment[23,24].

Conclusions

As women have become the fastest-rising population group at risk for infection, and due to longer survival of AIDS patients, with profound states of immunosuppression, the relative risk of invasive cervical cancer or of cervical intraepithelial neoplasm appears to increase. In addition, cervical intraepithelial neoplasia and invasive cervical cancer may be the first sign of HIV infection. These findings, plus the increased prevalence of cervical dysplasia to HIV infection, prompted the US Centers for Disease Control and Prevention to include cervical cancer as an AIDS-indicating diagnosis: the presence of cervical cancer plus the HIV seropositivity define the AIDS diagnosis regardless of the CD4 cell count[25]. As many of these patients are already in profound immunosuppression and their prognosis is poor, efforts should be focused on early diagnosis of HPV infection and cervical malignancy in HIV patients. Also, because relapse is more common in these patients, alternative therapeutic schemes should be considered in HIV-positive women with cervical carcinoma.

AIDS-RELATED ANORECTAL CANCER

Although carcinomas of the anorectal area are rare in the general population, it seems that their incidence in immunosuppressed patients is increased, with lesions ranging from epithelial atypias to invasive tumours[8,26]. Nevertheless, despite the status of profound immunosuppression of AIDS patients, the rarity of these malignancies makes it difficult to demonstrate an AIDS-related increase of their incidence.

Epidemiology

Homosexuality and receptive anal intercourse were recognized as important risk factors for anorectal cancer long before the AIDS epidemic, with a 25-fold increased incidence of anorectal cancer compared with heterosexual controls[27]. Homosexuals also have a high prevalence of anal HPV infection[28,29]. It seems that behavioural and environmental changes taking place before the outbreak of the AIDS epidemic have created a high-risk group for anorectal cancer. Nevertheless, it seems that HIV-infected individuals are at even higher risk of developing anorectal cancer. In a study of the malignancies diagnosed between 1980 and 1987 in San Francisco the incidence of invasive cancer and of *in situ* disease of the anorectal area was almost three times higher among HIV-infected patients[4].

Pathogenesis

The anatomy and histopathology of the anorectal mucosa is analogous with that of the female cervix, with a 'transforming zone'. In addition, cervical and anal cancers share many characteristics, the most crucial being the presence of HPV infection[30,31]. It has been demonstrated that cytological changes indicative of HPV infection and of dysplasia of the anorectal epithelium are found in high incidence of HIV-infected men[32]. The prevalence of HPV among these individuals increases inversely with the CD4 cell counts. In support of the direct influence of HIV infection on anal cancer is the observed close correlation of anal intraepithelial abnormalities with decreased immunocompetence[28,29,33] and the statistically significant association between a decreased CD4/CD8 ratio and the degree of dysplasia[32]. Also, high-grade lesions are more frequently found in HIV-infected men, whereas lower-grade lesions prevail in HIV-negative patients[34]. Finally, cohort studies have shown that HIV seropositivity with significantly low CD4 cell counts serves as an independent risk factor for the detection of HPV in anal epithelium[28].

Progress of the Disease

Low absolute CD4 T-lymphocyte cell counts ($<800/mm^3$) are associated in HIV-infected men with the detection of anal squamous intraepithelial lesions; the magnitude of the association increases significantly with decreasing absolute CD4 counts. In fact the risk for such lesions in HIV-seropositive homosexual men with CD4 counts less than $500/mm^3$ was increased almost three times compared with the risk with counts greater than $500/mm^3$ [35]. The CD4 cell count is also associated with the HPV genotype. In fact, in patients with low CD4 counts HPV-11, -16 and -18 were more often detected, which have an increased oncogenic potential[34].

As has already been demonstrated, the prevalence, extent and progression of anal carcinoma correlate with the degree of immunodeficiency. According to the model proposed by Palefsky *et al*, early HIV disease and relatively normal immune status are associated with only marginal HPV detection, with the use of highly sensitive methods (e.g. polymerase chain reaction technique), while advanced HIV disease correlates with enhanced HPV replication, and HPV DNA can be easily detected by hybridization techniques. At that level most of the patients develop low-grade anal neoplasia. Finally, when the individual has developed profound immunodeficiency, the dysplastic lesion progresses towards development of high-grade anal intraepithelial neoplasia. The above concept could be used as a model for other immunodeficiency-induced neoplasms as well[36].

Treatment

Although the relative risk of invasive anal cancer is increased among AIDS patients, the absolute risk in HIV-infected homosexual men is as low as 1 : 1000. In addition, most of these patients with anal dysplasia do not develop clinically apparent symptoms, mainly because of the currently poor outlook for these individuals. As survival of AIDS patients is improving, clinicians dealing with HIV-infected homosexual men should be aware of the potential for their patients to develop anal cancer. Digital examination of anorectal cancer should be standard medical procedure, and when anal cancer is suspected cytological examination should follow. Radiotherapy, the treatment of choice, is very often complicated by increased normal tissue radiosensitivity[37].

OTHER AIDS-RELATED NEOPLASMS

A few research groups have suggested an increased incidence of several tumours in HIV-infected individuals, though this is not generally accepted. These malignancies include basal cell carcinoma, cancer of the lung (various types), larynx and oropharynx, as well as testicular germ cell tumours. There are also reports of HIV-infected patients who developed gastric, colon and pancreatic adenocarcinoma, thymoma, thyroid carcinoma and glioblastoma.

It is not clear whether HIV-induced immunosuppression plays a role in the development or progression of these malignancies. An attractive yet unconfirmed concept is that HIV activity may accelerate carcinogenesis induced by common oncogenic factors such as tobacco, alcohol and Epstein–Barr virus infection. It is of particular interest that all these malignancies reported in HIV-infected patients occurred at a relatively early age and had an accelerated clinical course, compared with the general population.

HIV-infected patients presenting with malignant lesions should have the usual investigations. Normally they tolerate the standard chemotherapy doses well, as long as they have not had prior opportunistic infections. Radiotherapy should be used carefully because of the increased radiosensitivity of normal tissues[38–40].

CONCLUSIONS

While diagnosed in approximately 5% of all patients with HIV infection, AIDS-associated malignancies are of particular interest, mainly because they provide an attractive model for the study of the pathogenesis of neoplastic disease in immunocompromised individuals. The development of effective therapies for opportunistic infections may eventually have a favourable influence on the outlook for AIDS patients. Unfortunately, prolonging survival with HIV infection, without a simultaneous correction of immunocompetence, is expected to lead to a further increase in HIV-related malignancies. Therefore, clinicians dealing with HIV-infected individuals should be aware of the increased risk of malignancies in these patients, as early detection is crucial for successful treatment. In addition to early diagnosis, research should focus on the evolution of alternative therapeutic strategies required for the treatment and prevention of relapse in HIV-infected individuals with malignancies.

REFERENCES

1. Spector BD, Perry GS, Kensen JH. Genetically determined immunodeficiency disease (GDID) and malignancy: report from the immunodeficiency cancer registry. *Clin Immunol Immunopathol* 1978; 11: 12–19.
2. Hiddemann W. What's new in malignant tumours in acquired immunodeficiency disorders? *Pathol Res Pract* 1989; 185: 930–934.
3. Peters BS, Beck EJ, Coleman DG *et al.* Changing disease patterns in patients with AIDS in a referral center in the UK. The changing face of AIDS. *Br Med J* 1991; 302: 203–206.
4. Reynolds P, Saunders LD, Laypesky ME, Lemp GF. The spectrum of AIDS associated malignancies in San Francisco 1980–1987. *Am J Epidemiol* 1993; 137: 19–30.
5. Bernstein L, Hamilton AS. The epidemiology of AIDS-related malignancies. *Curr Opinion Oncol* 1993; 5: 822–830.
6. Fauci AS, Macher AM, Longo DL *et al.* AIDS: epidemiology, clinical, immunological and therapeutic considerations. *Ann Intern Med* 1984; 100: 92–106.
7. Pen I. Cancers of the anogenital region in renal transplant recipients: analysis of 65 cases. *Cancer* 1986; 58: 611–616.
8. Pen I. Tumors of the immunocompromised patients. *Annu Rev Med* 1988; 39: 63–73.
9. Hurlin PJ, Kaur P, Smith PP *et al.* Progression of human-papillomavirus-type-18-immortalized human keratinocytes to a malignant phenotype. *Proc Natl Acad Sci USA* 1991; 88: 570–574.
10. Kataja V, Syrjanen K, Syrjanen S *et al.* Prospective follow-up of genital HPV infections: survival analysis of the HPV typing data. *Eur J Epidemiol* 1990; 6: 9–14.
11. Schiffman MH, Bauer HM, Hoover RN *et al.* Epidemiologic evidence showing that human papillomavirus infection causes most cervical intraepithelial neoplasia. *J Natl Cancer Inst* 1993; 85: 958–964.
12. Schrager LK, Friedland GH, Maude D *et al.* Cervical and vaginal squamous abnormalities in women infected with human immunodeficiency virus. *J AIDS* 1989; 2: 570–575.
13. Adachi A, Fleming I, Burk RD *et al.* Women with human immunodeficiency virus infection and abnormal papanicolaou smears: a prospective study of colposcopy and clinical outcome. *Obstet Gynecol* 1993; 81: 472–477.

14. Feingold AR, Vermund SH, Burk RD *et al.* Cervical cytologic abnormalities and papillomavirus in women infected with human immunodeficiency virus. *J AIDS* 1990; 3: 896–903.
15. Laga M, Icenogle JP, Marsella R *et al.* Genital papillomavirus infection and cervical dysplasia: opportunistic complications of HIV infection. *Int J Cancer* 1992; 50: 45–48.
16. Kreiss JK, Kiviat NB, Plummer FA. Human immunodeficiency virus, human papillomavirus and cervical intraepithelial neoplasia in Nairobi prostitutes. *Sex Transm Dis* 1992; 19: 54–59.
17. Mandelblatt JS, Fahs M, Garibaldi K *et al.* Association between HIV infection and cervical neoplasia: implications for clinical care of women at risk for both conditions. *AIDS* 1992; 6: 173–178.
18. Ter Meulen J, Eberhard HC, Luande J *et al.* HPV infection, HIV infection and cervical cancer in Tanzania, East Africa. *Int J Cancer* 1992; 51: 515–521.
19 Spinillo A, Tenti P, Zappatore R *et al.* Langerhans' cell counts and cervical intraepithelial neoplasia in women with human immunodeficiency virus infection. *Gynecol Oncol* 1993; 48: 210–213.
20. Nuovo GJ, Babury R, Calayag PT. Human papillomavirus types and recurrent cervical warts in immunocompromised women. *Mod Pathol* 1991; 4: 632–636.
21. Marte C, Kelly P, Cohen M *et al.* Papanicolaou smear abnormalities in ambulatory care sites for women infected with the human immunodeficiency virus. *Am J Obstet Gynecol* 1992; 166: 1232–1237.
22. Maiman M, Fruchter RG, Guy L *et al.* Human immunodeficiency virus infection and invasive cervical carcinoma. *Cancer* 1993; 71: 402–406.
23. Iwasaka T, Hayashi Y, Yokoyama M *et al.* Interferon gamma treatment for cervical intraepithelial neoplasia. *Gynecol Oncol* 1990; 37: 96–102.
24. Levine AM. AIDS-related malignancies: the emerging epidemic. *J Natl Cancer Inst* 1993; 85: 1382–1397.
25. Centers for Disease Control. 1993 revised classification system for HIV infection and expanded surveillance case definition for AIDS among adolescents and adults. *MMWR* 1993; 41: 10–19.
26. Bender ME, Katz HI, Posalaky Z. Carcinoma in situ of the genitalia. *JAMA* 1980; 6: 95–106.
27. Daling JR, Weiss NS, Klopfenstein LL. Correlates of homosexual behavior and the incidence of anal cancer. *JAMA* 1982; 247: 1988–1990.
28. Caussy D, Goedert JJ, Palefsky J *et al.* Interaction of human immunodeficiency and papilloma viruses: association with anal epithelial abnormality in homosexual men. *Int J Cancer* 1990; 46: 214–219.
29. Melbye M, Palefsky J, Gonzales J *et al.* Immune status as a determinant of human papillomavirus detection and its association with analepithelial abnormalities. *Int J Cancer* 1990; 46: 203–206.
30. Scholefield JH, Sonnex C, Talbot IC *et al.* Anal and cervical intraepithelial neoplasia: possible parallel. *Lancet* 1989; ii: 765–769.
31. Melbye M, Sprogel P. Aetiological parallel between anal cancer and cervical cancer. *Lancet* 1991; 338: 657–659.
32. Frazer JH, Medley G, Crapper RM *et al.* Association between anorectal dysplasia, human papillomavirus and human immunodeficiency virus infection in homosexual men. *Lancet* 1986; ii: 657–660.
33. Palefsky JM, Gonzales J, Greenblatt RM *et al.* Anal intraepithelial neoplasia and anal papillomavirus infection among homosexual males with group IV disease. *JAMA* 1990; 263: 2911–2916.
34. Bernard C, Mougin C, Madoz L *et al.* Viral co-infection in human papillomavirus-

associated anogenital lesions according to the serostatus for the human immunodeficiency virus. *Int J Cancer* 1993; 52: 731–737.
35. Kiviat NB, Critchlow CW, Holmes KK *et al.* Association of anal dysplasia and human papillomavirus with immunosuppression and HIV infection among homosexual men. *AIDS* 1993; 7: 43–49.
36. Palefsky JM, Holly EA, Gonzales J. Natural history of anal cytologic abnormalities and papillomavirus infection among homosexual men with group IV HIV disease. *J AIDS* 1992; 5: 1258–1265.
37. Lipsey LR, Northfelt DW. Anogenital neoplasia in patients with HIV infection. *Curr Opinion Oncol* 1993; 5: 861–866.
38. Monfardini S, Vaccher E, Pizzocaro G *et al.* Unusual malignant tumours in 49 patients with HIV infection. *AIDS* 1989; 3: 449–452.
39. Behling CA, Wolf PL, Haghighi P. AIDS and malignant mesothelioma: is there a connection? *Chest* 1993; 103: 1268–1269.
40. Ravalli S, Chabon A, Khan A. Gastrointestinal neoplasia in young HIV antibody-positive patients. *Am J Clin Pathol* 1989; 91: 458–461.

10

AIDS-related Malignancies and the Respiratory System

David Mitchell
St Mary's Hospital, London, UK

INTRODUCTION

Pulmonary complications are well described and common in human immunodeficiency virus (HIV)-infected individuals and patients with acquired immunodeficiency syndrome (AIDS). In recent years the focus of attention has been directed towards patients with AIDS. In North American and European AIDS patients the most common opportunist infection involving the lung is *Pneumocystis* pneumonia, while in Africa tuberculosis is the most common opportunist. In both groups the most common AIDS-related pulmonary neoplasm is Kaposi's sarcoma (KS)[1–3]. Pulmonary problems are also common in HIV-infected individuals before the onset of an AIDS-defining diagnosis. For example, in a large prospective study over an 18-month period of over 1200 HIV-infected individuals before the onset of AIDS, 33% had an upper respiratory infection, 16% acute bronchitis and 5% sinusitis, whereas nearly 4% developed *Pneumocystis* pneumonia. Only five patients developed a pulmonary malignancy during this time.[4,5].

The aim of this chapter is to describe the clinical features of pulmonary malignant disease arising in AIDS patients within the context of pulmonary disease generally. First the pathophysiological consequences of HIV infection on the lung will be described. This will be followed by a brief description of the respiratory complications in HIV disease. An account will then be given of the respiratory malignancies seen in AIDS patients, the most common of which is KS.

AIDS and Malignancies: Current Concepts and Perspectives.
Edited by B.C. Golematis and V.T. DeVita Jr

PATHOPHYSIOLOGICAL CONSEQUENCES OF HIV INFECTION

Early reports described physiological abnormalities in HIV-infected individuals both with and without overt lung disease[6–8]. Several abnormalities were described including low arterial oxygen tension (PaO_2) (particularly in patients with *Pneumocystis* pneumonia)[7], reductions in the carbon monoxide diffusing capacity for the lung (TLCO)[6], the presence of restrictive defects with reductions in vital capacity[9,10] and finally evidence of airway disease particularly in the presence of endobronchial KS[11]. Initial studies of the pathophysiology of the lung in HIV disease utilized simple lung function testing. In one study of 48 HIV-seropositive individuals with respiratory symptoms, 32 (67%) had *Pneumocystis* pneumonia diagnosed at bronchoscopy. In seven patients TLCO was measured and was reduced to less than 60% of predicted normal in all seven. The total lung capacity was reduced in one patient and five patients had reductions in forced expiratory volume in 1 s (FEV_1) and forced vital capacity (FVC)[12]. In a larger study of 169 HIV-infected individuals belonging to all categories of HIV-related disease from asymptomatic status through to AIDS (none were intravenous drug users), abnormalities in TLCO, transfer coefficient (KCO) and FVC were seen in most of the categories of HIV-related disease. Asymptomatic patients and patients with persistent generalized lymphadenopathy were thought to have normal TLCO values which were greater than 83% of predicted normal, whereas patients with AIDS-related complex had mean TLCO values of 77% of predicted normal. Patients with KS but without evidence of pulmonary disease had a mean TLCO of 70% of predicted normal and patients with AIDS who did not have KS and had no evidence of pulmonary disease had mean TLCO reduced to 70% of predicted normal. Patients with *Pneumocystis* pneumonia had TLCO values of 50% of predicted normal and these improved to 63% upon recovery[6].

In a further study of 331 HIV-infected individuals reductions of TLCO were seen in HIV-seropositive asymptomatic individuals (85% predicted normal) as well as patients with the AIDS-related complex, whereas patients with *Pneumocystis* pneumonia had values of 50% of predicted normal[13]. A larger prospective study involving 474 HIV-seropositive individuals was done over an 18-month period to further define pathophysiological changes[14]. Table 10.1 shows the number of patients and demographic details in each category of HIV disease and spirometry. Lung function at presentation (TLCO, KCO, FVC) is expressed as a percentage of predicted normal for patients on entry into the study classified according to clinical diseases category (Figure 10.1). More profound reductions in TLCO were seen than in the other measurements and even completely asymptomatic patients had slight reductions in TLCO values (88% of predicted), with stepwise reductions in TLCO being seen in the other categories of HIV disease, including pulmonary KS. This

Table 10.1 Age range, percentage who smoked, percentage with mild and severe dyspnoea and spirometry in HIV-infected individuals according to clinical classification (HIV+ve, asymptomatic seropositive patients; PGL, persistent generalized lymphadenopathy; ARC, AIDS-related complex; non-lung KS, patients with Kaposi's sarcoma but not involving the lung; non-KS non-lung AIDs, AIDS patients without Kaposi's sarcoma and without opportunist lung infection; AC PCP, acute *Pneumocystis carinii* pneumonia; post PCP, patients >1 month after PCP; lung myco, AIDS patients with pulmonary mycobacterial infections; lung KS, lung involvement by Kaposi's sarcoma; lung pyog, AIDS patients with pyogenic bacterial pulmonary infection)

Group name	Clinical classification	CDC group	No. of patients	Age range (years)	Smoker SOB (% of patients)	Mild dyspnoea (% of patients)	Severe SOB (% of patients)	FEV_1 (% of patients)	PEFR (% of patients)
HIV+ve	Asymptomatic HIV seropositive	II	126	20–58	56	24	8	106	96
PGL	Persistent generalized lymphadenopathy	III	95	23–54	59	31	6	102	90
ARC	AIDS-related complex	IV subgroup A, B, C_2, E	92	19–59	57	39	6	96	87
KS	Non-pulmonary Kaposi's sarcoma (KS), mainly skin KS	IV subgroup D	35	23–57	34	6	11	95	86
Non-KS AIDS	Non-pulmonary AIDS without KS, i.e. opportunistic infection of other organs	IV subgroup C_1	19	22–50	40	30	5	96	86
Pulmonary AIDS	Pulmonary complications of AIDS		107						
Including									
acute PCP	Acute *P.carinii* pneumonia (PCP)	IV subgroup C_1	78	24–60	34	53	27	78	74
post PCP	3 months following recovery from PCP		42	24–60	31	36	9	95	84
lung KS	Lung Kaposi's sarcoma		11	26–53	45	27	9	87	88
lung myco	Lung mycobacterial infection		11	25–60	63	47	20	91	79
lung pyog	AIDS patients with pyogenic bacterial lung infections		7	29–44	29	66	0	101	84

Reproduced by permission from *Am Rev Respir Dis.*

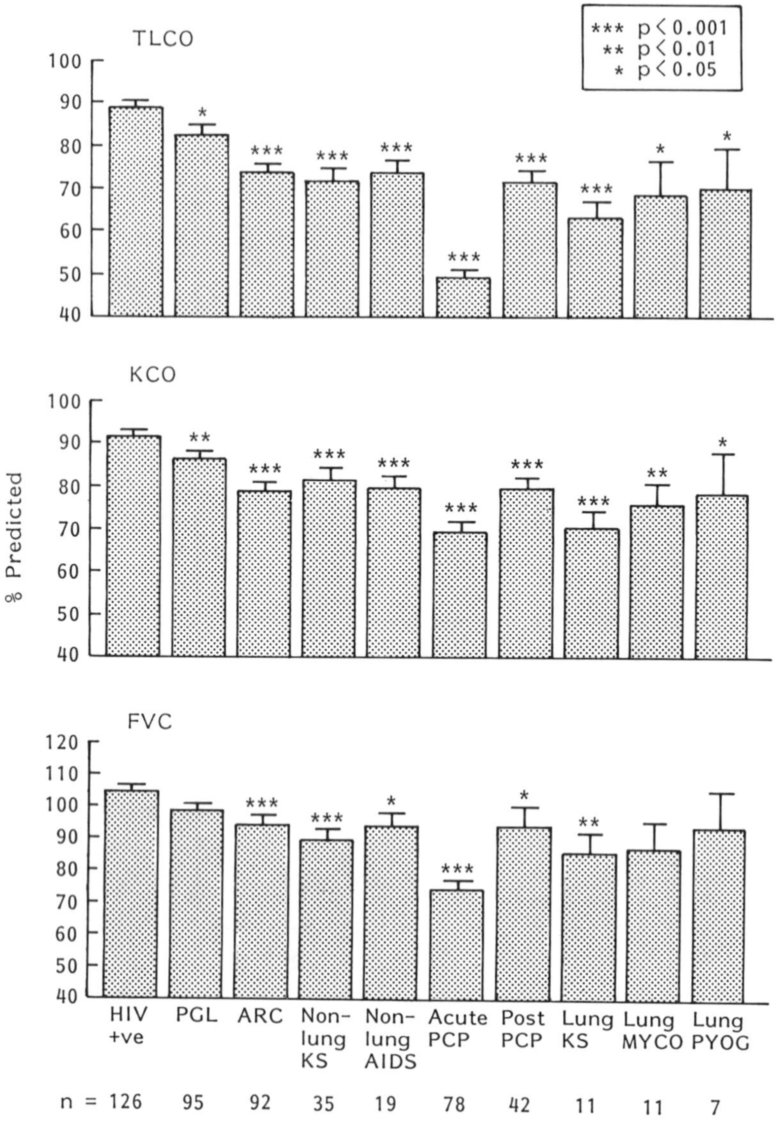

Figure 10.1 *Carbon monoxide transfer factor (TLCO), transfer coefficient (KCO) and forced vital capacity (FVC) as percentages of predicted values (means with SD) for asymptomatic HIV-seropositive patients (HIV+ve), persistent generalized lymphadenopathy (PGL), AIDS-related complex (ARC), non-lung Kaposi sarcoma (NON LUNG KS), non-lung non-KS AIDS (e.g., CMV infection at non-pulmonary site), acute* Pneumocystis carinii *pneumonia (ACUTE PCP), patients >1 month after PCP (POST PCP), mycobacterial lung infection (LUNG MYCO), lung Kaposi sarcoma (LUNG KS) and AIDS patients with pyogenic bacterial pulmonary infection (LUNG PYOG), expressed as mean ±SD (*$^{*}p < 0.05$, $^{**}p < 0.01$, $^{***}p < 0.001$).

study showed that over the 18-month follow-up period, these abnormalities were not progressive provided that patients did not change clinical diagnostic group. The exception to this observation was in patients with pulmonary KS where further deterioration in lung function occurred with time, presumably relating to progressive disease[14]. The lung function changes seen were not due to the effects of smoking or use of zidovudine and none of the subjects were intravenous drug users, which can result in defects in TLCO. The main conclusion of the study was that pathophysiological changes are seen in HIV-infected individuals even in the asymptomatic phase but these changes become more pronounced with the onset of pulmonary disease, either with opportunist infections or pulmonary neoplasm, namely KS. Although the main abnormality is seen with TLCO, reductions in both KCO and FVC as well suggest that the abnormalities are a product of both reductions in carbon monoxide diffusing capacity and loss of lung volume.

A further attempt to examine the pathophysiological abnormality in asymptomatic individuals was made in a small study of six HIV-seropositive patients who had TLCO measurements of less than 75% predicted normal on at least two separate occasions[15]. None had respiratory symptoms or any previous respiratory disease and all had normal chest radiographs and none of the individuals developed any respiratory illness over follow-up periods of 14 months, with the exception of one individual who could only be followed-up for two months. Two patients had persistent generalized lymphadenopathy, two patients had the AIDS-related complex and one patient had cutaneous KS. The final patient had cytomegalovirus (CMV) retinitis. All patients had simple lung function tests and in addition the alveolar membrane component (Dm) and the pulmonary vascular component (Vc) of the TLCO were measured. All patients had a simple exercise test to determine oxygen desaturation during exercise and pulmonary clearance of aerosol technetium-99-labelled pentetic acid (DTPA) was also measured. High-resolution computed tomography (CT) scans of the thorax were done to detect early subtle interstitial lung disease. Four of the patients were smokers. At the time of the study TLCO values ranged from 54% to 74% of predicted normal, all but one patient had reductions in Dm and all but two also had reductions in Vc, so both components of the TLCO measurement were affected. None of the patients had oxygen desaturation at rest and there was no desaturation on exercise. All patients had reductions in ^{99}Tc-labelled DTPA clearance measurements, reductions being more marked in smokers than non-smokers, and all patients but one had normal high-resolution CT scans of the thorax. A single patient had very subtle subpleural banding present in the prone position which could be interpreted as very early interstitial lung disease.

These studies show that there are physiological abnormalities in the lungs of HIV-infected individuals even in the absence of overt pulmonary disease, and these abnormalities could possibly be due to HIV infection itself. A low

TLCO value in an HIV-infected individual may have prognostic significance and it has been suggested that abnormal TLCO values in the absence of lung disease could act as surrogate markers for the severity of HIV-induced immunosuppression. In one study, 84 individuals who had regular lung function tests and who eventually developed AIDS were identified retrospectively from a cohort of HIV-infected individuals. None had evidence of active pulmonary disease at the time of initial pulmonary function testing. The relation between the time taken to progress to AIDS and the initial pulmonary function tests was determined by life table survival analysis. Patients with a TLCO value of less than 80% of predicted normal progressed more rapidly to AIDS with a median time of eight months when compared to a median time of 16.5 months for those with a TLCO value of greater than 80% of predicted. Reductions of other measurements of lung function (KCO, FVC) were not associated with the development of AIDS[16].

As a result of studies utilizing bronchoalveolar lavage, the underlying explanation for these pathophysiological changes is now becoming apparent[17–19]. Even in the asymptomatic phase of HIV infection HIV can be detected in bronchoalveolar lavage cells and many of these patients have a lymphocytic alveolitis predominantly of the CD8 phenotype. It has been shown that these cells can recognize and kill autologous HIV-infected macrophages[18,20]. It has also been shown that there is a correlation between reduction in TLCO, increases in DTPA clearance and the level of cytotoxic T-cells directed towards HIV in brochoalveolar lavage[19]. These data therefore suggest that early in the course of HIV infection pathophysiological changes occur within the lung during the asymptomatic phase involving chronic inflammatory changes, possibly relating to an immune response to HIV itself. Later in the course of HIV infection further pathophysiological changes occur in relation to the opportunist infections and malignancies that complicated HIV disease.

THE PULMONARY COMPLICATIONS OF HIV DISEASE AND AIDS

Pneumocystis Pneumonia

The causes of pulmonary disease in AIDS are listed in Table 10.2. Despite effective prophylaxis *Pneumocystis* pneumonia probably remains the most common serious opportunist pulmonary infection in AIDS patients[3,21]. *Pneumocystis carinii* is now classified as a fungus[22] and causes opportunist pneumonia in the face of diminished cell-mediated immunity when the peripheral blood CD4 lymphocyte count is low. Typically it causes a radiologically diffuse pneumonia (Figure 10.2) which histologically consists of a profuse intraalveolar foamy exudate containing the cysts and trophozoites of *Pneumocystis carinii* associated with a mild interstitial pneumonitis (Figure

Table 10.2 Spectrum of lung disease in AIDS

Common	Rare
Pneumocystis pneumonia	Herpes simplex/varicella zoster
	Adenovirus
Mycobacterium tuberculosis	
Mycobacterium avium–intracellulare	*Nocardia*
	Mycobacterium xenopi/kansasii etc.
Bacterial infections	
Streptococcus pneumoniae	*Candida/Aspergillus* spp.
Haemophilus influenzae	*Cryptococcus/Histoplasma*
Staphylococcus aureus	*Strongyloides stercoralis*
Moraxella catarrhalis	*Toxoplasma gondii*
Gram-negative bacteria	Cryptosporidia
Mycoplasma	
	Lymphoma
(Cytomegalovirus)	Non-specific interstitial pneumonitis
	Lymphocytic interstitial pneumonitis
Kaposi's sarcoma	Pulmonary drug reactions

10.3). The clinical onset is usually insidious, often with several weeks' history of dry cough and increasing breathlessness on exertion associated with fever and weight loss. Physical signs are usually not present unless the patient is in respiratory failure. The chest radiograph may be normal in early cases (10%) and in a further 10% atypical radiological features such as focal consolidation or nodular shadows may be seen. Pleural effusion and mediastinal adenopathy are most unusual[3]. As *Pneumocystis* pneumonia remains a common cause of pneumonia in AIDS patients in Europe and North America despite the use of prophylaxis, and as the clinical presentation is often typical it has been argued that an empirical approach to therapy can be adopted without further investigation[23]. However, as other pulmonary infections and neoplasms can mimic *Pneumocystis* pneumonia most authorities recommend establishing an aetiological diagnosis, either by induced sputum techniques or bronchoalveolar lavage taken during fibre-optic bronchoscopy to obtain material from the lung. The cysts of the fungus can then be identified by light microscopy using methenamine silver staining or immunofluorescent techniques with monoclonal antibodies. More recently several studies have been reported using the polymerase chain reaction to detect *Pneumocystis*[24]. The treatment of choice remains cotrimoxazole (sulphamethoxazole and trimethoprim in combination) given in high dose, initially intravenously for a period of three weeks. Other agents which are effective are dapsone and trimethoprim in combination, clindamycin and primaquine in combination or intravenous pentamidine. Adjuvant high-dose corticosteroids are used if

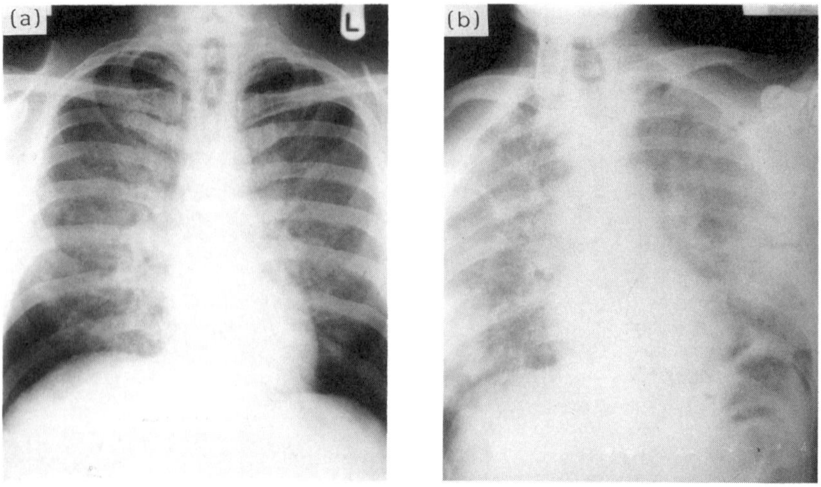

Figure 10.2 *Typical chest radiography appearance of* Pneumocystis *pneumonia: (a) moderate; (b) severe*

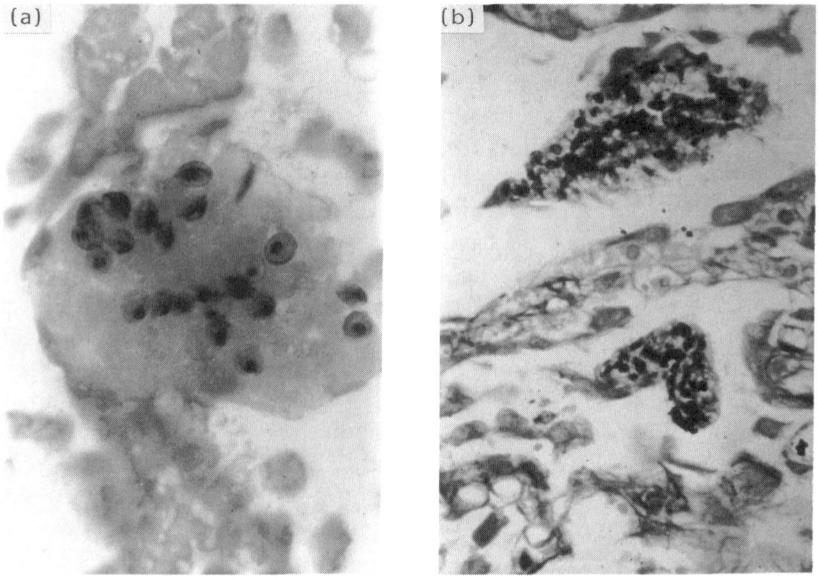

Figure 10.3 Pneumocystis *pneumonia: (a) bronchoalveolar lavage; (b) transbronchial lung biopsy showing clumps of cysts stained with methenamine—silver lying in the air spaces*

respiratory failure is present[3]. Endotracheal intubation and mechanical ventilation should be avoided for the management of respiratory failure in these patients if possible, owing to the very high mortality associated with this procedure in AIDS[25]. On recovery all patients should be offered prophylaxis against further episodes: the most effective agent is cotrimoxazole, taken orally. Nebulized pentamidine, dapsone and pyrimethamine in combination are also effective. Primary prophylaxis should be offered to patients with a low CD4 T-helper lymphocyte count (below $0.2 \times 10^9/l$) who will be susceptible to *Pneumocystis* pneumonia to prevent a first episode[14].

Bacterial Infection

This incidence of bacterial infection in HIV-infected individuals, in particular intravenous drug abusers, is high[26]. The spectrum of bacterial pathogens causing pneumonia is similar to that of acute community-acquired pneumonia in non-HIV-seropositive individuals. Chest radiograph appearances are often atypical and can resemble *Pneumocystis* pneumonia. The onset of bacterial pneumonia in AIDS patients is often rapid and severe and clinically similar to the pattern seen in non-HIV-infected individuals. Response to appropriate antibiotics is usually rapid[27] but relapse is common. The most common bacterial pulmonary infections in AIDS patients are caused by *Streptococcus pneumoniae*; other bacterial pathogens that cause pneumonia include *Haemophilus influenzae, Moraxella catarrhalis, Klebsiella pneumoniae, Staphylococcus aureus* and *Pseudomonas aeruginosa*[28,29]. Unlike patients with *Pneumocystis* pneumonia, pleural effusion is relatively common in AIDS patients with bacterial pneumonia[30]. Sinusitis and acute bronchitis, usually due to bacterial infection, are now recognized as being frequent in HIV-positive individuals[31–33]. Sinusitis may be acute or chronic and may relapse following appropriate antibiotic therapy.

HIV and Tuberculosis

The relationship between HIV infection and tuberculosis is well established[34–36]. Unlike the other opportunist infections of AIDS, tuberculosis is also infectious to normal individuals and so the prevalence of tuberculosis in the general population may be influenced by the prevalence of HIV disease in the same population. Tuberculosis complicating HIV disease may be due to reactivation, primary infection or secondary exogenous infection[37]. Tuberculosis can develop at any time during the course of HIV disease but atypical and extrapulmonary manifestations are particularly common when the CD4 lymphocyte count is low[38]. Diagnostic tests for tuberculosis in patients with HIV disease may be unhelpful as the tuberculin test is frequently negative in active disease[39,40]. The chest radiograph may be atypical[38] and sputum may be negative for acid-fast bacilli[41]. However, standard chemotherapy normally results in a good clinical response[42], although up to 20% of patients develop adverse reactions to medication[43]. In HIV-seropositive individuals who are also tuberculin test positive, isoniazid prophylaxis has been shown to provide protection against developing clinical tuberculosis[44]. As tuberculosis is infectious, contact tracing and case identification are extremely important and HIV-positive patients with tuberculosis need to be regarded as infectious. Multi-drug-resistant tuberculosis has recently been transmitted from an HIV patient to a health care worker[45]. Nosocomial transmission of tuberculosis between four HIV cases in the UK has recently been reported using restriction fragment length polymorphism (RFLP) analysis[46]. There has been recent concern regarding the emergence of drug-resistant tuberculosis in the USA. In New York City 33% of isolates were resistant to one or more drugs and outbreaks of multi-drug-resistant tuberculosis have now been reported in HIV-seropositive patients in the USA[47,48]. The prognosis for multi-drug-resistant tuberculosis in HIV-infected individuals is very poor, with a median survival of only two months[49–51], and treatment is extremely difficult[52], with the need for complex regimens of second-line drugs.

Mycobacterium avium–intracellulare (MAI)

MAI normally causes disseminated disease and this can include pneumonitis. MAI is the most common of the atypical mycobacterial infections in AIDS patients. It is a ubiquitous organism and the portal of entry is thought to be the gut. Disseminated disease occurs towards the end of the natural history of HIV infection when the CD4 lymphocyte count is very low (below $0.05 \times 10^9/l$) and may occur in up to 50% of AIDS patients prior to death[53]. Presentation is often with fever, weight loss, diarrhoea, anaemia and lymphadenopathy. Patients with disseminated MAI infection have reduced survival when compared with similar AIDS patients without disseminated MAI[54]. MAI is resistant to all first-line antituberculosis drugs but clinical response is seen with newer drug combinations which include, for example, rifabutin, ethambutol, ciprofloxacin and clarithromycin[55]. There is some evidence that prophylactic monotherapy and rifabutin may delay colonization and disseminated infection with MAI[56]. Disseminated infection with other atypical mycobacterial organisms, in particular *M. kansasii*, may occur and general response to therapy remains poor.

Pulmonary Virus Infections

Upper respiratory infections are generally more common in HIV-seropositive than seronegative individuals[4,57]. Both herpes simplex and herpes zoster may cause pneumonitis[58,59]. Clinical disease due to CMV is very common in AIDS patients and eventually occurs in up to 40% of HIV-infected patients[60]. CMV causes retinitis, colitis, adrenalitis, encephalitis and radiculopathy. Clinical disease usually responds favourably to specific antiviral therapy with ganciclovir or foscarnet. The role of CMV in causing pneumonitis remains uncertain. CMV can be isolated from bronchoalveolar lavage in up to 50% of samples from HIV-seropositive persons but probably only occasionally contributes to episodes of pneumonitis seen in these patients, as complete clinical resolution of pneumonitis usually occurs following antimicrobial therapies which are not effective against this virus. However, it occasionally causes pneumonitis either when the CD4 lymphocyte count is high or at around the time of seroconversion following HIV infection[61].

Fungi

Fungal infections causing pulmonary disease are increasingly recognized particularly in the late stages of AIDS and in patients who live in or travel to endemic areas. Pulmonary histoplasmosis has been described in European patients[62]. *Cryptococcus neoformans* has a worldwide distribution, being the most common cause of meningitis in AIDS. It may also cause pulmonary disease. Clinical response is usual to fluconazole; in some cases amphotericin B and flucytosine are required. Infection with *Penicillium marneffei* has been identified as a common opportunist infection in HIV-infected patients in Thailand and may cause pulmonary disease[63]. This infection has also been described in the UK[64]. Disseminated candidiasis with pulmonary involvement is relatively uncommon in AIDS patients.

Non-specific Interstitial Pneumonitis (NIP) and Lymphocytic Interstitial Pneumonitis (LIP)

NIP remains poorly understood, being characterized by diffuse alveolar damage with an interstitial inflammatory infiltrate consisting of chronic inflammatory cells[65]. Alveolar septal thickening with alveolar cell hyperplasia may also be present with interstitial fibrosis[66]. It is essentially a histological diagnosis lacking specific aetiological features and so requires a tissue biopsy for the diagnosis to be made. There are no specific radiographic features. It is now less frequently diagnosed as routine lung biopsy performed at diagnostic bronchoscopy is no longer performed routinely in most centres. In an earlier report[65], 38% of AIDS patients with episodes of clinical pneumonitis had NIP on transbronchial biopsies, no pathogens being isolated. Possible causes for these changes that were implicated included concomitant pulmonary KS, previous episodes of *Pneumocystis* pneumonia and intravenous drug usage. In a further study[67], 24 HIV-seropositive individuals who either had an AIDS-defining diagnosis but no clinical evidence of lung disease or CD4 lymphocyte counts of less than $0.2 \times 10^9/l$ but no chest symptoms underwent transbronchial biopsy to detect early *Pneumocystis* infection. None of the study group had *Pneumocystis* pneumonia but 11 of 23 transbronchial biopsies showed NIP. All these patients had normal chest radiographs, so it would appear that the condition can either be subclinical or may present with a respiratory illness. Symptoms are usually mild but can resemble *Pneumocystis* pneumonia, from which the condition has to be distinguished, and the diagnosis is made on the basis of typical histopathological features and the exclusion of other pathologies[68,69]. In a further study of 105 HIV-positive patients presenting with episodes of pneumonia, 36 had NIP. Eighteen of these patients had previous respiratory opportunist infections or were intravenous drug users, five had pulmonary KS, 20 had abnormal radiographs of which 14 showed interstitial infiltrates, four also had pleural effusions, three had alveolar shadowing, one patient had a nodular mass and 16 patients had normal chest radiographs[69]. Generally the clinical course was mild and, in some, spontaneous resolution occurred. It has been suggested that corticosteroids may lead to improvement. LIP on the other hand is usually part of a generalized non-malignant lymphoproliferative disorder and is most commonly seen in children and in individuals of Afro-Caribbean descent[70].

RESPIRATORY MALIGNANT DISEASE IN AIDS PATIENTS

Lymphoma

The incidence of non-Hodgkin's lymphoma in HIV-infected individuals is increased and the incidence is related to the duration of HIV infection[71]. Most lymphomas which also affect the lung are high-grade B-lymphocyte-derived tumours. The Epstein–Barr virus (EBV) may be involved in the development of these lymphomas. With loss of T-cell immune function, EBV-infected B-cells can proliferate, possibly allowing the activation of oncogenes[72,73]. Pulmonary involvement in AIDS patients from generalized lymphoma is unusual[73], but in one series of 35 HIV-infected patients who had generalized lymphoma, 11 had intrathoracic disease[74]. Of these 11 patients eight had pleural effusions, five had interstitial or alveolar shadows or an intrapulmonary mass, and three had hilar or mediastinal lymphadenopathy. Endobronchial involvement by lymphoma is very rare and only a handful of cases have been reported in patients with very low CD4 lymphocyte counts[75,76]. They present with fever, cough, dyspnoea and wheeze. Tracheal and carinal involvement was seen at bronchoscopy, and biopsy obtained with the rigid bronchoscope was necessary for adequate tissue diagnosis, fibre-optically obtained samples being insufficient in size. Primary intrathoracic lymphoma without evidence of disease at other organ sites is extremely rare, again with only a few case reports[77,78]. In one patient rigid bronchoscopy was necessary for diagnosis where fibre-optic bronchoscopic biopsies were non-diagnostic. In a second patient diagnosis was only established following left lower lobectomy following a non-diagnostic percutaneous CT-guided fine-needle biopsy. Pulmonary lymphoma in HIV infection as with lymphoma at other sites is difficult to treat and survival from diagnosis is not good.

Bronchogenic Carcinoma

Despite a number of reports it still remains uncertain if the incidence of lung cancer is genuinely increased in HIV-infected individuals. In a study of a large group of 1701 haemophiliacs over several years, the development of lung cancer was not different between HIV-infected and HIV-non-infected patients. Lung cancer developed in 0.09% of HIV-infected patients whereas it developed in 0.15% of HIV-non-infected individuals[79]. In a smaller study based on six HIV-seropositive individuals with adenocarcinoma of the lung, it was estimated that HIV infection carried a 14-fold increased risk for lung cancer; however, this study was not controlled for age, gender or smoking habits[80]. In a further report of seven HIV-seropositive individuals with adenocarcinoma, the HIV-seropositive individuals presented with more advanced disease, with more extensive chest radiograph abnormalities and more physical signs than a control HIV-seronegative group of patients[81]. In another study of 21 HIV-seropositive individuals with lung cancer, half of the patients were under the age of 40 and all patients but one were cigarette smokers. Eleven of these patients had adenocarcinoma, six patients had small cell carcinoma, three patients had squamous cell carcinoma, and one had mixed histology with adenosquamous features[82]. In another report of 19 HIV-positive patients with lung cancer, 16 were smokers and, when compared to HIV-seronegative historical control groups, the HIV-seropositive patients were younger, with a median age of 47, and had a shorter median survival of only three months[83]. Because of problems with bias and ascertainment in these small studies, it is not possible to reach a definite conclusion as to whether bronchogenic carcinoma is genuinely more common in HIV-infected persons than HIV-seronegative individuals, but on the evidence available it would seem that lung cancer in HIV-positive individuals tends to present at an earlier age, is likely to be more extensive at presentation, is strongly associated with smoking and tends to run a more rapid clinical course, with adenocarcinoma representing the predominant histological type.

Kaposi's Sarcoma

KS is the most common malignant condition of the respiratory system in AIDS patients and the most common non-infectious pulmonary complication of AIDS. The general features of KS epidemiology, natural history and pathogenesis are discussed in detail in other chapters of this book. In this section, the specific pulmonary aspects of KS will be described.

General Features of Kaposi's Sarcoma and the Lung

Epidemic AIDS-related KS has a tendency to originate at multi-centric sites, to affect many organ systems including the lung and to run an aggressive clinical course, so that although many patients with KS die of opportunist infections a proportion, particularly if it affects the lungs, may actually die of the tumour itself. Overall, KS is found in up to a quarter of reported cases of AIDS in Europe and North America[84]. KS is particularly common in AIDS patients belonging to the homosexual and bisexual risk groups. In the USA, 95% of all AIDS-related KS are in homosexual and bisexual men and about 40% of homosexual men with AIDS will develop KS at some stage, whereas only 4% of intravenous drug abusers with AIDS develop KS, and the condition is extremely rare in haemophilia complicated by AIDS[85,86]. The skin is the most frequent site to be involved and often the first, followed by widespread and multi-focal distribution of KS lesions involving nearly all organ systems, particularly the lymph nodes, the gastrointestinal tract and the lungs[87]. Despite a progressive decrease in the frequency of KS in HIV-infected individuals in recent years, pulmonary KS remains the most common non-infectious pulmonary complication of AIDS, being seen in African patients as well, where the male predominance is less marked than in European and US cases[88]. The incidence of pulmonary KS varies considerably depending on the AIDS population studied. In patients with cutaneous KS lesions, pulmonary KS probably contributes to respiratory disease in between 10% and 40% of cases[87–91], and is a cause of pleural effusion in between 10% and 40%[92–93].

Clinical Features of Pulmonary Kaposi's Sarcoma

Most patients with pulmonary KS have evidence of mucocutaneous or lymph node lesions, although primary pulmonary KS has been described[94,95]. Pulmonary KS may initially be asymptomatic and the clinical problem is frequently to decide if the respiratory symptoms and clinical findings are due solely to pulmonary KS or whether there is added pathology, in particular opportunist infection. At postmortem, intrathoracic KS lesions are found in 40%–80% of cases with cutaneous KS but in many of these cases the presence of pulmonary KS was not clinically manifested during life[96]. Within the thorax, KS can affect the pulmonary parenchyma, the bronchi and trachea, the pleura and the intrathoracic lymph nodes. KS may involve the upper oropharynx in up to 20% of cases, where it rarely causes clinical problems, but involvement of the lower pharynx and larynx may produce critical airway obstruction[97,98]. Cardiac involvement is rare, clinically, but up to 30% of patients with cutaneous KS are found to have asymptomatic subepicardial deposits at postmortem. Pericardial involvement with KS is very rare[99]. At postmortem the lungs and pleura are involved, with multiple red or purple nodules of variable sizes; small lesions tend to have a peribronchial and perivascular distribution[100]. Even though pulmonary KS is quite common, most morbidity and mortality due to lung disease result from opportunist infections, even though pulmonary KS may be present. However, pulmonary KS itself may produce respiratory failure due to progressive massive pulmonary consolidation, obstruction to the trachea or major bronchi by KS, pulmonary oedema due to lymphatic obstruction from KS involving the mediastinal lymph nodes or bilateral large pleural effusions. The majority of patients have cutaneous KS lesions which may have been treated, and although primary isolated pleuropulmonary KS is rare[94,95] symptomatic pulmonary KS often with lymph node and other visceral involvement may occur in the absence of obvious cutaneous lesions[89,101]. The majority of patients (40%–80%) presenting with symptomatic pulmonary KS have had previous opportunist infections[87,90,101,102]. Symptomatic pulmonary KS normally occurs when the CD4 count is low ($0.07–0.17 \times 10^9/l$)[24,28]. The most common symptom is progressive dyspnoea, which is found in all symptomatic cases, often associated with non-productive cough. Haemoptysis is unusual but in some series has occurred in up to 30%[101–103]. Pleural effusions which are often bilateral have been reported in between 10% and 50% of cases, whereas fever due entirely to pulmonary KS is relatively unusual, being more commonly associated with opportunist infection. Even so, more aggressive forms of KS involving the lung have been reported to cause fever on their own[101]. Physical examination is frequently normal unless respiratory failure is present, when crackles or signs of pleural effusion may be evident. Very rarely, stridor or monophonic wheeze may be present if there is major airway involvement.

Diagnosis

Chest X-rays frequently show non-specific features. In one review 62% had bilateral interstitial alveolar infiltrates, 15% had bilateral nodular infiltrates, 9% had unilateral changes, 26% had hilar or mediastinal lymph node involvement, 42% had a pleural effusion and 25% had septal lines[97]. The presence of septal lines and/or coarse nodular densities is suggestive of the diagnosis[87,104–106], and the presence of mediastinal lymph node enlargement or pleural effusion is also suggestive of the diagnosis, both features being very unusual in *Pneumocystis* pneumonia (Figure 10.4).

Routine pulmonary function tests show abnormalities in most patients with pulmonary KS which are generally non-specific. These include reduced lung volumes (FEV_1 and FVC) and reductions in TLCO. Airflow obstruction may be evident if there is extensive airway involvement[14,91,103]. These changes, although sensitive for the presence of pulmonary KS, are completely non-specific and are also found in pulmonary opportunist infections as well

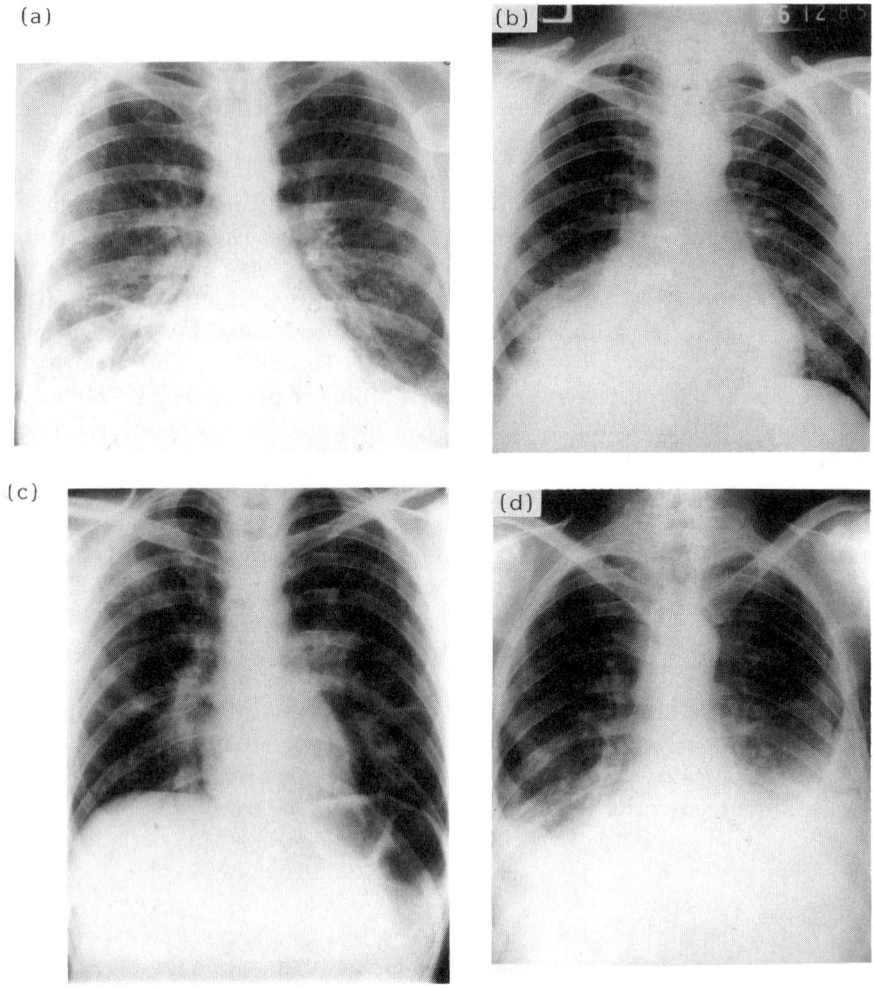

Figure 10.4 *Kaposi's sarcoma. (a) Chest radiograph showing diffuse reticulonodular shadows. (b) KS involving right middle lobe. Patient presented with haemoptysis. (c) Pulmonary KS and* Pneumocystis *pneumonia: ill-defined nodular shadows. (d) Chest radiograph showing pleural effusions in patients with pulmonary KS*

as asymptomatic individuals. In one study[91] there was a relationship between the extent of endobronchial involvement with KS as judged at bronchoscopy with the degree of lung function abnormality, in particular, reductions in FEV_1 and FVC, and the extent of changes on chest X-ray.[91] In this prospective study of 140 consecutive HIV-seropositive patients requiring diagnostic bronchoscopy for respiratory symptoms or chest X-ray abnormalities, 39 (21%) had cutaneous KS. Nineteen of the 39 (49%) had endobronchial KS lesions seen at bronchoscopy. All patients in this series with endobronchial KS also had cutaneous lesions. All had dyspnoea and cough. Four patients of the 39 also had *Pneumocystis* pneumonia. Eight patients had localized (trachea or one segmental bronchus only) KS lesions seen at bronchoscopy and 11 had extensive (more than one segmental bronchus) lesions. Four of the patients with localized lesions had a normal chest X-ray; patients with extensive lesions had more widespread chest X-ray abnormalities. All patients had reductions in TLCO (localized: 51% predicted normal; extensive, 45% predicted normal) whereas patients with extensive lesions had reductions in FEV_1 and FVC as well (localized: FEV_1, 92% predicted normal; FVC, 89% predicted normal; extensive: FEV_1, 56% predicted normal; FVC, 59% predicted normal)[91].

Changes seen on CT have included pulmonary nodules, pleural effusions and peribronchovascular changes, but these probably do not add much to diagnosis[107], whereas gallium citrate scans can distinguish between pulmonary infection and pulmonary KS as gallium is not taken up by the KS lesions[108].

Fibre-optic bronchoscopy is probably the most sensitive direct diagnostic technique for pulmonary involvement by KS but only 45% of patients with pulmonary involvement have visible endobronchial lesions[91,97,109]. Lesions tend to occur in the major airways involving the trachea, the main bronchi and the segmental bronchi, and may also be seen at the segmental orifices. The lesions are red or purple and are usually flat. Occasionally raised lesions produce functional airflow obstruction. As the majority of patients have lesions at other sites and indeed may have biopsy confirmation of the presence of KS, bronchoscopic biopsy is frequently unnecessary. Endobronchial lesions can be biopsied with safety although in one series 30% had haemorrhage[110]. Diagnostic yield from endobronchial biopsy is generally poor, possibly because of the submucosal location of the lesions (10–20%).

Similarly, transbronchial biopsy produces low diagnostic yields, possibly because of the patchy distribution of KS within the lung parenchyma. Also, on the small samples obtained from the lung by biopsy, it may be difficult for the histopathologist to give an unequivocal diagnosis. The main value of bronchoscopy with bronchoalveolar lavage, with or without added transbronchial biopsy, in patients suspected of pulmonary KS is in excluding concomitant opportunist infections or, if lung biopsy is done, other non-infectious complications of pulmonary AIDS such as NIP.

In the majority of patients bronchoscopy provides supportive evidence that pulmonary disease is due to KS, as evidenced by the presence of endobronchial lesions, and concomitant opportunist infections can be excluded. However, if endobronchial lesions are not present and it is necessary to confirm the diagnosis, it may occasionally be necessary to perform either thoracoscopic or open lung biopsy. In patients with mediastinal lymphadenopathy, where the diagnosis cannot be made by other means,

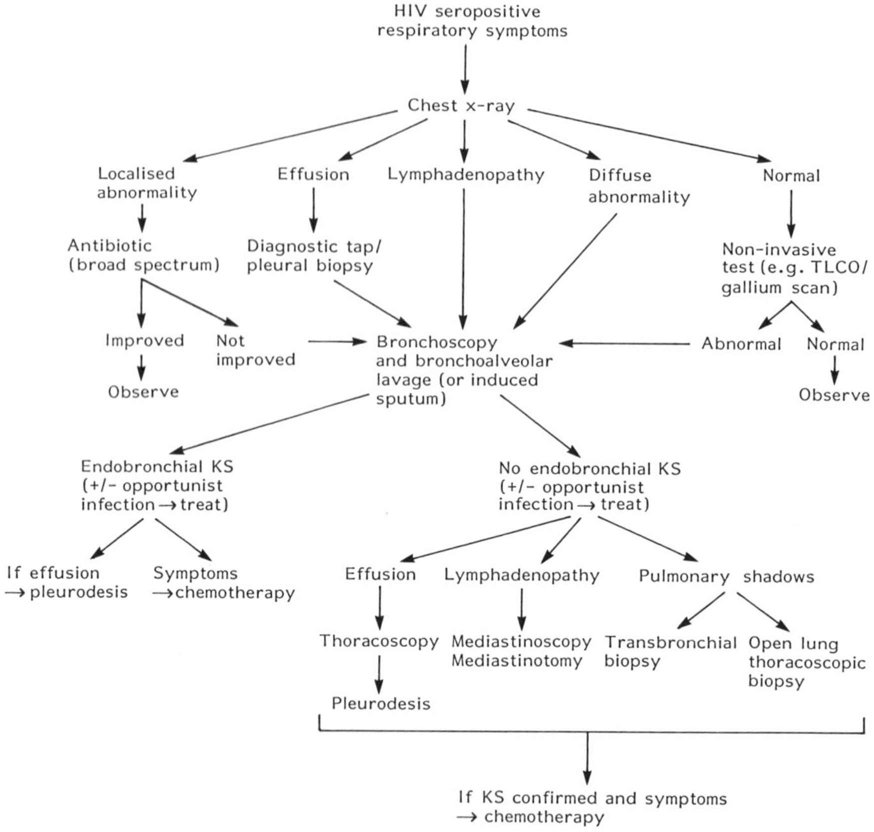

Figure 10.5 *Diagnostic algorithm for pulmonary diseases and KS in HIV-seropositive individuals*

mediastinoscopy may be necessary. Thoracoscopy may be required for the diagnosis of recurrent pleural effusions where the other causes cannot be excluded by routine laboratory investigations including culture.

Alveolar haemorrhage has been described at postmortem and in open lung biopsy samples from patients with pulmonary KS, and it has been suggested that haemosiderin-containing macrophages in lavage fluid obtained at bronchoscopy is suggestive of pulmonary KS[111]. In one study, six of nine patients with pulmonary KS had evidence of haemorrhage in the lavage fluid which was not present in 75 other patients with diagnoses including tuberculosis and CMV. However, in a further study[112], 16 of 23 patients with KS had occult alveolar haemorrhage, and a further 40 patients had alternative diagnoses including *Pneumocystis* pneumonia or bacterial pneumonia. Eighteen of these patients also had evidence of occult alveolar haemorrhage as evidenced by the presence of haemosiderin-containing macrophages. Pleural effusion aspirate due to pulmonary KS normally reveals serosanguineous fluid although clear fluid may be obtained and transudates have been reported in hypoalbuminaemic patients. Closed-needle pleural biopsy rarely provides diagnostic information as the parietal pleural is normally not involved in pulmonary KS.

A diagnosis of pulmonary involvement by KS is usually suggested by the presence of KS lesions on other sites; Figure 10.5 shows a scheme for diagnosis.

Treatment

Pulmonary KS is often seen in the context of other HIV-related diseases within the same patient, in particular the opportunist infections that characterize AIDS, so that in treating these patients general measures will include treating any concomitant opportunist infection in the lung or at other sites. Prophylactic measures to prevent *Pneumocystis* pneumonia, tuberculosis and severe pneumococcal infection should be taken as most patients with pulmonary KS have low CD4 peripheral blood lymphocyte counts and are therefore particularly susceptible to these infections. Similarly most patients with pulmonary KS will be on antiretroviral therapy with zidovudine or another agent.

Pulmonary KS is generally difficult to treat as it often represents more aggressive systemic disease or late-stage disease. Treatment of pleural effusions, which may be large, can be problematic. They may be due to either KS involving the visceral pleura or to lymphatic obstruction. They may also occur as a late manifestation of extensive parenchymal disease; chemical pleurodesis is not always successful and radiotherapy is of limited value only[97]. Radiotherapy has been used to a limited extent for palliative treatment of extensive pulmonary KS[113,114]. Improvements in symptoms such as severe haemoptysis and breathlessness have been reported and radiotherapy may be of particular value in patients who tolerate chemotherapy poorly.

Chemotherapy

Early studies showed that it was possible to palliate symptoms due to respiratory involvement with single-agent etoposide, vincristine, vinblastine or doxorubicin[115,116]. Interferon α, which has been used successfully to treat cutaneous lesions of KS, is not so effective for visceral disease and the toxicity from the high doses required is generally unacceptable[117,118]. The prognosis for patients with pulmonary KS without treatment is very poor, with a mean survival of only three months from diagnosis[100]. Combination chemotherapy with bleomycin, vincristine and doxorubicin has resulted in improved results. In a more recent study, 20 patients with pulmonary KS were treated with two weekly cycles of bleomycin 10 mg/m^2 and vincristine 2 mg. Doxorubicin 20 mg/m^2 was added to this regimen for patients with severe disease. Twelve patients had a partial or complete response and their median survival was 12 months. The eight patients who did not respond had a median survival of only six months. In this study, short survival was associated with pleural effusion or a CD4 lymphocyte count of less than 0.1×10^9/l[102,119]. A further study employed vincristine and bleomycin with zidovudine and produced partial or complete responses in about 80% of patients treated[120].

However, treatment responses using chemotherapy are relatively short lived and combination chemotherapy provides palliation only. It should be used only for symptomatic pulmonary KS, namely progressive breathlessness with cough. A major problem with chemotherapy in this context is with myelotoxicity resulting in further immune suppression and therefore likelihood of severe opportunist infections. Over half of patients with pulmonary KS in fact die as a result of overwhelming infection and/or drug-induced complications, so that a decision to treat with chemotherapy must be carefully considered with these aspects in mind and weighed against the severity of symptoms which are to be treated[87,101,102,116,120,121]. There are several reports of the effects of combination chemotherapy on pulmonary KS, but precise evaluation of these results is difficult as different regimens are used. Furthermore pulmonary KS is difficult to stage, adding further difficulties to comparison of results[87,101,102,116,120,121]. A general conclusion from these studies is that major improvements in symptoms occur in the majority of patients treated but complete X-ray resolution is less frequently observed. Beneficial effects tend to be short lived, so that chemotherapy has to be repeated normally every three to four weeks to maintain improvement.

Median survival rates reported with chemotherapy range between six and nine months. In a recent study[101] 30 AIDS patients with symptomatic pulmonary KS were evaluated following careful classification and staging, all patients had proven pulmonary KS. They received adriamycin 30 mg/m^2, bleomycin 10 mg/m^2 and vincristine 2 mg intravenously every four weeks. All patients complained of breathlessness, most also had cough and half had chest pain. All patients were taking cotrimoxazole or dapsone for prophylaxis against *Pneumocystis* pneumonia, and zidovudine dosage was either reduced or the drug stopped for 10 days of each chemotherapy cycle to minimize toxicity. Two patients died during the first chemotherapy cycle. In the remaining 28 patients, dyspnoea and PaO_2 improved, whereas in 11 there was no improvement in the chest X-ray appearance and in 17 there was minimal improvement only. The median survival from starting chemotherapy was 6.5 months; the longest survival was for 23 months. The cause of death was identified in 25 patients: 12 died of respiratory failure due to pulmonary KS, 10 died from respiratory infection and three died from extrapulmonary opportunist infections. Poor prognostic features were absence of cutaneous KS, previous opportunist infection, CD4 lymphocyte count less than $0.1x10^9/l$, leucocyte count less than $3.5 \times 10^9/l$, haemoglobin less than 10 g/dl and absence of radiological response. Survival was not associated with previous treatment of cutaneous KS, presence of pleural effusion, degree of hypoxaemia, platelet count or the use of adjuvant steroids during the first court of chemotherapy or to the extent of improvement in PaO_2 after the first course of chemotherapy. Twenty-four of 28 patients had at least one episode of neutropenia, which was associated with a bacterial infection in 16 cases. Three patients had a febrile reaction to bleomycin, two developed peripheral neuropathy (vincristine) and one developed asymptomatic cardiomyopathy (adriamycin). The authors concluded that chemotherapy resulted in good symptomatic improvement despite absence of radiological improvement, high incidence of neutropenia and bacterial infection related to chemotherapy and poor overall survival, with about half dying of pulmonary KS itself rather than other causes such as infection[101].

CONCLUSION

Pulmonary KS may be difficult to diagnose as it may be associated with other pulmonary disorders, in particular pulmonary opportunist infections. Combination chemotherapy provides effective palliation for symptomatic disease but the effects are short lived and median survival remains poor despite treatment. Chemotherapy is often limited by myelotoxicity, which may in the future be partially circumvented by the use of haematological growth factors administered with chemotherapy such as granulocyte colony-stimulating factor and granulocyte–macrophage colony-stimulating factor[122,123].

REFERENCES

1. Murray JF, Mills J. Pulmonary infectious complications of human immunodeficiency virus infection. *Am Rev Respir Dis* 1990; 141: 1356–1372.
2. Mitchell DM, Miller RF. Recent developments in the management of the pulmonary complications of HIV disease. *Thorax* 1992; 47: 381–390.
3. Miller RF, Mitchell DM. *Pneumocystis carinii* pneumonia. AIDS and the Lung. Update 1992. *Thorax* 1992; 47: 305–314.
4. Wallace JM, Rao AV, Glassroth J *et al.* Respiratory illnesses in persons with HIV infection. *Am Rev Respir Dis* 1993; 148: 1523–1529.
5. Pulmonary Complications of HIV Infection Study Group. The prospective study of pulmonary complications of HIV infection. *J Clin Epidemiol* 1993; 46: 497–507.
6. Shaw RJ, Roussak C, Forster SM *et al.* Lung function abnormalities in patients infected with the human immunodeficiency virus with and without overt pneumonitis. *Thorax* 1988; 43: 436–404.
7. Stover DE, White DA, Roman PA *et al.* Spectrum of pulmonary diseases associated with AIDS. *Am J Med* 1985; 74: 429–437.

8. Suffredini AF, Ognibene FP, Lack EE. Nonspecific interstitial pneumonitis: a common cause of pulmonary disease in AIDS. *Ann Intern Med* 1987; 107: 7–13.
9. Coleman DL, Dodek PM, Golden JA *et al.* Correlation between serial pulmonary function tests and fibre-optic bronchoscopy in patients with pneumocystis pneumonia and AIDS. *Am Rev Respir Dis* 1984; 129: 491–493.
10. Murphy M, Fox C, Travis W *et al.* AIDS may present as severe restrictive lung disease. *Am J Med* 1989; 86: 237–240.
11. Meduri GU, Stover DE, Lee M *et al.* Pulmonary Kaposi's sarcoma in AIDS: clinical, radiological and pathological manifestations. *Am J Med* 1986; 81: 11–18.
12. Rosen MJ, Tow TW, Teirstein AS *et al.* Diagnosis of pulmonary complications of AIDS. *Thorax* 1985; 40: 571–575.
13. Camus F, de Picciotto C, Gerbe J *et al.* Pulmonary function tests in HIV-infected patients. *AIDS* 1993; 7: 1075–1079.
14. Mitchell DM, Fleming JP, Pinching AJ *et al.* Pulmonary function in HIV infection: a prospective 18 month study of serial lung function in 474 patients. *Am Rev Respir Dis* 1992; 146: 745–751.
15. French PD, Cunningham DA, Fleming J *et al.* Low carbon monoxide transfer factor (TLCO) in HIV infected patients without lung disease. *Resp Med* 1992; 86: 253–256.
16. Nieman RB, Fleming J, Coker RJ *et al.* Reduced carbon monoxide transfer factor (TLCO) in HIV-1 infection as a predictor for faster progression to AIDS. *Thorax* 1993; 48: 481–485.
17. Clarke JR, Fleming J, Nieman R *et al.* Effect of HIV-1 and cytomegalovirus in broncho-alveolar lavage cells on the transfer factor for lung carbon monoxide in AIDS patients. *AIDS* 1991; 5: 1333–1338.
18. Plata F, Autran B, Martins LP. AIDS virus specific cytotoxic T-lymphocytes in lung disorders. *Nature* 1987; 328: 348–351.
19. Meigan M, Guillon JM, Denis M. Increased lung epithelial permeability in HIV infected patients with isolated cytoxic T-lymphocyte alveolitis. *Am Rev Respir Dis* 1990; 40: 65–91.
20. Guillon JM, Autran B, Denis M. Human immunodeficiency virus related lymphocyte alveolitis. *Chest* 1988; 94: 1264–1270.
21. Pitkin AD, Grant AD, Foley NM, Miller RF. Changing patterns of respiratory disease in HIV positive patients in a referral centre in the United Kingdom between 1986–7 and 1990–1. *Thorax* 1993; 48: 204–207.
22. Edman JC, Kovacs JA, Masur H *et al.* Ribosomal RNA sequences show *Pneumocystis carinni* to be a member of the fungi. *Nature* 1988; 334: 519–522.
23. Tu JV, Biem HJ, Detsky AS. Bronchoscopy versus empirical therapy in HIV infected patients with presumptive *Pneumocystis carinii* pneumonia: a decision analysis. *Am Rev Respir Dis* 1993; 148: 370–377.
24. Miller RF, Mitchell DM. AIDS and the lung: update 1995. *Pneumocystis carinii* pneumonia. *Thorax* 1995; 50: 191–200.
25. Jeffrey AA, Bullen C, Miller RF. Intensive care management of *Pneumocystis carinii* pneumonia. *Crit Care III* 1993; 9: 258–260.
26. Selwyn PA, Feingold AR, Harte D. Increased risk of bacterial pneumonia in HIV-infected intravenous drug users without AIDS. *AIDS* 1988; 2: 267–272.
27. Janoff EN, Breiman RF, Daley CU, Hopewell PC. Pneumococcal disease during HIV infection: epidemiologic, clinical and immunologic perspectives. *Ann Intern Med* 1992; 117: 314–324.
28. Levine SJ, White DA, Fels AOS. The incidence and significance of *Straphylococcus aureus* in respiratory cultures from patients infected with HIV. *Am Rev Respir Dis* 1990; 141: 89–93.

29. Baron AD, Hollander H. *Pseudomonas aeruginosa* bronchopulmonary infection in late human immunodeficiency virus disease. *Am Rev Respir Dis* 1993; 148: 992–996.
30. Joseph J, Strange C, Sahn SA. Pleural effusions in hospitalised patients with AIDS. *Ann Intern Med* 1993; 118: 856–859.
31. Sample S, Lenahan GF, Secowonska MH. Allergic diseases and sinusitis in acquired immune deficiency syndrome. *J Allergy Clin Immunol* 1989; 83: 190.
32. Zurco JJ, Feuerstein I, Lebovics R, Lane AC. Sinusitis in HIV-infection. *Am J Med* 1992; 93: 157–162.
33. Godofsky EW, Zinreich J, Armstrong M *et al*. Sinusitis in HIV-infected patients: a clinical and radiographic review. *Am J Med* 1992; 93: 163–170.
34. Fitzgerald JM, Gryzbowski S, Allen EA. The impact of human immunodeficiency virus infection on tuberculosis and its control. *Chest* 1991; 100: 191–200.
35. Styblo K, Enarson DA. The impact of infection with human immunodeficiency virus on tuberculosis. In Mitchell DM (ed.) *Recent Advances in Respiratory Medicine 5*. Edinburgh: Churchill Livingstone, 1991; pp. 147–162.
36. Harries AD. Tuberculosis and human immunodeficiency virus infection in developing countries. *Lancet* 1990; 335: 387–389.
37. Selwyn PA, Hartel D, Lewis VA. A prospective study of the risk of tuberculosis among intravenous drug users with human immunodeficiency virus infection. *N Engl J Med* 1989; 320: 545–550.
38. Chaisson RE, Schecter GF, Thener CP. Tuberculosis as a manifestation of the acquired immunodeficiency syndrome. *Am Rev Respir Dis* 1987; 136: 570–574.
39. Sunderam G, McDonald RJ, Maniatis T. Tuberculosis as a manifestation of the acquired immunodeficiency syndrome (AIDS). *JAMA* 1986; 256: 362–366.
40. Pesanti EL. The negative tuberculin test: tuberculin, HIV and anergy panels. *Am J Respir Crit Care Med* 1994; 149: 1699–1709.
41. Long R, Maycher B, Scalcini M. The chest roentgenogram in pulmonary tuberculosis patients seropositive for human immunodeficiency virus type I. *Chest* 1991; 99: 123–127.
42. Brindle RJ, Nunn PP, Githui W *et al*. Quantitative bacillary response to treatment in HIV-associated pulmonary tuberculosis. *Am Rev Respir Dis* 1993; 147: 958–961.
43. Small PM, Schecter GF, Goodman PC *et al*. Treatment of tuberculosis in patients with advanced human immunodeficiency virus infection. *N Engl J Med* 1991; 324: 289–294.
44. Pape JW, Jean SS, Ho JL *et al*. Effect of isoniazid prophylaxis on incidence of active tuberculosis and progression of HIV infection. *Lancet* 1993; 342: 268–272.
45. Centres for Disease Control. Transmission of multidrug-resistant tuberculosis from an HIV-positive client in a residential substance-abuse treatment facility—Michigan. *MMWR* 1991; 40: 129–131.
46. Kent RJ, Uttley AHC, Stoker NG *et al*. Transmission of tuberculosis in a British Centre for patients infected with HIV. *Lancet* 1994; 308: 639–640.
47. Edlin BR, Tokars JI, Grieco MH *et al*. An outbreak of multidrug-resistant tuberculosis among hospitalized patients with the acquired immunodeficiency syndrome. *N Engl J Med* 1992; 326: 1514–1521.
48. Fischl MA, Uttamchandani RB, Daikos GL *et al*. An outbreak of tuberculosis caused by multidrug resistant tubercle bacilli among patients with HIV infection. *Ann Intern Med* 1992; 117: 177–183.
49. Frieden TR, Sterling T, Pablos-Mendez A *et al*. The emergence of drug resistant tuberculosis in New York City. *N Engl J Med* 1993; 328: 521–526.
50. Fischl MA, Daikos GL, Uttamchandani RB *et al*. Clinical presentation and outcome of patients with HIV infection and tuberculosis caused by multiple drug resistant bacilli. *Ann Intern Med* 1992; 117: 184–190.

51. Pearson ML, Jereb JA, Friedan TR *et al.* Nosocomial transmission of multidrug-resistant *Mycobacterium* tuberculosis: a risk to patients and health care workers. *Ann Intern Med* 1992; 117: 191–196.
52. Iseman MD. Treatment of multidrug resistant tuberculosis. *N Engl J Med* 1993; 329: 784–791.
53. Masur H. Recommendations in prophylaxis and therapy for disseminated *Mycobacterium avium* complex disease in patients infected with HIV. *N Engl J Med* 1993; 329: 898–904.
54. Horsburgh CR, Havlik JA, Ellis DA *et al.* Survival of patients with AIDS and disseminated *Mycobacterium avium* complex infection with and without anti-mycobacterial chemotherapy. *Am Rev Respir Dis* 1991; 144: 557–559.
55. Kemper CA, Meng TC, Nussbaum J *et al.* Treatment of *Mycobacterium avium* complex: bacteraemia in AIDS with a four drug oral regimen. *Ann Intern Med* 1992; 116: 466–472.
56. Nightingale SD, Cameron DW, Gordin FM *et al.* Two controlled trials of Rifabutin prophylaxis against *Mycobacterium avium* complex infection in AIDS. *N Engl J Med* 1993; 329: 828–833.
57. Hoover DR, Graham NMH, Bacellar H. Epidemiologic patterns of upper respiratory illness and *Pneumocystis carinii* pneumonia in homosexual men. *Am Rev Respir Dis* 1991; 183: 604–605.
58. Murray J, Mills J. State of the art: pulmonary infections, complications of HIV part I. *Am Rev Respir Dis* 1990; 141: 1356–1372.
59. Murray J, Mills J. State of the art: pulmonary infections, complications of HIV part II. *Am Rev Respir Dis* 1990; 141: 1582–1598.
60. Drew WL. Cytomegalovirus infection in patients with AIDS. *Clin Infect Dis* 1992; 14: 608–615.
61. Squire SB, Lipman MCI, Bagdades EK *et al.* Severe cytomegalovirus pneumonitis in HIV infected patients with higher than average CD4 counts. *Thorax* 1992; 47: 301–304.
62. Miller RF, Lucas SB, Pinching AJ. Disseminated histoplasmosis in patients with acquired immunodeficiency syndrome. *Genitourin Med* 1994; 70: 132–137.
63. Supparatpingo K, Khamwan C, Baosoung V *et al.* Disseminated *Penicillium marneffei* infection in South East Asia. *Lancet* 1994; 344: 110–113.
64. Pitkin AD, Grant AD, Foley NM, Miller RF. Changing patterns of respiratory disease in HIV positive patients in a referral centre in the United Kingdom between 1986–7 and 1990–1. *Thorax* 1993; 48: 204–207.
65. Suffredini A, Ognibene F, Lack E. Non-specific interstitial pneumonitis: a common cause of pulmonary disease in the acquired immunodeficiency syndrome. *Ann Intern Med* 1987; 107: 7–13.
66. Ramaswamy G, Jagadha V, Tchertkoff V. Diffuse alveolar damage and interstitial fibrosis in acquired immunodeficiency syndrome patients without concurrent pulmonary infection. *Arch Pathol Lab Med* 1985; 109: 408–412.
67. Ognibene FP, Masur H, Rogers P *et al.* Non-specific interstitial pneumonitis without evidence of *Pneumocystis carinii* in asymptomatic patients infected with HIV. *Ann Intern Med* 1988; 109: 874–879.
68. Stover DE, White DA, Romano PA *et al.* Spectrum of pulmonary diseases associated with the acquired immune deficiency syndrome. *Am J Med* 1985; 78: 429–437.
69. Simmons JT, Suffredini AF, Lack EE *et al.* Non-specific interstitial pneumonitis in patients with AIDS: radiological features. *AJR* 1987; 149: 265–268.
70. Teirstein A, Rosen M. Lymphocytic interstitial pneumonia. *Clin Chest Med* 1988; 9: 467–471.

71. Tirelli U, Franceschi S, Carbone A. Malignant tumours in patients with HIV infection. *Br Med J* 1994; 308: 1148–1153.
72. Zeigler JL, Beckstead JA, Volberding PA *et al.* Non-Hodgkin's lymphoma in 90 homosexual men. *N Engl J Med* 1984; 311: 565–570.
73. Kaplan LD, Abrams DI, Feigal E *et al.* AIDS-associated non-Hodgkin's lymphoma in San Francisco. *JAMA* 1989; 261: 719–724.
74. Sider L, Weiss JA, Smith MD. Varied appearance of AIDS-related lymphoma in the Chest. *Radiology* 1989; 171: 629–632.
75. Chaouat A, Fraisse P, Kessler R *et al.* A life threatening tracheal localization of lymphoma in a patient with AIDS. *Chest* 1993; 103: 1297–1299.
76. Keys TC, Judson MA, Reed CE, Sahn SA. Endobronchial HIV associated lymphoma. *Thorax* 1994; 49: 525–526.
77. Poelzleitner D, Huebsch P, Mayerhofer S *et al.* Primary pulmonary lymphoma in a patient with the acquired immune deficiency syndrome. *Thorax* 1989; 44: 438–439.
78. Cottrill CP, Moxham J, Gallimore AP *et al.* AIDS related primary intrathoracic lymphoma. *Genitourin Med* 1992; 68: 235–240.
79. Rabkin CS, Hilgartner MW, Hed Berg KW *et al.* Incidence of lymphomas and other cancers in HIV-infected and HIV-uninfected patients with haemophilia. *JAMA* 1992; 267: 1090–1094.
80. Braun MA, Killam DA, Remick SC, Ruckdeschal J. Lung cancer in patients seropositive for human immundeficiency virus. *Radiology* 1990; 175: 341–343.
81. Karp J, Profeta G, Marantz PR, Karpel JP. Lung cancer in patients with immunodeficiency syndrome. *Chest* 1993; 103: 410–413.
82. Fraire AE, Awe RJ. Lung cancer associated with human immunodeficiency virus infection. *Cancer* 1992; 70: 432–436.
83. Sidhar KS, Flores MR, Raub WA, Saldana M. Lung cancer in patients with human immunodeficiency virus infection compared to historical control subjects. *Chest* 1992; 102: 170–173.
84. Centres for Disease Control. Update: acquired immunodeficiency syndrome (AIDS)—United States. *MMWR* 1986; 35: 17–21.
85. Haverkar HW, Drotman DP, Morgan M. Prevalence of Kaposi's sarcoma among patients with AIDS. *N Engl J Med* 1985; 313: 1518.
86. Jarlais DC, Marmor M, Thomas P. Kaposi's sarcoma among four different AIDS risk groups. *N Engl J Med* 1984; 310: 1119.
87. Garay S, Belenko M, Fazzini E, Schinella R. Pulmonary manifestations of Kaposi's sarcoma. *Chest* 1987; 91: 39–43.
88. Pozniak A, Latif A, Neill P *et al.* Pulmonary Kaposi's sarcoma in Africa. *Thorax* 1992; 47: 730–733.
89. Ognibene F, Steis R, Macher A *et al.* Kaposi's sarcoma causing pulmonary infiltrates and respiratory failure in the acquired immunodeficiency syndrome. *Ann Intern Med* 1985; 102: 471–475.
90. Meduri G, Stover D, Lee M *et al.* Pulmonary Kaposi's sarcoma in the acquired immune deficiency syndrome. *Am J Med* 1986; 81: 11–18.
91. Mitchell DM, McCarty M, Fleming J, Moss F. Bronchopulmonary Kaposi's sarcoma in patients with AIDS. *Thorax* 1992; 47: 726–729.
92. Cadranel J, Chouaid C, Denis M *et al.* Causes of pleural effusion in 75 HIV-infected patients. *Chest* 1993; 104: 655.
93. O'Brien R, Cohn D. Serosanguineous pleural effusions in AIDS-associated Kaposi's sarcoma. *Chest* 1989; 96: 460–466.
94. Talavera W, Wasser L, Villamena P. Primary pleuropulmonary Kaposi's sarcoma in AIDS (abstract). *Am Rev Respir Dis* 1988; 137: A287.
95. Bach MC, Bagwell SP, Fanning JP. Primary pulmonary Kaposi's sarcoma in the

acquired immunodeficiency syndrome: a cause of persistent pyrexia. *Am J Med* 1988; 85: 274–275.

96. Stover D, White D, Romano P *et al.* Spectrum of pulmonary disease associated with acquired immune deficiency syndrome. *Am J Med* 1985; 78: 429–437.
97. O'Brien RF. Pulmonary and pleural Kaposi's sarcoma in AIDS. *Semin Respir Med* 1989; 10: 12–20.
98. Greenberg JE, Fischl MA, Berger JR. Upper airway obstruction secondary to acquired immunodeficiency syndrome-related Kaposi's sarcoma. *Chest* 1985; 88: 638–640.
99. Silver MA, Macher AM, Reichert C. Cardiac involvement by Kaposi's sarcoma in acquired immunodeficiency syndrome (AIDS). *Am J Cardiol* 1984; 53: 983–986.
100. White D, Matthay R. Non-infectious pulmonary complications of infection with human immunodeficiency virus. *Am Rev Respir Dis* 1989; 140: 1763–1787.
101. Candranel J, Kammoun S, Chevret S *et al.* Results of chemotherapy in 30 AIDS patients with symptomatic pulmonary Kaposi's sarcoma. *Thorax* 1994; 49: 101–103.
102. Gill P, Akil B, Colletti P *et al.* Pulmonary Kaposi's sarcoma: clinical findings and results of therapy. *Am J Med* 1989; 87: 57–61.
103. Miller R, Tomlinson M, Cottrill C *et al.* Bronchopulmonary Kaposi's sarcoma in patients with AIDS. *Thorax* 1992; 47: 721–725.
104. Naidich D, Tarras M, Garay S *et al.* Kaposi's sarcoma: CT–radiographic correlation. *Chest* 1989; 96: 723–728.
105. Sivit C, Schwartz A, Rockoff S. Kaposi's sarcoma of the lung in AIDS: radiologic–pathologic analysis. *AJR* 1987; 148: 25–28.
106. Zibrak J, Silvestri R, Costello P *et al.* Bronchoscopic and radiologic features of Kaposi's sarcoma involving the respiratory system. *Chest* 1986; 90: 476–479.
107. Wolff S, Kuhlman J, Fishman E. Thoracic Kaposi's sarcoma in AIDS: CT findings. *J Comput Assist Tomogr* 1993; 17: 60–62.
108. Woolfenden J, Carrasquillo J, Larsen S. Acquired immunodeficiency syndrome. Ga-67 citrate imaging. *Radiology* 1987; 162: 383–387.
109. Hamm PG, Judson MA, Aranda CP. Diagnosis of pulmonary Kaposi's sarcoma with fibre-optic bronchoscopy and endobronchial biopsy. *Cancer* 1987; 59: 807–810.
110. Pitchenik AE, Fischl MA, Saldanda MJ. Kaposi's sarcoma of the tracheobronchial tree. *Chest* 1985; 87: 122–124.
111. Touboul JL, Mayaud CM, Fouret P. Pulmonary lesions in Kaposi's sarcoma, intra-alveolar haemorrhage and pleural effusion. *Ann Intern Med* 1985; 103: 808.
112. Hugues-Davies L, Kocjan G, Spittle M, Miller R. Occult alveolar haemorrhage in bronchopulmonary Kaposi's sarcoma. *J Clin Pathol* 1992; 45: 536–537.
113. Meyer J. Whole-lung irradiation for Kaposi's sarcoma. *Am J Clin Oncol* 1993; 16: 371–376.
114. Doyal M, Johnstone P, Watkins E. Role of radiation therapy in management of pulmonary Kaposi's sarcoma. *South Med J* 1993; 86: 285–288.
115. Volberding PA. Kaposi's sarcoma and the acquired immunodeficiency syndrome. *Med Clin North Am* 1986; 70: 665–675.
116. Laubenstein L, Krigel R, Odajnyk C *et al.* Treatment of epidemic Kaposi's sarcoma with etoposide or a combination of doxorubicin, bleomycin and vinblastin. *J Clin Oncol* 1984; 2: 1115–1120.
117. Krigel R, Slywotzky C, Lonbert M. Treatment of epidemic Kaposi's sarcoma with a combination of interferon-alpha 2b and etoposide. *J Biol Response Mod* 1988; 7: 359–364.
118. Shepherd F, Evans W, Garvey B. Combination chemotherapy and interferon in

the treatment of Kaposi's sarcoma associated with the acquired immunodeficiency syndrome. *Can Med Assoc J* 1988; 139: 635–639.
119. Gill P, Rarick M, Espina B *et al.* Advanced acquired immune deficiency syndrome-related Kaposi's sarcoma. *Cancer* 1990; 65: 1074–1078.
120. Gelmann E, Longo D, Lane H *et al.* Combination chemotherapy of disseminated Kaposi's sarcoma in patients with the acquired immune deficiency syndrome. *Am J Med* 1987; 82: 456–462.
121. Gill P, Rarick M, McCutchan J *et al.* Systemic treatment of AIDS-related Kaposi's sarcoma: results of a randomized trial. *Am J Med* 1991; 90: 427–433.
122. Gill P, Bernstein-Singer M, Espina B *et al.* Adriamycin, bleomycin and vincristine chemotherapy with recombinant granulocyte–macrophage colony-stimulating factor for the treatment of AIDS-related Kaposi's sarcoma. *AIDS* 1992; 6: 1477–1481.
123. Sloand E, Kumar P, Pierce P. Chemotherapy for patients' pulmonary Kaposi's: benefit of filgrastim (G-CSF) in supporting dose administration. *South Med J* 1993; 86: 1219–1224.

11

Disorders of the Kidneys in AIDS Patients

Theodoros D. Mountokalakis

Athens Medical School, Sotiria Hospital, Athens, Greece

INTRODUCTION

The epidemic of acquired immunodeficiency syndrome (AIDS) appeared in North America and Western Europe in the late 1970s. Its subsequent spread worldwide not only had a tremendous social and ethical impact, but also led to considerable changes in the everyday practice of medicine. Since human immunodeficiency virus (HIV) preferentially invades and depletes circulating CD4 lymphocytes, it is not unexpected that infections and neoplasms are the dominant clinical manifestations of the disease. However, during the last few years it has become increasingly evident that infection with the virus may result in multisystem involvement beyond the immune system. Although parenchymal involvement of solid abdominal organs, such as the liver, the spleen and the pancreas, has been well described in patients with AIDS[1], less attention has been paid to the renal sequelae of this disease. It is noteworthy that because of the fact that a variety of non-specific renal and electrolyte abnormalities occur in patients with AIDS[2], and perhaps, because of the general assumption that the kidney is not a 'target' organ for the replication or dissemination of HIV, the first reports about the existence of a specific AIDS-associated nephropathy, only a few years after the first description of the syndrome, were treated with scepticism. Today, as the doubt over the new clinicopathological entity fades and the number of AIDS patients with renal disease increases, recognition of the spectrum of renal disorders complicating HIV infection becomes particularly important.

AIDS and Malignancies: Current Concepts and Perspectives.
Edited by B.C. Golematis and V.T. DeVita Jr

WHAT IS AIDS-ASSOCIATED NEPHROPATHY?

The term AIDS-associated nephropathy was used for the first time in 1984 to describe a particular form of rapidly progressive focal and segmental glomerulosclerosis (FSGS) occurring in clusters of blacks with AIDS in New York and Miami[3–5]. Following the advent of serological studies to detect HIV infection, the term has been changed to HIV-associated nephropathy (HIVAN)[6].

Not long after the report of the first cases, a controversy was established when workers from San Francisco, the city with the highest number of AIDS cases per capita in the USA, were unable to confirm in their patients, consisting mainly of homosexual or bisexual white men, the occurrence of the specific nephropathy reported from New York and Miami[7]. Because intravenous drug abuse was common among patients with HIVAN, the group in San Francisco suggested that the nephropathy seen in the black patients with AIDS might be ascribed almost exclusively to heroin-associated nephropathy (HAN), a form of focal glomerulosclerosis recognized in intravenous drug addicts several years before AIDS[8]. However, an analysis of specific risk factors for renal disease in HIV infection demonstrated that although heroin addicts were clearly a majority, a considerable proportion of patients with HIVAN (47%) comprised non-addicts[9]. Moreover, FSGS associated with clinical manifestations similar to those observed in adults with HIVAN was also described in children[10], in whom intravenous drug abuse can be unquestionably excluded. Advocates of the new type of nephropathy provided criteria to separate the two entities both on clinical and pathological basis. They indicated that renal size is normal to large and progression to end-stage renal disease is rapid in HIVAN, whereas shrinkage of kidney size and a gradual deterioration of renal function over years characterize the natural history of HAN[6]. On the other hand, a logical assumption would be that HIV infection superimposed to drug addiction can exert an additive effect in inducing a more fulminant progression to end-stage renal disease[11].

The characteristic glomerular lesion in HIVAN is similar to other forms of FSGS, including HAN. More specifically, the histological pattern is one of the so-called 'collapsing variants' of FSGS[12]. This term emphasizes the fact that the endocapillary space is reduced by implosive retraction of the glomerular capillary walls ('collapse'), resulting in the loss of patency of glomerular capillary lumina. Glomerular capillaries are often crowned by a row of hypertrophic visceral epithelial cells with numerous Schiff-positive protein resorption droplets in their vacuolized cytoplasm[13]. Mesangial hyperplasia is believed to predominate in early lesions when changes of FSGS are minor[13], while hypocellularity of the glomerular mesangium characterizes the typical forms of the disease[9,14]. Tubular degeneration, microcytic dilatation of renal tubules, and prominent interstitial inflammation characterized by a lymphocytic and plasma cell infiltrate, oedema and fibrosis are common features[3]. Routine immunofluorescence reveals immunoglobulin M (IgM), C3, and C1 localized predominantly to segments of glomerular sclerosis and less frequently to the mesangium[15]. Tubuloreticular inclusions involving glomerular endothelial cells, interstitial capillary endothelial cells, interstitial leucocytes, electron-dense deposits, and effacement of foot processes are demonstrated by electron microscopy[15].

A common initial clinical presentation of HIVAN is the nephrotic syndrome. Patients have massive proteinuria of greater than 3.5 g/day, oedema and serum albumin less than 2.5 g/dl accompanied by either normal glomerular filtration rate or varying degrees of renal insufficiency. Occasionally, patients with HIVAN present with microscopic or gross haematuria associated with mild proteinuria. Typically, the clinical course of HIVAN is one of a rapid deterioration of renal function leading to end-stage renal disease in a few weeks or months. In contrast to other forms of glomerulosclerosis, severe hypertension is rare. Mortality in patients with HIVAN and end-stage renal disease is high in spite of renal replacement therapy[6,13].

Of all HIVAN cases reported until 1989, more than 70% were blacks, and only about 13% were whites[6]. During the last decades, epidemiological studies have provided evidence that black race is a risk factor for FSGS and, in particular, for the more malignant forms of the disease, including hypertensive nephrosclerosis[16] and HAN[17]. More recently, a similar strong black racial predilection was reported in the so-called 'collapsing variant' of idiopathic FSGS, which is also characterized by a rapid progression to renal failure[12]. These observations have prompted the suggestion that genetic factors may be important in the pathogenesis of the lesion. An increased prevalence of certain human leucocyte antigen (HLA) haplotypes has been reported among patients with HAN and idiopathic FSGS[18]. Up to now, such genetic analyses have not been reported in HIVAN.

Is there a causative relationship between HIV and the particular nephropathy seen in HIV-infected patients? Though not specific of HIV infection, ultrastructural changes described in HIVAN, such as tubuloreticular inclusions in glomerular capillary endothelial cells[15], are generally regarded as morphological markers of viral infection[13]. In addition, using *in situ* hybridization and immunohistochemistry, Cohen *et al.*[19] demonstrated HIV p24 antigen and proviral HIV DNA localized to glomerular and tubular epithelium in kidneys from patients with HIVAN, but not from those who had HIV without renal disease. More recently, Kimmel *et al.*[20] microdissected renal biopsy material obtained from HIV-infected patients with and without typical HIVAN and performed DNA polymerase chain reaction (PCR). They detected proviral nucleic acid within glomeruli, tubules and infiltrating inflammatory cells, but not within interstitial cells. These findings are consistent with the presence of intact provirus within renal cells. Alternatively, they may be the result of vascular proximity, or contamination by circulating HIV-infected lymphocytes or HIV-infected inflammatory cells[21]. Further evidence supporting a direct infection of glomerular cells by HIV was provided by experiments in which homogeneous cultures of human glomerular capillary endothelial, mesangial and epithelial cells were exposed to HIV *in vitro*. HIV was found to infect and replicate in glomerular endothelial and mesangial cells, but not in glomerular epithelial cells[22]. However, because pretreatment with DEA–dextran used in these studies may obviate receptor-mediated viral interactions, these results have been criticized as possibly representing a model of transfection rather than infection[12].

In addition to the potential direct effects of viral infection on renal cells, HIV-1 regulatory gene products or envelope may be toxic to glomerular epithelial or tubular cells or may act indirectly in the pathogenesis of HIVAN through host cytokine dysregulation[12,21]. Evidence in support of the existence of such molecular triggering mechanisms has been provided by studies using transgenic models of HIVAN[23]. Moreover, other factors that modulate the susceptibility of glomerular cells to infection, such as other viruses, drug abuse, genetic predisposition, immune factors, or growth factors, may be involved in the clinical expression of renal disease. Thus, Foster *et al.*[24] suggested that FSGS and tubular epithelial cell injury can be caused by non-HIV viral infection in children with congenital immune deficiencies. Also, experimental findings indicate an important role of the fibroblast growth factor family in the pathogenesis of HIVAN[25].

That HIV *per se* may play an important role in HIVAN is further indicated by the fact that HIVAN can be seen in asymptomatic seropositive patients as the initial or only manifestation of HIV infection. The first observation by D'Agati *et al.*[26] that HIVAN can be clinically manifested months to years before the diagnosis of AIDS has been subsequently confirmed by others[27–30]. What is more, some of the investigators state that as many as 50% of patients with HIVAN currently are either asymptomatic or show early signs of AIDS-related syndrome[27]. Recently, Bass *et al.*[30] reported a case of a young, heterosexual man who presented with a focal segmental membranous glomerulopathy and was later found to be HIV positive. The patient died from cerebral infarction associated with HIV vasculitis 16 months after his initial presentation. Because of the above observations, screening for HIV have been proposed as a component of the evaluation of patients with nephrotic syndrome of unknown origin in areas with a high prevalence of HIV infection[6].

Although HIV infection has been postulated to be causally related to HIVAN, only a few studies have been concentrated on the effectiveness of antiviral agents in slowing down the usually rapid progression of HIVAN to end-stage renal failure. Although the limited knowledge of the natural history of HIVAN makes difficult the demonstration of the effectiveness of any therapeutic intervention, observations published during the last few years suggest that zidovudine therapy may result in clinical improvement in

HIV-infected patients with renal disease[31–34]. Thus, Babut-Gay *et al.*[31] noted that the administration of zidovudine in a patient with HIVAN and the nephrotic syndrome resulted in considerable reduction of proteinuria which lasted for 11 months. On the other hand, Lam and Park[33] reported regression of renal failure, but not change in proteinuria, in a patient with HIVAN on zidovudine therapy. It is noteworthy that in this patient discontinuation of zidovudine therapy resulted in a new deterioration of renal function. Finally, in a retrospective analysis of 11 patients with histologically proven HIVAN, Michel *et al.*[34] reported a beneficial effect on renal function in three out of six patients treated with zidovudine. The effectiveness of the antiretrovial agent was found to be more marked in the patients treated at an earlier stage of the renal disease.

WHAT ELSE MAY BE AN AIDS-ASSOCIATED NEPHROPATHY?

Although FSGS is the most common renal disease, other forms of glomerular disease have also been described in patients with HIV infection. Thus, as early as in the original report from San Francisco, a variety of acute and chronic glomerular and tubulointerstitial changes, including FSGS, but also proliferative glomerulonephritis, IgM/IgG nephropathy, interstitial fibrosis and end-stage renal disease, were described in 11 patients in whom renal tissue was examined[7]. In a more recent multicentric study from Paris hospitals[35] FSGS was found in 84% of 29 black patients, but only in 11% of 31 white patients. A second major glomerular lesion consisting of the immune-complex type of glomerulonephritis was present in 37% of patients (22 out of 60 biopsies). Six patients of both ethnic groups were diagnosed to have acute proliferative postinfectious glomerulonephritis, four white patients presented with a diffuse proliferative form of glomerulonephritis with mesangial IgA deposits, and 10 patients had diffuse proliferative glomerulonephritis and IgG mesangiocapillary deposits, resembling lupus nephritis. The latter changes were present in 45% of white and 20% of black patients. Other glomerulonephritides, including membranous glomerulonephritis[36], membranoproliferative glomerulonephritis[37], and minimal change disease[38] have been noted by other groups, in patients with HIV infection.

Typical IgA-associated nephritis has been repeatedly reported in association with HIV positivity[39–42]. A recent review of the literature disclosed 18 reported cases[43]. Since IgA nephritis is the commonest glomerulonephritis all over the world, the coexistence of IgA nephritis with HIV infection could be coincidental. On the other hand, the demonstration of tubuloreticular inclusions in endothelial cells and nuclear bodies in interstitial cells[40], as well as the presence of IgA immune complexes in HIV-positive patients with IgA nephritis[42,44,45], raise the possibility that IgA nephritis may develop as a consequence of HIV infection in susceptible individuals.

As already mentioned, not only IgA nephritis, but also other glomerulonephritides with pathological characteristics consistent with an immune-mediated pathogenesis, can be seen in patients with HIV infection. Obviously, these pathological findings may be related to infectious complications of HIV infection manifested at postinfectious glomerulonephritis. Thus, in the French collaborative study[35], the infectious agent responsible for all six cases of acute postinfectious glomerulonephritis seen in patients with HIV infection was identified as *Staphylococcus aureus*. On the other hand, HIV-related circulating immune complexes are common in patients with HIV infection[45]. Therefore, the possibility that circulating immune complex deposition and/or the formation of *in situ* complexes may underlie the pathogenesis of glomerulonephritis in HIV-infected patients cannot be ruled out. This hypothesis is further supported by the fact that HIV-associated antigen–antibody complexes have been identified from both the circulation and eluates of renal tissue, and that HIV genome has been demonstrated in the renal tissue of HIV-infected patients with proliferative glomerulonephritis consistent with immune-mediated disease[46]. If this hypothesis is true, then the term HIVAN must be extended beyond the typical pattern of FSGS with heavy proteinuria and rapid progression to end-stage renal disease, to include HIV-associated immune-mediated glomerulonephritis[46], and perhaps other types of renal disease.

In a review of the literature, Bourgoignie[13] calculated that mesangial hyperplasia accounted for 27% of the glomerular pathology reported from both autopsies and biopsies in patients with HIV infection. This figure contrasted with the corresponding incidence of 83% of FSGS. Whether mesangial hyperplasia represents a distinct form of renal disease associated with HIV infection or merely corresponds to an early stage of the typical FSGS remains controversial. Observations in non-HIV-infected paediatric patients with FSGS suggest that mesangial hypercellularity may be a morphological feature of early disease[47]. A hypothesis proposed by Bourgoignie[13] is that the renal lesion in HIVAN begins with mesangial hyperplasia resulting in modest proteinuria with normal or slightly decreased renal function, and progresses to nephrotic syndrome and irreversible renal failure complicating FSGS.

OTHER RENAL ABNORMALITIES IN PATIENTS WITH AIDS

In addition to renal diseases which may be causally related to the infection with HIV virus, a variety of electrolyte and acid–base disturbances, as well as other renal disorders, can be seen in HIV-infected patients. These abnormalities may be coincidental to HIV infection, may be related to its complications or may be due to various diagnostic or therapeutic interventions.

Typically, electrolyte and acid–base abnormalities occur in patients with

Table 11.1 Disorders of the kidneys in patients with AIDS

- Renal disease probably associated with HIV-infection
  - HIV-associated nephropathy
    - Focal and segmental glomerulosclerosis
  - HIV-associated immune-mediated renal disease
    - IgA nephropathy
    - Other immune-complex mediated glomerulonephritides
- Other coincidental glomerular disease
  - Post-infectious (e.g. post-staphylococcal) glomerulonephritis
  - Heroin-associated nephropathy
  - Diabetes mellitus
  - Other
- Fluid and electrolyte derangements
  - Hyponatraemia
  - Hypo- and hyperkalaemia
  - Hypo- and hypercalcaemia
  - Hypo- and hyperuricaemia
  - Hypomagnesaemia
  - Metabolic alkalosis
  - Type IV renal tubular acidosis (hyporeninaemic hypoaldosteronism)
- Acute renal failure
  - Acute tubular necrosis
    - Hypovolaemia, sepsis
    - Drug-induced
      - Antibiotics, antifungal, or antiviral agents
      - Radiocontrast material
      - Non-steroid anti-inflammatory drugs
  - Acute (allergic) interstitial nephritis
    - Trimethoprim-sulphamethoxazole and other agents
  - Obstructive nephropathy
    - Sulfadizine-related crystalluria
    - Chemotherapy-induced hyperuricosuria
  - Due to AIDS-associated or incidental glomerular disease
- Infections of the kidney
  - Microabscesses from bacterial infection
  - Tuberculosis (including atypical mycobacterial)
  - Cytomegalovirus lesions
  - *Pneumocystis carinii* infection
  - Fungal diseases (cryptococcal, aspergillous and other)
- Infiltrative disease of the kidney
  - Lymphomas
  - Kaposi's sarcoma
  - Multiple myeloma
  - Amyloidosis
- HIV infection acquired during renal replacement therapy
  - Regular dialysis patients
  - Transplanted patients

the fully developed clinical syndrome of HIV infection, whereas the frequency and severity of these abnormalities seem to be very low in patients with AIDS-related complex[2]. Hyponatraemia is the most common electrolyte disorder in patients with AIDS. In the majority of cases it is due to sodium and volume depletion associated with gastrointestinal losses or malnutrition. Renal sodium wasting due to drug toxicity or other causes of tubular dysfunction, inappropriate secretion of ADH associated with pulmonary or central nervous system infections, and dilutional hyponatraemia as a result of excess free-water intake in the presence of renal insufficiency are other potential causes of low serum sodium concentration in AIDS[13]. Both hypo- and hyperkalaemia can be observed in patients with AIDS. Hyperkalaemia may be the consequence of adrenal insufficiency or of hyporeninaemic hypoaldosteronism. Adrenal necrosis related to cytomegalovirus (CMV) mycobacterium, or cryptococcal infection is a frequent autopsy finding, but overt adrenal insufficiency is relatively rare in AIDS patients[48–50]. Hyperkalaemia is also a common side effect of pentamidine, an antiparasitic agent used to treat *Pneumocystis carinii* pneumonia. As many as 100% of patients with AIDS receiving pentamidine for more than six days develop this complication[51,52]. Recent experiments suggest that this agent may act on the distal nephron in a manner similar to potassium-sparing diuretics[53].

Volume depletion and sepsis are important causes of acute renal failure in patients with AIDS. In addition, many of the various antimicrobial agents used in these patients can cause acute tubular necrosis or acute interstitial nephritis. Nephrotoxicity is the most common side effect of pentamidine[54]. Renal failure is usually reversible with dosage reduction[55]. Trimethoprim–sulphamethoxazole can produce acute interstitial nephritis, but it is generally regarded as less nephrotoxic than pentamidine[55]. Acute renal failure can also be induced by various antibiotics, such as aminoglycosides, antifungal agents, such as amphotericin B, or antiviral agents, such as foscarnet[56], as well as by radiocontrast material. In most cases, renal failure is mild and can be reversed if the nephrotoxic agent is discontinued. Finally, acute renal failure can be caused by obstruction due to hyperuricosuria secondary to chemotherapy for AIDS-associated lymphomas, or to crystalluria related to sulphadiazine therapy for toxoplasmosis in patients with AIDS[57].

The kidneys of patients with AIDS are subject to a variety of opportunistic infections. Pyogenic infections, *Mycobacterium tuberculosis*, often resistant to conventional therapy, renal involvement from disseminated extrapulmonary *Mycobacterium avium–intracellulare*[58] or *Pneumocystis carinii* infection[59], candida microabscesses, cryptococcal lesions or aspergilloma[60], and CMV lesions may all occur in these patients.

An increased incidence of lymphomas has been known to be associated with HIV infection. Among patients with AIDS-related lymphomas imaging studies reveal renal involvement in 6–12% of cases[61]. Renal lesions usually appear as bilateral, discrete parenchymal masses rather than the diffuse increase of renal size that is usually seen in non-AIDS patients with renal lymphoma[62]. Renal involvement can occur as secondary to retroperitoneal or generalized lymphomas or even as a primary renal lymphoma[63]. As a rule, invasion of the kidney by Kaposi's sarcoma is microscopic and as a consequence it is usually found at autopsy[64]. Amyloidosis and multiple myeloma with IgA κ deposits[65] are other causes of renal infiltration reported in patients with AIDS.

RENAL REPLACEMENT THERAPY IN PATIENTS WITH AIDS

In HIV-infected patients with reversible acute renal failure, temporary dialysis therapy permits recovery of renal function and, therefore, prolongs life[27]. In contrast, patients with HIVAN and irreversible renal failure have a very poor prognosis on dialysis. In one series of 43 patients with AIDS and end-stage renal disease, 31 were haemodialysed, but only five of them survived more than three months[66]. In a prospective study, 51 patients with HIV infection and irreversible renal failure, including 31 patients with HIVAN and 20 chronic haemodialysis patients with superimposed HIV infection, were followed to evaluate survival on outpatient dialysis[67]. All 11 patients who developed AIDS on haemodialysis died after a mean of 93 days from diagnosis. In contrast, 12 asymptomatic HIV carriers were alive after a mean follow-up on chronic haemodialysis of 488 days, and five haemodialysed patients with AIDS-related complex were alive after a mean of 564 days. These data demonstrate the importance of severity of disease in the outcome of dialysis treatment. In general, after AIDS is diagnosed, survival rarely exceeds one month, while in earlier stages of HIV infection haemodialysis provides many months to years of survival. Home peritoneal dialysis may be a good alternative. Advantages include the lack of blood exposure, provision of better nutrition, and possibly a more favourable effect on immune function. A possible disadvantage is the increased risk of peritonitis[11].

Several ethical issues are raised in patients with HIV infection and end-stage renal disease. Because in patients with HIVAN under chronic haemodialysis patient survival is dependent upon the stage of HIV infection, a crucial question is whether dialysis should be performed in patients who have already developed AIDS or should be reserved only for HIV carriers and patients with AIDS-related complex. In view of the increasing incidence of HIV infection in some dialysis centres, another important dilemma is whether renal replacement treatment should be discontinued after the diagnosis of AIDS in a patient on chronic dialysis. Most physicians think that there are no grounds to provide therapy that is unlikely to give medical benefit, and, therefore, that chronic dialysis should be performed only on asymptomatic HIV-seropositive patients or patients with early stages of HIV infection[11]. However, a patient with AIDS may wish to survive only a few more days, for personal reasons[68]. On ethical grounds, decisions about withholding treatment should not be based on convenience or prejudice, but should be reached after considering both medical issues and patient preference[11]. A third question arises regarding renal transplantation: should patients with asymptomatic HIV infection or with AIDS-related complex be excluded from transplantation? Although there have been exceptional cases of functioning grafts several years after transplantation in asymptomatic HIV carriers, because of the generally poor outcome of these patients most surgeons will not perform transplantation in an HIV-seropositive recipient[13].

REFERENCES

1. Tanowitz HB, Simon D, Wittner M. Gastrointestinal manifestations. *Med Clin North Am* 1992; 76: 45–62.
2. Vaziri ND, Barbari A, Licorish K *et al.* Spectrum of renal abnormalities in acquired immune-deficiency syndrome. *J Natl Med Assoc* 1985; 77: 369–375.
3. Rao TKS, Filippone EJ, Nicastri AD *et al.* Associated focal and segmental glomerulosclerosis in the acquired immunodeficiency syndrome. *N Engl J Med* 1984; 310: 669–673.
4. Pardo V, Aldana M, Colton RM *et al.* Glomerular lesions in the acquired immunodeficiency syndrome. *Ann Intern Med* 1984; 101: 429–434.
5. Gardenswartz MH, Lerner CW, Seligson GR *et al.* Renal disease in patients with AIDS: a clinicopathologic study. *Clin Nephrol* 1984; 21: 197–204.
6. Rao TKS, Friedman EA. AIDS (HIV)-associated nephropathy: does it exist? An in-depth review. *Am J Nephrol* 1989; 9: 441–453.
7. Mazbar SA, Schoenfeld PY, Humphreys MH. Renal involvement in patients infected with HIV: experience at San Francisco General Hospital. *Kidney Int* 1990; 37: 1325–1332.
8. Rao TKS, Nicastri AD, Friedman EA. Natural history of heroin-associated nephropathy. *N Engl J Med* 1974; 290: 19–23.
9. Pardo V, Meneses R, Ossa L *et al.* AIDS-related glomerulopathy: occurrence in specific risk groups. *Kidney Int* 1987; 31: 1167–1173.
10. Strauss J, Abitbol C, Zilleruelo G *et al.* Renal disease in children with the acquired immunodeficiency syndrome. *N Engl J Med* 1989; 321: 625–630.
11. Stone HD, Appel RG. Human immunodeficiency virus-associated nephropathy: current concepts. *Am J Med Sci* 1994; 307: 212–217.
12. D'Agati V. The many masks of focal segmental glomerulosclerosis. *Kidney Int* 1994; 46: 1223–1241.
13. Bourgoignie JJ. Renal complications of human immunodeficiency virus type I. *Kidney Int* 1990; 37: 15571–15584.
14. Chander P, Soni A, Suri A *et al.* Renal ultrastructural markers in AIDS-associated nephropathy. *Am J Pathol* 1987; 126: 513–526.
15. D'Agati V, Suh JL, Carbone L *et al.* Pathology of HIV-associated nephropathy: a detailed morphologic and comparative study. *Kidney Int* 1989; 35: 1358–1370.
16. Hall WD, Saunders EJ, Shulman NB (eds). *Hypertension in Blacks: Epidemiology, Pathophysiology and Treatment*. Chicago: Yearbook Medical Publishers, 1985.
17. Cunningham EE, Zielezny MA, Venuto RC. Heroin-associated nephropathy, a nation wide problem. *JAMA* 1983; 250: 2935–2967.

18. Haskell LP, Glicklich D, Senitzer D. HLA association in heroin-associated nephropathy. *Am J Kidney Dis* 1988; 12: 45–50.
19. Cohen AH, Sun NCJ, Shapshak P, Imagawa DT. Demonstration of human immunodeficiency virus in renal epithelium in HIV-associated nephropathy. *Mod Pathol* 1989; 2: 125–128.
20. Kimmel PL, Fereira-Centeno A, Farkas-Szallasi T *et al.* Viral DNA in microdissected renal biopsy tissue from HIV infected patients with nephrotic syndrome. *Kidney Int* 1993; 43: 1347–1352.
21. Rappaport J, Kopp JB, Klotman PE. Host virus interaction and the molecular regulation of HIV-1: role in the pathogenesis of HIV-associated nephropathy. *Kidney Int* 1994; 46: 16–27.
22. Green DF, Resnick L, Bourgoignie JJ. HIV infects glomerular endothelial and mesangial but not epithelial cells in vitro. *Kidney Int* 1992; 41: 956–960.
23. Kopp JB, Klotman ME, Adler SH *et al.* Progressive glomerulosclerosis and enhanced renal accumulation of basement membrane components in mice transgenic for human immunodeficiency virus type 1 genes. *Proc Natl Acad Sci USA* 1992; 89: 1577–1581.
24. Foster S, Hawkins E, Hanson CG, Shearer W. Pathology of the kidney in childhood immunodeficiency: AIDS-related nephropathy is not unique. *Pediatr Pathol* 1991; 11: 63–74.
25. Ray PE, Bruggeman LA, Weeks BS *et al.* bFGF and its low affinity receptors in the pathogenesis of HIV-associated nephropathy in transgenic mice. *Kidney Int* 1994; 46: 759–772.
26. D'Agati V, Suh J, Carbone L, Appel G. HTLVIII associated nephropathy: a comparative pathologic study. *Kidney Int* 1987; 31: 336.
27. Bourgoignie JJ, Meneses R, Ortiz C *et al.* The clinical spectrum of renal disease associated with human immunodeficiency virus. *Am J Kidney Dis* 1988; 12: 131–137.
28. Rao TKS, Mallis LR, Friedman EA. Nephropathy as the initial manifestation of human immunodeficiency virus. *Kidney Int* 1988; 33: 205.
29. Bates WD, Muller N, van der Wal BW, Jacobs JC. HIV-associated nephropathy: an initial presentation in a HIV-positive patient. *S Afr Med J* 1994; 84: 223–224.
30. Bass PS, Garrett PJ, Ellison DW *et al.* AIDS presenting as focal segmental membranous glomerulopathy. *J Clin Pathol* 1994; 47: 179–181.
31. Babut-Gay ML, Echard M, Kleichnecht D, Mayrier A. Zidovudine and nephropathy with human immunodeficiency virus (HIV) infection. *Ann Intern Med* 1989; 111: 856–857.
32. Cook PP, Appel RG. Prolonged clinical improvement in HIV-associated nephropathy with zidovudine therapy. *J Am Soc Nephrol* 1990; 1: 842.
33. Lam M, Park J. HIV-associated nephropathy: beneficial effect of zidovudine therapy. *N Engl J Med* 1990; 323: 1775–1776.
34. Michel C, Dosquet P, Ronco P *et al.* Nephropathy associated with infection by human immunodeficiency virus: a report on 11 cases including 6 treated with zidovudine. *Nephron* 1992; 62: 434–440.
35. Nochy D, Glotz D, Dosquet P *et al.* Renal disease associated with HIV infection: a multicentric study of 60 patients from Paris hospitals. *Nephrol Dial Transplant* 1993; 8: 11–19.
36. Guerra IL, Abraham AA, Kimmel PL *et al.* Nephrotic syndrome associated with chronic persistent hepatitis B in an HIV antibody positive patient. *Am J Kidney Dis* 1987; 10: 385–388.
37. Kenneth KK, Factor SM. Membranoproliferative glomerulonephritis and plexogenic pulmonary arteriopathy in a homosexual man with acquired immunodeficiency syndrome. *Hum Pathol* 1987; 18: 1293–1296.

38. Singer DRJ, Jenkins AP, Gupta S, Evans DJ. Minimal change nephropathy in the acquired immunodeficiency syndrome. *Br Med J* 1985; 291: 868.
39. Kenouch S, Delahousse M, Mery JP, Nochy D. Mesangial IgA deposits in two patients with AIDS-related complex. *Nephron* 1990; 54: 338–340.
40. Katz A, Bargman JM, Miller DC *et al.* IgA nephritis in HIV-positive patients: a new HIV-associated nephropathy? *Clin Nephrol* 1992; 38: 61–68.
41. Kimmel PL, Phillips TM, Ferreira-Centeno A *et al.* Idiotypic IgA nephropathy in patients with HIV infection. *N Engl J Med* 1992; 327: 702–706.
42. Schoeneman MJ, Ghali V, Lieberman K, Reisman L. IgA nephritis in a child with human immunodeficiency virus: a unique form of human immunodeficiency virus-associated nephropathy? *Pediatr Nephrol* 1992; 6: 46–49.
43. Beaufils H, Jouanneau C, Katlama C *et al.* HIV-associated IgA nephropathy: a post-mortem study. *Nephrol Dial Transplant* 1995; 10: 35–38.
44. Nishanian P, Huskins KR, Stehn S *et al* A simple method for improved assay demonstrates that HIV p24 antigen is present as immune complexes in most sera from HIV-infected individuals. *J Infect Dis* 1990; 162: 21–28.
45. Lighfoote MM, Folks TM, Redfield R *et al.* Circulating IgA immune complexes in AIDS. *Immunol Invest* 1985; 14: 341–345.
46. Kimmel PL, Phillips TM, Fereira-Centeno A *et al.* HIV-associated immune-mediated renal disease. *Kidney Int* 1993; 44: 1327–1340.
47. Southwest Pediatric Nephrology Study Group. Focal segmental glomerulosclerosis in children with idiopathic nephrotic syndrome. *Kidney Int* 1985; 27: 442–449.
48. Tapper ML, Rotterdam HZ, Lerner CW *et al.* Adrenal necrosis in the acquired immunodeficiency syndrome. *Ann Intern Med* 1984; 100: 239–241.
49. Guenthner EE, Rabinowe SL, van Niel A *et al.* Primary Addison's disease in a patient with the acquired immunodeficiency syndrome. *Ann Intern Med* 1984; 100: 847–848.
50. Greene LW, Cole W, Greene JB *et al.* Adrenal insufficiency as a complication of the acquired immunodeficiency syndrome. *Ann Intern Med* 1984; 101: 497–498.
51. Lachaal M, Venuto RC. Nephrotoxicity and hyperkalemia in patients with the acquired immunodeficiency syndrome treated with pentamidine. *Am J Med* 1989; 87: 260–263.
52. Peltz S, Hashmi S. Pentamidine-induced severe hyperkalemia. *Am J Med* 1989; 87: 698–699.
53. Kleyman TR, Roberts C, Ling BN. A mechanism for pentamidine-induced hyperkalemia: inhibition of distal nephron sodium transport. *Ann Intern Med* 1995; 122: 103–106.
54. Glatt AE, Chirgwin K, Landesman SH. Treatment of infections associated with human immunodeficiency virus. *N Engl J Med* 1988; 318: 1439–1448.
55. Sattler FR, Cowan R, Nielsen DM, Ruskin J. Trimethoprim-sulfamethoxazole compared with pentamidine for treatment of *Pneumocystis carinii* pneumonia in the acquired immunodeficiency syndrome: a prospective noncrossover study. *Ann Intern Med* 1988; 109: 280–287.
56. Cacoub O, Deray G, Baumelou A *et al.* Acute renal failure induced by foscarnet: 4 cases. *Clin Nephrol* 1988; 29: 315–318.
57. Christin S, Baumelou A, Bahri S *et al.* Acute renal failure due to sulfadiazine in patients with AIDS. *Nephron* 1990; 55: 233–234.
58. Pitchenik AE, Fertel D. Tuberculosis and nontuberculous mycobacterial disease. *Med Clin North Am* 1992; 76: 121–152.
59. Bargman JM, Wagner C, Cameron R. Renal cortical nephrocalcinosis: a manifestation of extrapulmonary *Pneumocystis carinii* infection in the acquired immunodeficiency syndrome. *Am J Kidney Dis* 1991; 17: 712–715.

60. Halpern M, Szabo S, Hochberg E *et al.* Renal aspergilloma: an unusual cause of infection in a patient with the acquired immunodeficiency syndrome. *Am J Med* 1992; 92: 437–440.
61. Miller FH, Parikh S, Gore RM *et al.* Renal manifestations of AIDS. *RadioGraphics* 1993; 13: 587–596.
62. Townsend RR. CT of AIDS-related lymphoma. *AJR* 1991; 156: 969–974.
63. Tsang K, Kneafsey P, Gill J. Primary lymphoma of the kidney in the acquired immunodeficiency syndrome. *Arch Pathol Lab Med* 1993; 117: 541–543.
64. Krown SE, Myskowski PL, Paredes J. Kaposi's sarcoma. *Med Clin North Am* 1992; 76: 239–252.
65. Thomas MA, Ibels LS, Wells JV *et al.* IgA kappa multiple myeloma and lymphadenopathy syndrome associated with AIDS virus infection. *Aust NZ J Med* 1986; 16: 402–404.
66. Rao TKS, Friedman EA, Nicastri AD. The types of renal disease in the acquired immunodeficiency syndrome. *N Engl J Med* 1987; 316: 1062–1068.
67. Ortiz C, Meneses R, Jaffe D *et al.* Outcome of patients with human immunodeficiency virus on maintenance hemodialysis. *Kidney Int* 1988; 34: 248–253.
68. Pennell JP, Bourgoignie JJ. Should AIDS patients be dialyzed? *Trans Am Soc Art Organs* 1988; 34: 907–911.

12

AIDS and the Haemophilic Patient

Christine A. Lee

The Haemophilia Centre, Royal Free Hospital, London, UK

BACKGROUND OF THE AIDS EPIDEMIC IN PATIENTS WITH HAEMOPHILIA

The first cases of acquired immunodeficiency syndrome (AIDS) in haemophilic patients were described in 1982[1]. In the UK it is likely that patients first became infected in 1979: a patient was reported who became infected as a result of transfusion with factor VIII concentrate of US donor origin[2]. This patient was treated in August 1979 and this was followed by a typical seroconversion illness in September and October of the same year. Retrospective testing of stored serum showed that he seroconverted in December. In a well-documented cohort in London the dates of seroconversion were shown to be between 1979 and 1985, when heated concentrates first became available (Figure 12.1)[3]. It is probable that in the USA seroconversions occurred a year earlier[4] (Figure 12.2) and overall in the world there were some late seroconversions occurring in 1986 following treatment with heated concentrate. The advent of virally inactivated therapeutic materials has successfully prevented further transmission of human immunodeficiency virus (HIV) and there have been no new seroconversions since 1986.

MORBIDITY AND MORTALITY FROM HIV INFECTION

AIDS has significantly changed the life expectancy for individuals with haemophilia[5]. From 1968 to 1989 2792 haemophilia A deaths were reported in

AIDS and Malignancies: Current Concepts and Perspectives.
Edited by B.C. Golematis and V.T. DeVita Jr

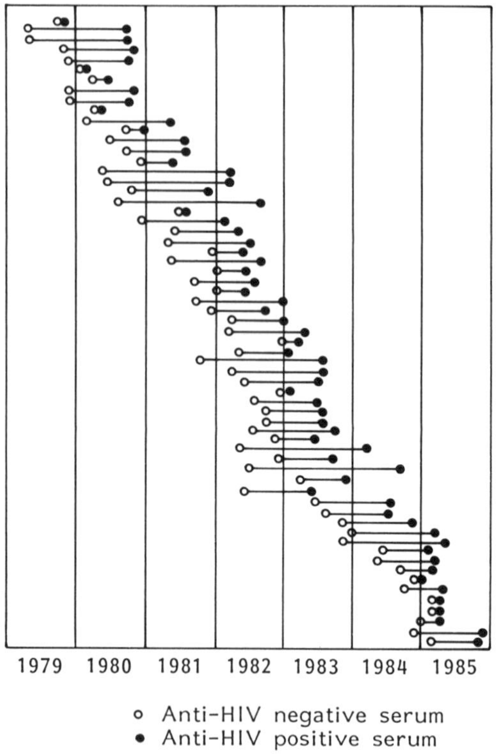

Figure 12.1 *Dates of seroconversion of 63 haemophiliacs*

the USA. The death rate increased from 0.5 to 1.3 per 1 000 000 individuals (Figure 12.3).

From 1979–1981 to 1987–1989 mortality increased in all age groups above 9 years of age (Figure 12.4). The median age at death decreased from 57 years in 1979–1981 to 40 years in 1987–1989. The percentage of deaths due to haemorrhage or diseases of the circulatory system decreased markedly as a result of the increase in deaths associated with HIV infection or infections other than HIV infection (Table 12.1).

When more detailed analysis is made in smaller populations of patients it is clear that there is an increasing morbidity and mortality from hepatitis C (HCV) infection which is superimposed on human immunodeficiency virus (HIV) infection. All individuals who became infected with HIV from clotting factor concentrates must also have been infected with HCV. In the cohort of patients with HIV infection at the Royal Free Hospital, London, of 111 men by 1 January 1995, 61 were alive and 50 had died. Forty-nine men had developed AIDS (43 dead, six alive)[6]. Kaplan–Meier progression rates to AIDS and death by 15 years from seroconversion were 56% and 59% respectively. The median

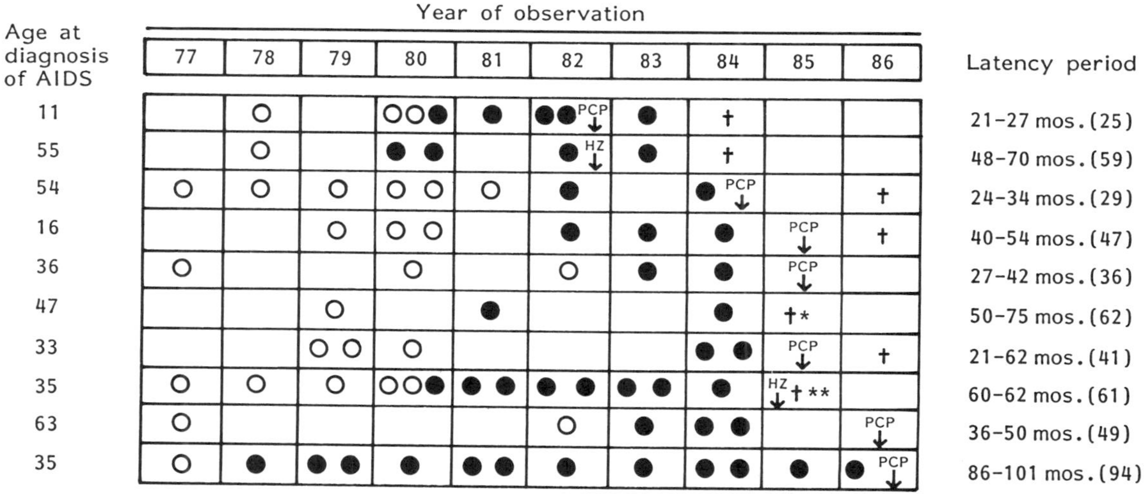

Figure 12.2 *Relationship of seroconversion to clinical disease in 10 haemophiliacs. (Reproduced by permission from Eyster* et al.[4]*)*

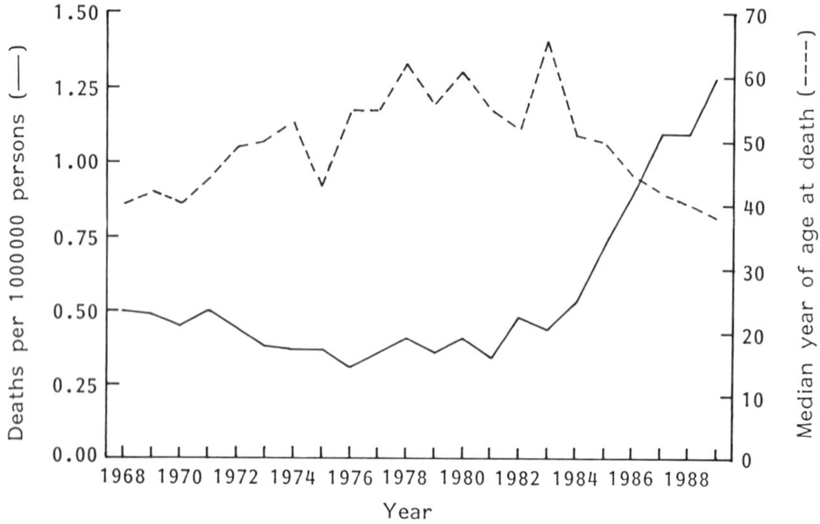

Figure 12.3 *Haemophilia A death rates and median age at death by year, USA, 1968–1989. From: Chorba TL, Holman RC, Strine TW* et al[5]. *Changes in longevity and causes of death among persons with haemophilia.* Am J Haematol *1994; 45: 112–121. Copyright © 1994. (Reprinted by permission of John Wiley & Sons, Inc.)*

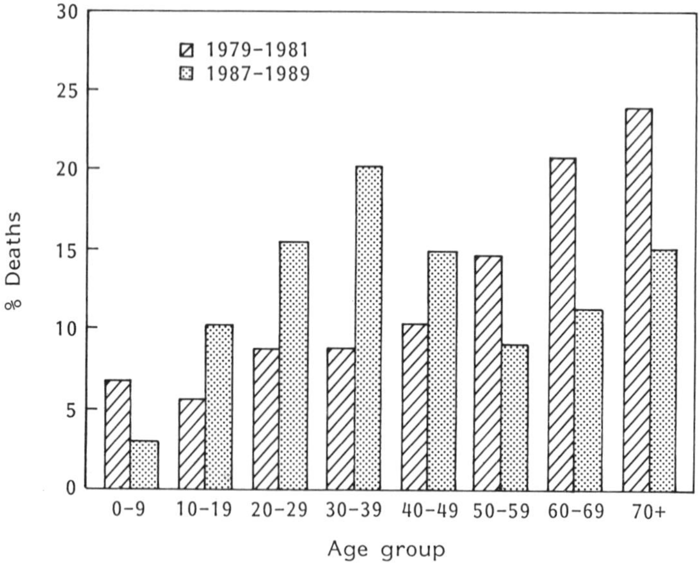

Figure 12.4 *Percentage of haemophilia A deaths by age group, USA, 1979–1981. From: Chorba TL, Holman RC, Strine TW* et al.[5] *Changes in longevity and causes of death among persons with haemophilia.* Am J Haematol *1994; 45: 112–121. Copyright © 1994. (Reprinted by permission of John Wiley & Sons, Inc.)*

Table 12.1 Cause of death on death certificates for persons with haemophilia A, USA, 1987–1989

Cause of death on death certificate	Number and percentage[a] of persons ($N=853$)
HIV-related disease	470 (55.1)
Circulatory disease	263 (30.8)
Haemorrhage	196 (23.0)
Infections other than pneumocystosis or HIV	139 (16.3)
Respiratory disease	128 (15.0)
Non-congenital intrinsic liver disease	111 (13.0)
Injury or poisoning	94 (11.0)
Endocrine, nutritional or metabolic disease	86 (10.1)
Neoplasm	60 (7.0)
Mental disorder or nervous system disease	60 (7.0)
Digestive system disease	45 (5.3)
Genitourinary disease or complication of pregnancy or childbirth	45 (5.3)
Cutaneous, musculoskeletal, or connective tissue disease, congenital anomaly, or perinatal condition	29 (3.4)

[a]Percentage of haemophilia A deaths. Persons may have had more than one cause of death listed. From: Chorba TL, Holman RC, Strine TW *et al.*[5] Changes in longevity and causes of death among persons with haemophilia. *Am J Haematol* 1994; 45: 112–121. Copyright © 1994. (Reprinted by permission of John Wiley & Sons, Inc.)

to the development of AIDS was 14.2 years. Table 12.2 shows the clinical details of the CD4 count of the remaining 61 patients.

The progression of HCV disease in HIV-infected patients is hastened by coinfection with HIV[7,8]. This is reflected in this small cohort of patients where of the 50 patients who have died, 41 deaths were AIDS-related, one was caused by haemorrhage, four were due to liver failure, and four to other non-HIV-related causes. Five of these patients (four patients who died from AIDS and one from other causes) died from liver failure, making a total of nine patients with liver failure. Furthermore, transaminases remain normal in only four (7%) (Table 12.2). Thus as efforts to increase life expectancy of haemophilic patients with HIV progress, substantial morbidity and mortality from HCV infection are likely to arise[6].

CD4 COUNTS ARE RELATED TO DISEASE PROGRESSION

The relationship between the time since seroconversation in a man with haemophilia is shown in Figure 12.5. We have previously shown in this cohort of patients that patients, on average, develop AIDS by a CD4 count to $50/\mu l$ unless they are protected by prophylactic treatment[3]. Thus it is possible

Table 12.2 Clinical and immunological status of 61 patients alive at 1 January 1995

	Number of patients (%)
Total	61 (100)
CD4 count (cells μl)	
⩾500	8 (13)
200⩽ CD4<500	32 (52)
50⩽ CD4<200	9 (15)
<50	12 (20)
Clinical status	
AIDS	6 (10)
Non-AIDS	55 (90)
AST concentration[a]	
Normal	4 (7)
Intermittently abnormal	32 (55)
Persistently abnormal	22 (38)

[a]AST concentration for past 5 years not available in 3 patients, so percentages based on total of 58 patients. Copyright © by the Lancet Ltd. (Reproduced by permission from Lee CA, Sabin CA, Phillips AN *et al.*[6] Morbidity and mortality from transfusion-transmitted disease in haemophilia. *Lancet* 1995; 345: 1309.)

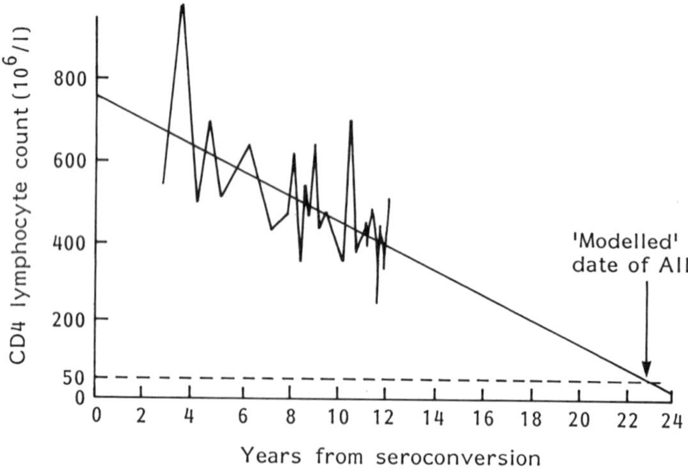

Figure 12.5 *Serial CD4 lymphocyte counts for an HIV-infected man. (Reproduced by permission from Phillips* et al.[9]*)*

using a linear regression slope to 'model' the time at which any individual may develop AIDS or a CD4 count of 50/μl (Figure 12.5). Using this approach for all individuals, it was thus possible to make Kaplan–Meier estimates of the probability of remaining AIDS free up to 25 years after seroconversion (Figure 12.6). The model predicted that 25% (95% confidence interval 16–34%)

would survive for 20 years after seroconversion and 18% (11–25%) for 25 years.

The extent to which these estimates can be applied to the non-haemophilic individual is uncertain. After differences in age have been accounted for there is no published data that shows different rates of progression in different exposure groups. There are differences between the various groups, e.g. Kaposi's sarcoma (KS) does not occur in haemophilic patients and HCV infection is more likely in haemophilia.

This long predicted survival of 20 years for a quarter of patients with HIV infection reflects the small group of patients who have very stable CD4 counts (Figure 12.7). The slow average loss of CD4 cells is clearly seen. Twenty-year survival free of AIDS seems highly plausible for these men.

THE EFFECT OF AGE

It was first shown by Eyster *et al.* in 1987 that older age at the time of seroconversion was associated with an increased risk for AIDS in haemophilic patients (Figure 12.8)[4] and there have been many studies which have confirmed these findings[3,10,11]. This observation is made possible by the study of haemophilic populations because the age range for seroconversion is so wide.

In order to understand the significance of changes in CD4 count during HIV infection amongst patients of different ages, the CD4 count by age should be appreciated in anti-HIV-negative haemophilic individuals (Figure 12.9). When the mean CD4 count by years from seroconversion according to four age categories is plotted after the age of 10 years, the decline of CD4 count is the same in all three age groups. After adjustment for the CD4 count the relative risk of developing AIDS for each 10-year increase in age is 1.31. Thus older patients are at higher risk of progression to AIDS than their younger counterparts even if the CD4 count is the same[12].

p24 ANTIGENAEMIA

A study of 96 haemophilic patients in 1987 showed that the decline of p24 antibody and the appearance of HIV antigen are predictive of HIV disease[13]. In another study of 88 haemophilic patients a high titre of p24 antibody response at the time of seroconversion was associated with a longer time to the development of HIV-related disease. In this study higher titres of gp120 at seroconversion also correlated with more rapid clinical deterioration[14]. The significance of this study is that it would suggest the possibility of postexposure immunotherapy with a p24 construct to boost the p24 antibody response. Several studies have shown in patients with haemophilia that the

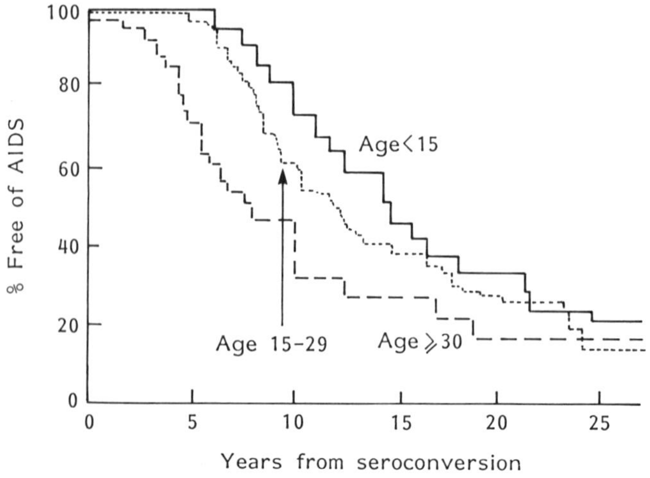

Figure 12.6 *Kaplan–Meier estimates of the percentage of patients surviving free of AIDS by years from seroconversion. (Reproduced by permission from Phillips* et al.[9]*)*

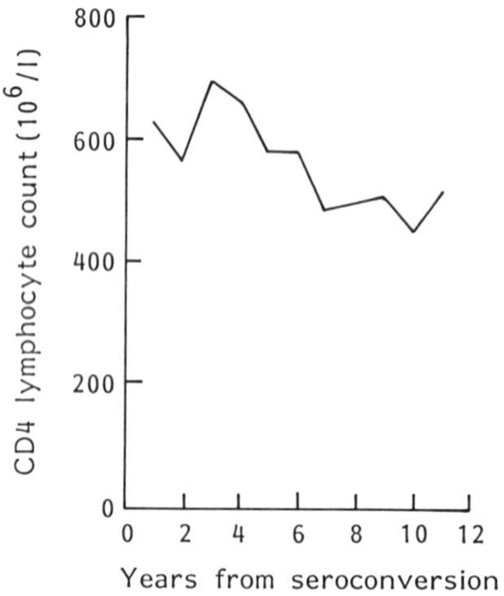

Figure 12.7 *Geometric mean CD4 lymphocyte count by years from seroconversion in 25 patients for whom the modelled time of AIDS is more than 20 years after seroconversion. (Reproduced by permission from Phillips* et al.[9]*)*

presence of p24 antigenaemia is associated with a markedly increased progression to AIDS[11,13,14]. It has been shown that CD4 lymphocyte counts declined more rapidly in p24-positive patients than those who were negative (Figure 12.10). Since p24 antigenaemia reflects increased viral load, it can be seen that increased viral replication is associated with a progressive decrease in the CD4 count.

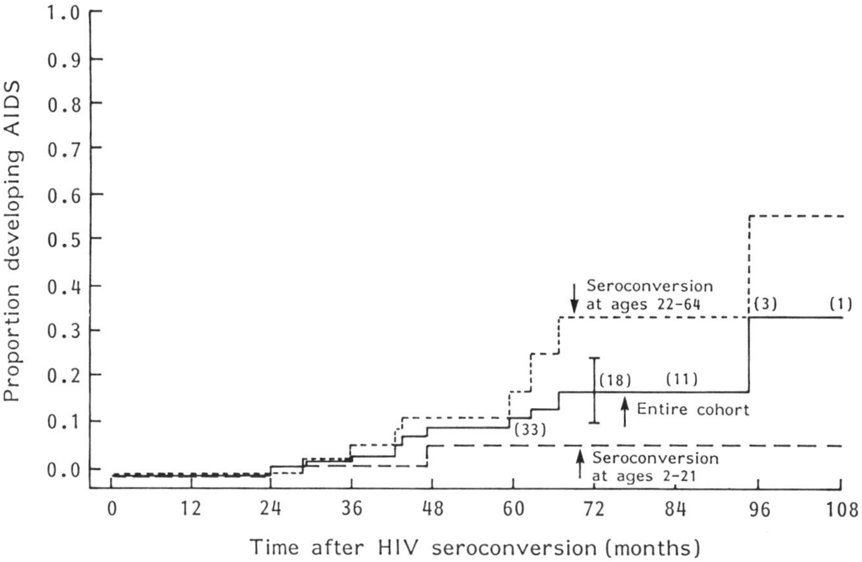

Figure 12.8 *Actuarial incidence of AIDS according to age. (Reproduced by permission from Eyster* et al.[4]*)*

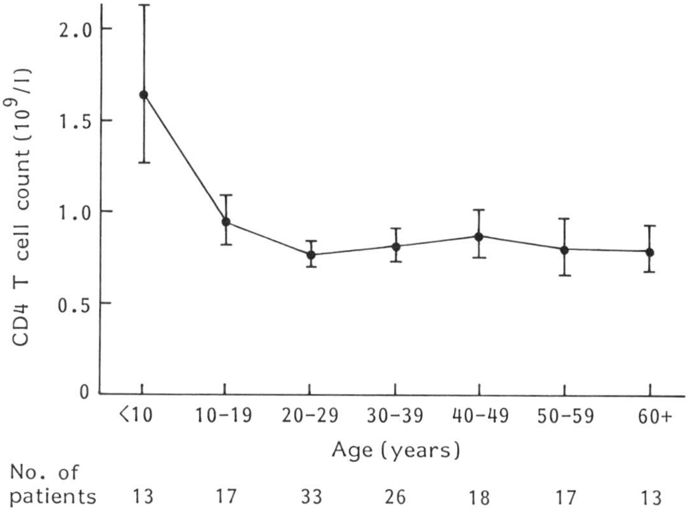

Figure 12.9 *CD4[+] count for 137 anti-HIV-negative haemophiliacs. (Reproduced by permission from Phillips* et al.[12]*)*

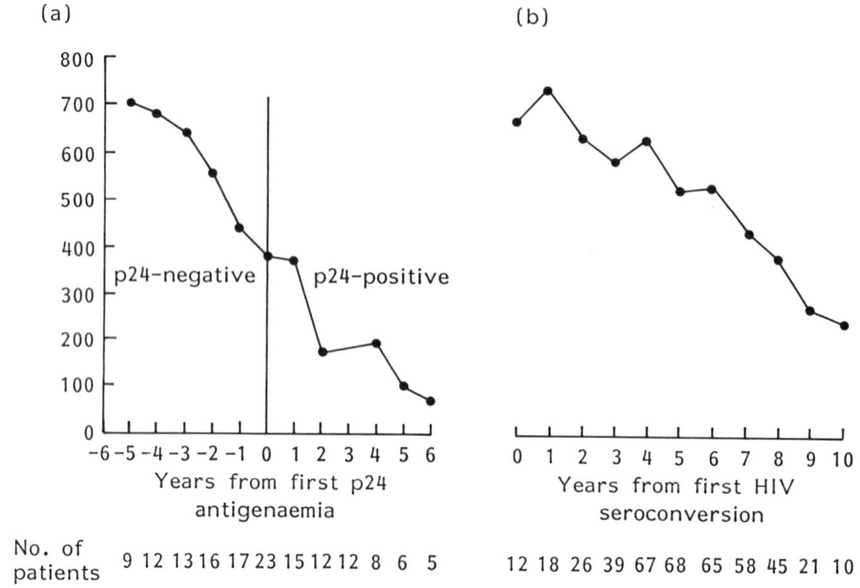

Figure 12.10 *Median CD4 lymphocyte count: (a) years from the first p24 antigen-positive test; (b) years from the first anti-HIV-positive test in patients persistently p24 antigen negative. (Reproduced by permission from Phillips* et al.[13]*)*

EARLY PREDICTORS OF DISEASE PROGRESSION

The immune response at the time of seroconversion determines the ultimate prognosis in HIV infection. Since the time of seroconversion is known for many haemophilic patients it has been possible to study this in haemophilia. In a cohort of 18 infected individuals in Edinburgh[15], in 1988 the human leukocyte antigen (HLA) haplotype A1 B8 DR3 predicted those individuals who progressed rapidly to AIDS (Table 12.3). Similarly, a study of French patients with haemophilia showed that the HLA haplotype HLA-B35 was associated with progression to AIDS[16]. Thus the nature and degree of the immune response determine the pathogenesis of HIV disease.

Serum β_2-microglobulin (s-b2m) is a small 12k peptide which is normally associated with HLA-A,B,C (class I) molecules. When lymphoid cells are activated s-b2m is shed and consequently, during infections, elevated levels of s-b2m are measured. It can be shown by measuring the s-b2m at specific levels of CD4, e.g. 500/μl and 200/μl, that the s-b2m level predicts individuals who will develop AIDS (Figure 12.11)[17]. A variety of studies in non-haemophilic patients have also demonstrated that s-b2m levels predicts AIDS largely independent of CD4 counts[18–23].

It has also been established that CD8 counts and IgA levels measured close

Table 12.3 Clinical state of haemophilic patients who seroconverted 1984–1989

Case no.	HLA-A1 B8 DR3	Year of birth	No. of phials of contaminated factor VIII received	AIDS state (CDC category) 1984	1985	1986	1987	1988	1989
1	–	1965	23	II	II	II	II	II	II
2	–	1959	9	II	III	III	IVc$_2$	IVc$_2$	IVc$_2$
3	–	1962	81	II	II	II	II	II	IVc$_1$
4	–	1946	20	II	II	II	II	II	II
5	–	1963	20	II	II	II	II	II	II
6	–	1947	10	II	II	IVc$_2$	IVc$_2$	IVc$_2$	IVc$_2$
7	–	1950	60	II	II	II	II	II	II
8	–	1944	20	III	III	III	III	III	III
9	–	1946	60	II	II	II	II	II	II
10	–	1941	10	II	II	II	II	II	II
11	+	1948	81	II	II	II	IVc$_2$	IVd	IVd[a]
12	+	1962	43	II	III	IVa	IVa	IVa	IVa
13	+	1954	51	II	II	IVc[b]	IVc	IVc	IVc
14	+	1941	109	II	II	IVa	IVa	IVa	IVa
15	+	1969	30	III	III	III	III	III	III
16	+	1942	50	II	II	IVa	IVa	IVa	IVc$_1$,c
17	+	1970	54	I	IVa	IVb,c$_1$	IVd[a]		
18	+	1945	20	II	II	II	IVa[a]		

[a]Died
[b]Thrombocytopenia
(Reproduced by permission from Cuthbert *et al.*[15])

to the time of seroconversion are good predictors of HIV disease progression. Individuals with high CD8 counts and high IgA levels experienced a more rapid decline of CD4 cell count than those with low baseline levels[14]. In a study of 202 haemophilic children in Europe rising IgA concentrations were markers of disease progression[25]. Similarly in a study of haemophilic patients in Edinburgh the IgA-specific immune response rose gradually in the year after exposure in most individuals. In one patient who was symptomatic at the time of seroconversion there was a much greater and prolonged IgA response[15] (Figure 12.12). Thus the process of CD4 depletion seems to be related to raised CD8 counts and raised IgA levels. It is also possible that the raised CD8 and IgA levels reflect viral load in these patients. This would be supported by the study from Edinburgh where 18 individuals who seroconverted to HIV received higher amounts of clotting factor concentrate than those who remained HIV negative[15]. Furthermore the amount of clotting factor received in this group of patients correlates with the disease progression (Figure 12.3).

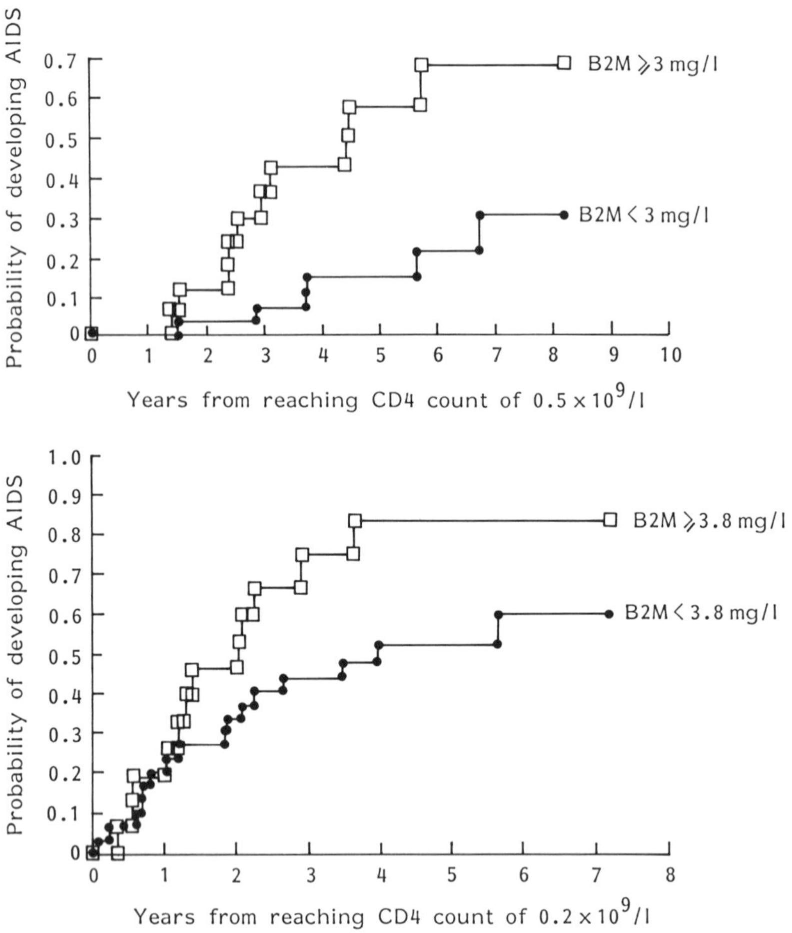

Figure 12.11 *Kaplan–Meier plot of progression to AIDS from a CD4⁺ of 0.5 x 10^9/l and 0.2 x 10^9/l. (Reproduced by permission from Sabin* et al.[17]*)*

CYTOMEGALOVIRUS AS A COFACTOR

It has been demonstrated in a group of haemophilic patients that evidence of previous cytomegalovirus (CMV) infection will predict those individuals who are likely to progress more rapidly to AIDS. Such an observation is possible in haemophilic individuals who, in contrast to homosexuals, are not universally seropositive for CMV IgG, a marker of previous infection. The influence of CMV acts independently of CD4 count—those individuals who are CMV positive develop AIDS at a higher CD4 count (Figure 12.13)[26]. Thus additional mechanisms mediated by CMV such as a functional deficit in

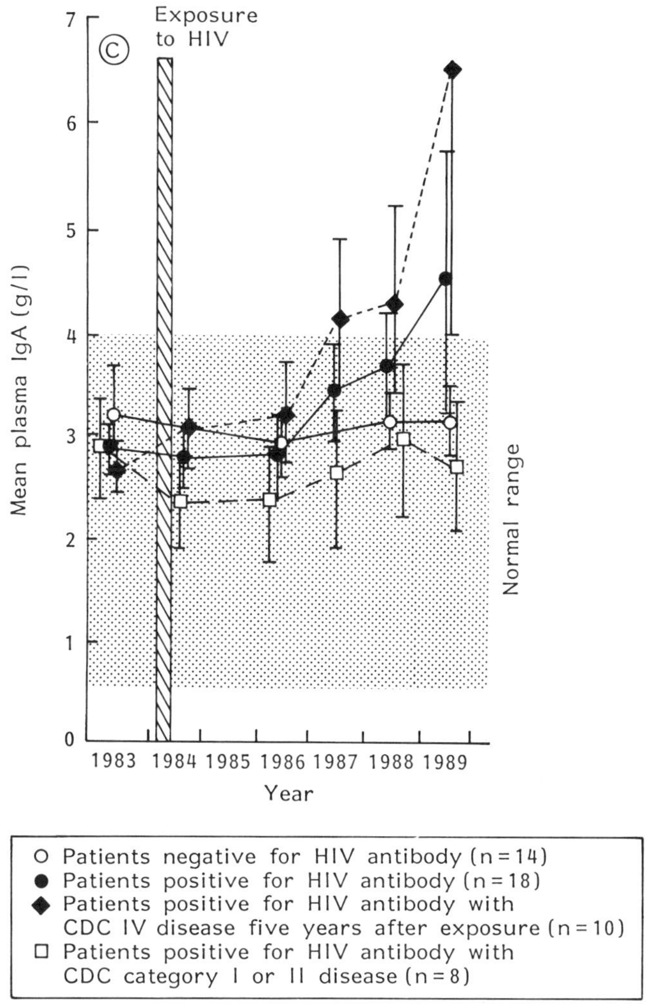

Figure 12.12 *IgA concentration in members of Edinburgh haemophilic cohort. (Reproduced by permission from Cuthbert* et al.[15]*)*

surviving CD4 lymphocytes, or entry of HIV into other cell types, may facilitate the onset of AIDS. For example, CMV may expand the trophic range of HIV disease, perhaps via the induction of Fc receptors, or may have a bystander effect by causing secretion of cytokines that can drive HIV replication in other cells. However, although CMV continues to exert a cofactor effect in this group of patients[26] (Figure 12.14), others have looked at haemophilic individuals and have failed to demonstrate this effect.

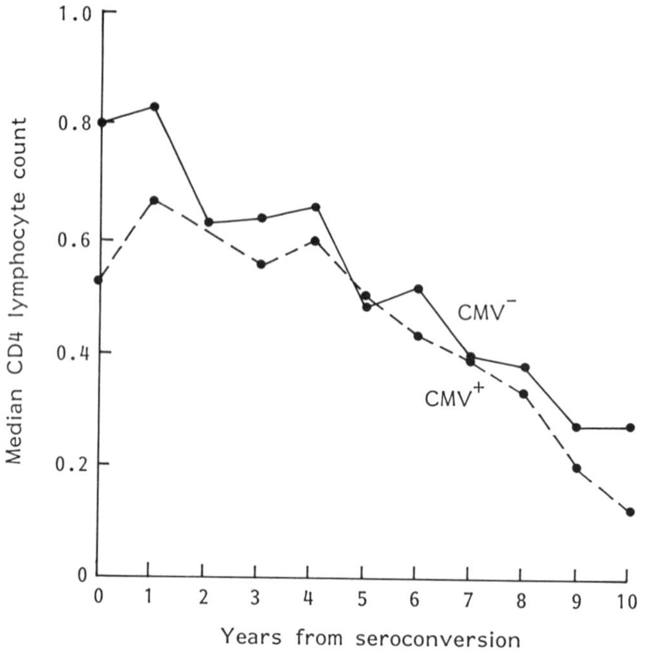

Figure 12.13 *Decline in CD4⁺ lymphocyte counts from the time of HIV seroconversion by CMV serostatus. (Reproduced by permission from Webster* et al.[26]*)*

THROMBOCYTOPENIA

The association of immune-mediated thrombocytopenia (ITP) with HIV disease was first recognized by Ratnoff[27] in 1983 in patients with haemophilia. He described this in five multiply transfused patients with haemophilia. Although ITP rarely results in bleeding complications in HIV-infected homosexuals or intravenous drug abusers, there may be a significant risk when ITP complicates haemophilia[28]. The mechanism of HIV-associated thrombocytopenia is thought to be due to deposition of immune complexes and complement on platelets and/or a specific antiplatelet antibody[29]. Treatment has included intravenous immunoglobulin, steroids, zidovudine, interferon, and splenectomy. A review of 17 haemophilic patients who underwent splenectomy for thrombocytopenia showed a permanent response rate of 90%[30]. Furthermore it has been shown that splenectomy in haemophilic patients has no adverse effect on the progression of HIV disease in these patients[31].

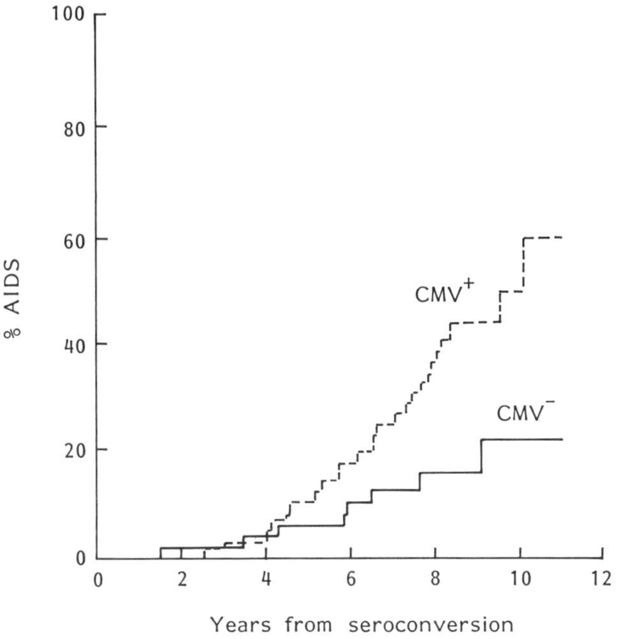

Figure 12.14 *Kaplan–Meier survival analysis for HIV-1-infected haemophiliacs by CMV serostatus. (Reproduced by permission from Webster* et al.[26]*)*

LIVER DISEASE AND HIV INFECTION

Haemophilic patients who were infected with HIV as a result of treatment with unsterilized clotting factor concentrate must also have been infected with HCV. Two large studies have shown that coinfection with HIV could accelerate the development of liver failure[7,8]. Viral replication of hepatitis C is increased in the presence of HIV (probably because of immune deficiency). From 1978 to 1993 concentrations of hepatitis C RNA in coinfected haemophilic patients increased 58 times compared with a trebling in those infected with HCV alone[32] (Figure 12.15). The relative risk of developing liver failure in hepatitis C infection increased 21-fold after HIV infection[8]. In our centre 10 of 11 deaths in liver failure occurred in HIV-infected individuals.

Patients infected with HCV who develop cirrhosis are at increased risk of developing hepatocellular carcinoma. A worldwide questionnaire sent to 11 801 patients with haemophilia identified 10 cases of hepatocellular carcinoma—a risk 30 times higher than normal[33].

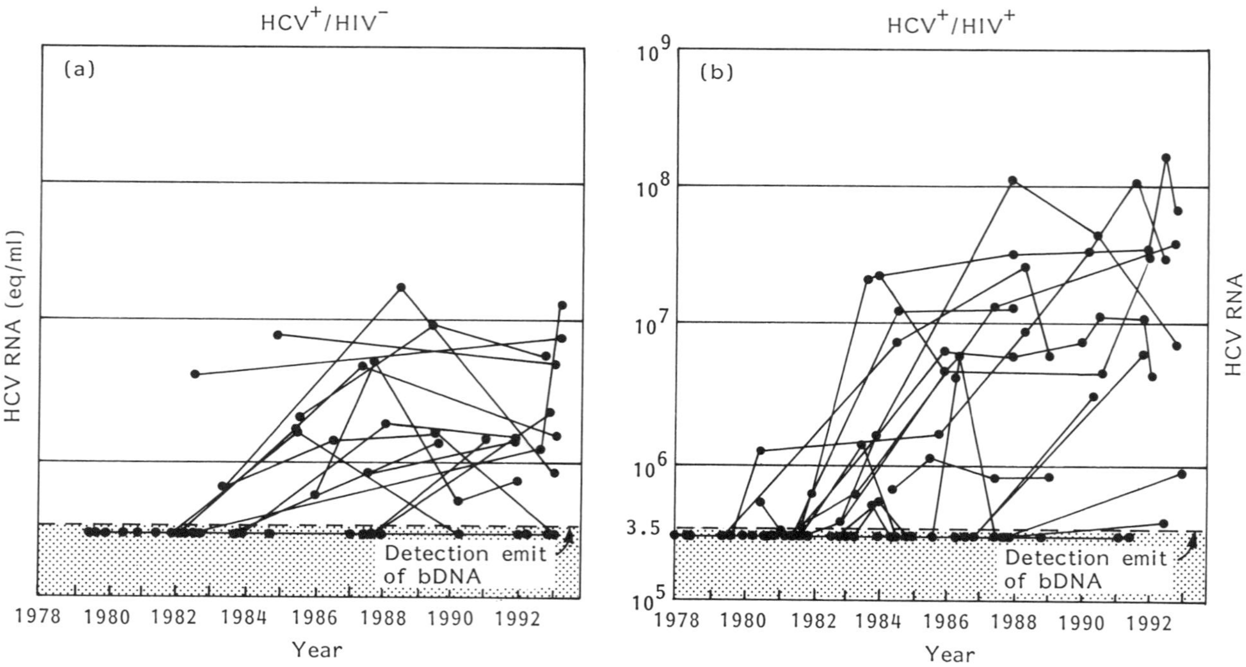

Figure 12.15 *Serial HCV RNA levels on 17 HCV-positive/HIV-negative subjects (a) and 17 HCV-positive/HIV-positive subjects (b). (Reproduced by permission from Eyster* et al.[32]*)*

LYMPHOMAS AND OTHER CANCERS

The most extensive assessment of the occurrence of malignancy in haemophilic patients and the relationship to HIV infection was published by the National Cancer Institute's Multicenter Hemophilia Cohort Study in 1992[34]. A total of 1701 patients with haemophilia and related clotting disorders from 15 haemophilia treatment centres were enrolled and followed up. The cut-off point for data analysis was March 1991 and 1065 subjects (63%) were seropositive for HIV-1. These individuals seroconverted during the years 1978–1986. Incident cancers were ascertained at follow-up visits and from clinical records. The cancer diagnoses were verified at the National Cancer Institute by examination of biopsy specimens (when available) and review of pathology reports. For calculation of cancer incidence in HIV-positive subjects, person-years at risk of cancer were determined between the estimated date of seroconversion and the date of follow-up. Since individuals with AIDS and/or cancer continued to be at risk for subsequent cancer, observation time after the development of these conditions was included in the person-years-at-risk calculation. The beginning of the observation period for the HIV-negative individuals was the median date of seroconversion of the HIV-positive individuals, i.e. 1 October 1982.

As of March 1991 there were 1065 HIV-positive patients with 8243 years of follow-up and 636 HIV-negative individuals with 4400 years of follow-up. From October 1982 there were 12 cases of non-Hodgkin lymphoma (NHL) and two cases of KS. All these tumours occurred in individuals who were HIV positive. However, it is significant that the cases of KS occurred in a homosexual man from New York City, and in a man from the Mediterranean region.

All the 12 HIV-associated NHL were classified histologically as intermediate or high grade (Table 12.4). Ten of these tumours were extranodal (83%) but only one was localized to the central nervous system. There was only one patient with a lymphoma who had been treated with zidovudine. Lymphoma was the initial AIDS-indicative diagnosis for 11 of 12 subjects and comprised 6.6% of AIDS-defining diagnoses for the 168 individuals with AIDS in the cohort. One individual had a T-cell lymphoma, which was not diagnostic of AIDS.

There were two cases of basal cell carcinoma of the skin and eight other cancers amongst the HIV-positive individuals, but the seronegative individuals had a comparable experience, with three cases of basal cell carcinoma and five cases of other cancers in the same period.

The age-specific incidence in the general population would have expected to have 0.01 cases of KS, 0.5 cases of NHL, and 8.4 cases of other cancers. Thus the observed cases were 200, 24, and 0.9 times the expected numbers respectively. For the HIV-negative subjects there would have been expected

Table 12.4 Frequencies of incident cancers in 1065 HIV-positive (+) and 636 HIV-negative (–) haemophilia patients, October 1982 to March 1991

Morphological classification	HIV+	HIV–
Non-Hodgkin lymphoma		
Immunoblastic	1	...
Burkitt's lymphoma	2	...
Small non-cleaved cell, non-Burkitt's lymphoma	2[a]	...
High-grade lymphoma, not otherwise specified	2	...
Large-cell diffuse T-cell lymphoma of uncertain classification	1[b]	...
Kaposi's sarcoma	2	...
Hodgkin's disease		
Nodular sclerosis	1	1
Mixed cellularity	1	...
Melanoma	1	1
Lymphoblastic leukaemia	1	...
Lung carcinoma	1	1
Oropharyngeal carcinoma	2	...
Cervical carcinoma *in situ*	1	...
Bladder carcinoma	...	1
Ependymona	...	1
Basal cell carcinoma of the skin	2	3

[a]Includes one tumour that may have been polyclonal.
[b]Lymphoepithelioid non-Hodgkin lymphoma versus Hodgkin's disease.
(Copyright © *JAMA* 26 February 1992; vol. 267(8), p. 1093, Rabkin *et al.*)[34]

0.3 cases of NHL and 5.2 cases of other cancers, an observed-to-expected risk ratio of 0 and 1.0 (Table 12.5).

Increasing duration of HIV infection was associated with an exponential rise in the incidence of NHL and on average lymphoma incidence doubled every 2.4 years (Table 12.4). The estimated 12-year cumulative incidence of NHL for HIV-positive subjects was 2.1%. In contrast to NHL other cancers showed no consistent trend in incidence after HIV seroconversaion (Table 12.6).

Although the incidence of NHL increased exponentially with increasing duration of HIV infection there was not a strong association with CD4 depletion, suggesting the importance of other factors in progression of HIV disease (Figure 12.16).

The histological subtypes of NHL that are associated with HIV include immunoblastic, small non-cleaved tumours and large-cell tumours. Infection with HIV may stimulate B-cell expansion, and activation of Epstein–Barr virus may be an important event which precedes lymphomagenesis[35].

Whereas in homosexual men there is an increase of up to 40 000-fold[36] of KS, in these haemophilic men the observed cases were only 24 times expected.

Table 12.5 Incident rates per 100 person-years on non-Hodgkin lymphoma and other cancers in HIV-positive (+) haemophilia patients by years from HIV seroconversion

	Non-Hodgkin lymphoma				Other cancers[a]		
HIV + (years)	Person-years	Cases	Rate	Cumulative risk (±SE)	Cases	Rate	Cumulative risk (±SE)
0–1	2118	0	0.00	0 ...	2	0.09	0.19 (±0.1)
2–3	2089	3	0.14	0.29 (±0.2)	5	0.24	0.67 (±0.3)
4–5	1925	2	0.10	0.50 (±0.2)	1	0.05	0.77 (±0.3)
6–7	1508	3	0.20	0.92 (±0.3)	0	0.00	0.77 (±0.3)
8–9	531	4	0.75	2.13 (±0.7)	0	0.00	0.77 (±0.3)
10–11	70	0	0.00	2.13 (±0.7)	0	0.00	0.77 (±0.3)
Total	8241	12	0.15	...	8	0.10	

[a]Excludes non-Hodgkin lymphoma, Kaposi's sarcoma, and basal cell carcinoma.
(Copyright © *JAMA* 26 February 1992 vol. 267(8). Rabkin *et al.*)[34]

Table 12.6 Incidence rates per 100 person-years and relative risk of non-Hodgkin lymphoma in HIV-positive haemophilia patients by 10-year age groups

Age group (years)	Person-years	Cases	Rate	US rate[a]	Relative risk
0–9	641	0	0.00	0.001	0
10–19	2197	2	0.09	0.002	49
20–29	2575	3	0.12	0.003	42
30–39	1705	4	0.23	0.007	32
40–49	649	1	0.15	0.014	11
50–59	319	1	0.31	0.025	12
>60	147	1	0.68	0.049	14

[a]Estimates from the Surveillance, Epidemiology, and End Results Program for males, all races, 1983–1987.
(Copyright © *JAMA* 26 February 1992 vol. 267(8). Rabkin *et al.*)[34]

Mediterranean ancestry is suggested as a risk factor for KS in immunosuppressed transplant recipients[37]. Since in the Multicenter Hemophilia Cohort study the two cases of KS occurred in a homosexual man from New York and a man from the Mediterranean, this supports the idea that a cofactor is required for immunodeficiency-related KS.

However, total cancer incidence was not increased compared to HIV-negative individuals with haemophilia or the general population. This is an important observation because treatment may alter immune function in the absence of HIV infection and it is therefore clear that these immune changes are not associated with an increased risk of cancer.

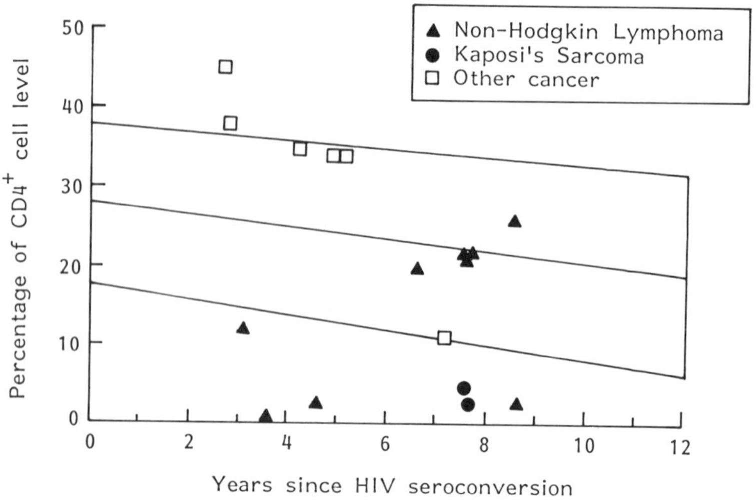

Figure 12.16 *Percentage of CD4+ T-lymphocytes near time of cancer diagnosis in 17 patients who are positive for human immunodeficiency virus (HIV) and have non-Hodgkin lymphoma, Kaposi's sarcoma or other cancer. From: Chorba TL, Holman RC, Strine TW* et al[5]. *Changes in longevity and causes of death among persons with haemophilia.* J Haematol *1994; 45: 112–121. Copyright © 1994. (Reprinted by permission of John Wiley & Sons, Inc.)*

HIV INFECTION AND THE TREATMENT OF HAEMOPHILIA

The development of neutralizing anti-factor VIII antibodies is one of the most serious complications of haemophilia treatment. Several authors have documented the loss of such antibodies in individuals infected with HIV[38,39]. Amongst 77 patients with inhibitors who were identified among a large group of HIV-infected patients with haemophilia, 13 of the high-responder patients were rechallenged with factor VIII concentrates after several years of treatment with other plasma products. Seven of the 13 patients were in the advanced stages of HIV infection at the time of rechallenge. Inhibitor titres measured less than 1 BU in five of these seven, reflecting the loss of antibody with advancing HIV disease[40]. There was a lack of anamnestic response in all 13 individuals—the clinical details and the outcome of the rechallenge are shown in Table 12.7. This observation reflects the loss in humoral immunity in individuals with HIV infection[41].

Clotting factor concentrates differ in the viral inactivation process as well as the level of purity achieved. Presently available concentrates include intermediate purity, with a specific activity of 1–50 U/mg, high-purity products made using chromatography with a specific activity of 100–2000 U/mg, and

Table 12.7 Characteristics of 13 HIV-infected inhibitor patients rechallenged with factor VIII

Patient no.	Age at inhibitor diagnosis (years)	Highest documented inhibitor titre (BU)	Age (years) and date at time of rechallenge	Date and result of most recent inhibitor assay
1	31	14.5	46.3; 3/89	4/89; negative
2	5	1151	17.9; 2/88	4/88; negative
3	5	19	17.8; 5/89	3/90; negative
4	19	66	38.8; 12/89	7/90; 0.6 BU
5	7	42	16.8; 4/89	2/89; 0.9 BU
6	4	18	16.1; 6/89	4/91; 0.9 BU
7	0.08	26	11.3; 12/88	4/91; 0.5 BU
8	9	14	19.8; 11/88	5/90; negative
9	42	32	57.7; 3/87	11/87; negative
10	4	344	13.1; 4/87	2/89; negative
11	2	63	6.1; 9/86	6/87; negative
12	5	26	16.9; 9/89	1/91; negative
13	8	25	14.2; 5/85	11/88; negative

From: Bray GL, Kroner BL, Arkin S *et al.*[40] loss of high-responder inhibitors in patients with severe haemophilia A and human immunodeficiency virus type 1 infection: a report from the multi-center hemophilia cohort study. *Am J Haematol* 1993; 42: 375–379. Copyright © 1993. (Reprinted by permission of John Wiley & Sons, Inc.)

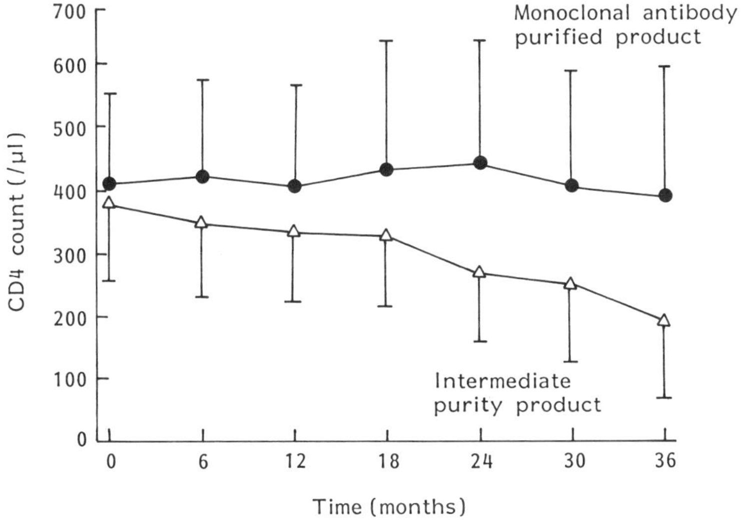

Figure 12.17 *Six-monthly CD4 counts. (Reproduced by permission from Seremetis SV, Aledort LM, Bergman GE* et al.[46] *Three-year randomised study of high-purity or intermediate-purity factor VIII concentrate in symptom-free HIV seropositive hemophiliacs: effects on immune status.* Lancet *1993; 342: 700–703. © by the Lancet Ltd.)*

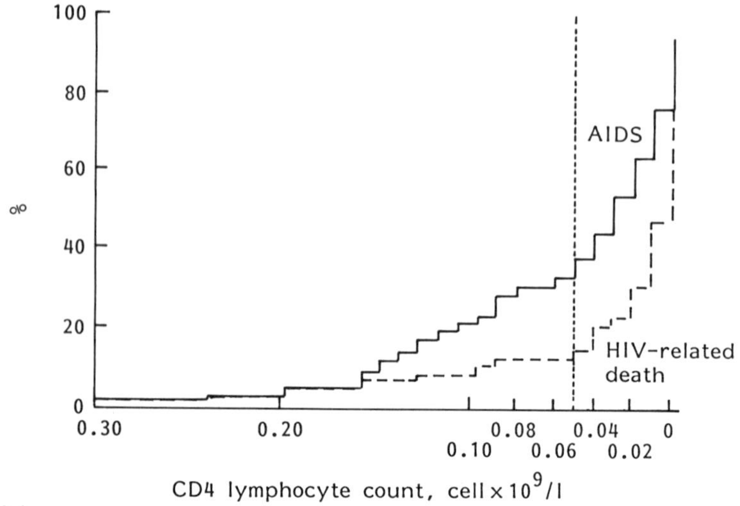

No. at risk

AIDS	73	60	36	29	25	21	15	4
Death	74	61	44	38	36	33	29	11

Figure 12.18 *Kaplan–Meier plots to AIDS and death according to CD4 count. (Reproduced by permission from Phillips* et al.[51]*)*

very high-purity concentrates made by monoclonal and recombinant technology with a specific activity of 2000–3000 U/mg.

A number of clinical studies suggested that monoclonal purified products had a beneficial effect on the decline of CD4 count in HIV-positive patients[42–44]. None of these studies had a control group, but de Biasi[45] was able to show convincingly that there was a significant improvement in the decline of CD4 count in patients treated with a monoclonal product compared to those treated with intermediate product. A further randomized study comparing the use of monoclonal purified product with intermediate-purity product has also demonstrated stabilization of the CD4 fall in those receiving the purer concentrate[46] (Figure 12.17). A retrospective analysis in a large cohort of haemophilic patients in the USA has also shown that those receiving the high-purity concentrates had a slower decline in CD4 count[47]. It would seem that this beneficial effect is not shown by chromatographically purified concentrates[48] but recombinant products do show the beneficial effect[49]. A retrospective study has also shown an improvement in CD4 decline following a switch to monoclonal products[50]. Since it has been demonstrated that survival is dependent on CD4 rather than length of time from seroconversion[51] (Figure 12.18) it is likely that the stabilization of CD4 counts following treatment with high-purity products will translate into decreased morbidity and increased survival.

CONCLUSIONS

HIV infection has had an enormous impact on patients with haemophilia. It is reassuring that there have been no new seroconversions following treatment with clotting factor concentrate since 1986 worldwide. Thus children born after 1986 are free from infection and have the benefit of ever more pure clotting factor concentrate. Since the time that individuals became infected with HIV is largely known and because patients with haemophilia undergo regular follow-up for their bleeding disorder, much about the natural history of HIV disease has been learnt from these patients. It seems likely that the latent period to the development of severe HIV disease may exceed 20 years in a substantial number of individuals and much will continue to be learnt from the study of these patients which can be applied to other risk groups.

REFERENCES

1. Anonymous. *Pneumocystis carinii* pneumonia among persons with haemophilia A. *MMWR* 1982; 31: 365–367.
2. Lee CA, Webster A, Griffiths PD, Kernoff PBA. Symptomless HIV infection after more than ten years. *Lancet* 1990; 335: 425–426.
3. Lee CA, Phillips A, Elford J *et al.* The natural history of human immunodeficiency virus infection in a haemophilic cohort. *Br J Haematol* 1989; 73: 228–234.
4. Eyster ME, Gail MH, Ballard JO *et al.* Natural history of human immunodeficiency virus infections in hemophiliacs: effects of T-cell subsets, platelet counts, and age. *Ann Intern Med* 1987; 107: 1–6.
5. Chorba TL, Holman RC, Strine TW *et al.* Changes in longevity and causes of death among persons with hemophilia A. *Am J Hematol* 1994; 45: 112–121.
6. Lee CA, Sabin CA, Phillips AN *et al.* Morbidity and mortality from transfusion-transmitted disease in haemophilia. *Lancet* 1995 345: 1309.
7. Eyster ME, Diamondstone LS, Lien JM *et al.* Natural history of hepatitis C virus infection in multitransfused hemophiliacs: effect of coinfection with human immunodeficiency virus. The Multicenter Hemophilia Cohort Study. *J AIDS* 1993; 6: 602–610.
8. Telfer P, Sabin C, Devereux H *et al.* The progression of HCV-associated liver disease in a cohort of haemophilic patients. *Br J Haematol* 1994; 87: 555–561.
9. Phillips AN, Sabin CA, Elford J *et al.* Use of CD4 lymphocyte count to predict long term survival free of AIDS after HIV infection. *Br Med J* 1994; 309: 309–313.
10. Darby SC, Rizza CR, Doll R *et al.* Incidence of AIDS and excess of mortality associated with HIV in haemophiliacs in the United Kingdom: report on behalf of the directors of haemophilia centres in the United Kingdom. *Br Med J* 1989; 298: 1064–1068.
11. Goedert JJ, Kessler CM, Aledort LM *et al.* A prospective study of human immunodeficiency virus type 1 infection and the development of AIDS in subjects with hemophilia. *N Engl J Med* 1989; 321: 1141–1148.
12. Phillips AN, Lee CA, Elford J *et al.* More rapid progression to AIDS in older HIV-infected people: the role of CD4+ T-cell counts. *J AIDS* 1991; 4: 970–975.

13. Phillips AN, Lee CA, Elford J *et al.* p24 antigenaemia, CD4 lymphocyte counts and the development of AIDS. *AIDS* 1991; 5: 1217–1222.
14. Cheingsong-Popov R, Panagiotidi C, Bowcock S *et al.* Relation between humoral responses to HIV gag and env proteins at seroconversion and clinical outcome of HIV infection. *Br Med J* 1991; 302: 23–26.
15. Cuthbert RJG, Ludlam CA, Tucker J *et al.* Five year prospective study of HIV infection in the Edinburgh haemophiliac cohort. *Br Med J* 1990; 301: 956–961.
16. Sahmoud T, Laurian Y, Garzengel C *et al.* Progression to AIDS in French haemophiliacs association with HLA-B35. *AIDS* 1993; 7: 497–500.
17. Sabin CA, Phillips AN, Lee CA *et al.* Beta-2 microglobulin as a predictor of prognosis in HIV-infected men with haemophilia: a proposed strategy for use in clinical care. *Br J Haematol* 1994; 86: 366–371.
18. Bhalla RB, Safai B, Pahwa S, Schwartz MK. $Beta_2$ microglobulin as a prognostic marker for development of AIDS. *Clin Chem* 1985; 31: 1411–1412.
19. Moss AR, Bacchetti P, Osmond D *et al.* Seropositivity of HIV and the development of AIDS or AIDs related condition: three-year follow-up of the San Francisco General Cohort. *Br Med J* 1988; 296: 745–750.
20. Fahey JL, Taylor JMG, Detels R *et al.* The prognostic value of cellular and serologic markers in infection with human immunodeficiency virus type 1. *N Engl J Med* 1990; 322: 166–172.
21. Hofmann B, Wang Y, Cumberland WG *et al.* Serum-$beta_2$-microglobulin level increases in HIV infection: relation to seroconversion, CD4 T-cell fall and prognosis. *AIDS* 1990; 4: 207–214.
22. Chevret S, Roquin H, Ganne P, Lefrere JJ. Prognostic value of an elevated CD8 lymphocyte count in HIV infection: results of a prospective study of 152 asymptomatic HIV-positive individuals. *AIDS* 1992; 6: 1349–1352.
23. Schwartlander B, Bek B, Skarabis H *et al.* Improvement of the predictive value of CD4+ lymphocyte count by β_2-microglobulin, immunoglobulin A and erythrocyte sedimentation rate. *AIDS* 1993; 7: 318–321.
24. Phillips AN, Sabin CA, Elford J *et al.* CD8 lymphocyte counts and serum immunoglobulin A levels early in HIV infection as predictors of CD4 lymphocyte depletion during 8 years of follow-up. *AIDS* 1993; 7: 975–980.
25. Aronstam A, Congard B, Evans DI *et al.* HIV infection in haemophilia: a European cohort. *Arch Dis Child* 1993; 68: 521–524.
26. Webster A, Phillips AN, Lee CA *et al.* Cytomegalovirus (CMV) infection, $CD4^+$ lymphocyte counts and the development of AIDS in HIV-1-infected haemophiliac patients. *Clin Exp Immunol* 1992; 88: 6–9.
27. Ratnoff OD, Menitove JE, Aster RH, Lederman MH. Coincident classic haemophilia and 'idiopathic' thrombocytopenia purpura in patients with concentrates of anti-haemophilic factor (factor VIII). *N Engl J Med* 1983; 308: 439–442.
28. Ragni MV, Bontempo FA, Myers DJ *et al.* Hemorrhagic sequelae of immune thrombocytopenic pupura in human immunodeficiency virus-infected haemophiliacs. *Blood* 1990; 75: 1267–1272.
29. Karpatkin S. Immunologic thrombocytopenia purpura in HIV seropositive homosexuals, narcotic addicts and haemophiliacs. *Semin Haematol* 1988; 23: 219–229.
30. Leissinger CA, Andes WA. Role of splenectomy in the management of hemophilic patients with human immunodeficiency virus-associated immunopathic thrombocytopenic purpura. *Am J Haematol* 1992; 40: 207–209.
31. Brown SA, Majumdar G, Harrington C *et al.* Effect of splenectomy on HIV-related thrombocytopenia and progression of HIV infection with patients with severe haemophilia. *Blood Coagul Fibrinolysis* 1994; 5: 393–397.
32. Eyster ME, Fried MW, Di Bisceglie AM, Goedert JJ. Increasing hepatitis C virus

RNA levels in haemophiliacs: relationship to human immunodeficiency virus infection and liver disease. *Blood* 1994; 84: 1020–1023.
33. Colombo M, Mannucci PM, Brettler DB *et al.* Hepatocellular carcinoma in hemophilia. *Am J Hematol* 1991; 37: 243–246.
34. Rabkin CS, Hilgartner MW, Hedberg KW *et al.* Incidence of lymphomas and other cancers in HIV-infected and HIV-uninfected patients with hemophilia. *JAMA* 1992; 267: 1090–1094.
35. Neri A, Barriga F, Inghirami G *et al.* Epstein–Barr virus infection precedes clonal expansion in Burkitt's and acquired immunodeficiency syndrome-associated lymphoma. *Blood* 1991; 77: 1092–1095.
36. Rabkin CS, Biggar RJ, Horm JW. Increasing incidence of cancers associated with the human immunodeficiency virus epidemic. *Int J Cancer* 1991; 47: 692–696.
37. Harwood AR, Osoba D, Hofstader SL *et al.* Kaposi's sarcoma in recipients of renal transplants. *Am J Med* 1979; 67: 759–765.
38. Leyva WH, Knutsen AP, Joist JH. Disappearance of a high responder factor VIII inhibitor in a haemophiliac with AIDS. *Am J Clin Pathol* 1988; 89: 414–418.
39. Ragni MV, Ruben FL, Winkelstein A *et al.* Antibody responses to immunization of patients with haemophilia with and without evidence of human immunodeficiency virus (human T-lymphotropic type III) infection. *J Lab Clin Med* 1987; 109: 545–549.
40. Bray GL, Kroner BL, Arkin S *et al.* Loss of high-responder inhibitors in patients with severe hemophilia A and human immunodeficiency virus type 1 infection: a report from the multi-center hemophilia cohort study. *Am J Hematol* 1993; 42: 375–379.
41. Lane HC, Masur H, Edgar LC *et al.* Abnormalities of B cell activation and immunoregulation in patients with the acquired immunodeficiency syndrome. *N Engl J Med* 1983; 309: 453–458.
42. Brettler DB, Forsberg AD, Levine PH *et al.* Factor VIII:C concentrate purified from plasma using monoclonal antibodies: human studies. *Blood* 1989; 73: 1859–1863.
43. Goldsmith JM, Deutsche J, Tang M, Green D. CD4 cells in HIV-1 infected haemophiliacs: effect of factor VIII concentrates. *Thromb Haemost* 1991; 66: 415–419.
44. Fukutake K, Ikematsu S, Fujimaki M *et al.* Multicenter study on the influence of long-term continuous use of purified factor VIII preparation on the immunological status of HIV infected and non-infected hemophilia A patients. *XIXth International Congress of the World Federation of Hemophilia,* 1990; pp. 34 (Abstract).
45. de Biasi R, Rocino A, Miraglia E *et al.* The impact of a very high purity factor VIII concentrate on the immune system of human immunodeficiency virus-infected hemophiliacs: a randomised, prospective, two-year comparison with an intermediate purity concentrate. *Blood* 1991; 78: 1919–1922.
46. Seremetis SV, Aledort LM, Bergman GE *et al.* Three-year randomised study of high-purity or intermediate-purity factor VIII concentrates in symptom-free HIV seropositive haemophiliacs: effects on immune status. *Lancet* 1993; 342: 700–703.
47. Hilgartner MW, Buckley JD, Operskalski EA *et al.* Purity of factor VIII concentrates and serial CD4 counts: the transfusion safety study group. *Lancet* 1993; 341: 1373–1374.
48. Mannucci PM, Gririgeri A, de Biasi R *et al.* Immune status of asymptomatic HIV-infected hemophiliacs: randomised, prospective, two-year comparison of treatment with a high-purity or an intermediate-purity factor VIII concentrate. *Thromb Haemost* 1992; 67: 310–313.
49. Mannucci PM, Brettler DB, Aledort LM *et al.* Immune status of human immunodeficiency virus seropositive and seronegative haemophiliacs infused for 3.5 years with recombinant factor VIII. *Blood* 1994; 83: 1958–1962.

50. Sabin C, Pasi J, Phillips A *et al.* CD4+ counts before and after switching to monoclonal high-purity VIII concentrate in HIV-infected haemophilic patients. *Thromb Haemost* 1994; 72: 214–217.
51. Phillips AN, Elford J, Sabin C *et al.* Immunodeficiency and the risk of death in HIV infection. *JAMA* 1992; 268: 2662–2666.

13

Opportunistic Infections in AIDS Patients

Marc Allan Tack and Kenneth H. Mayer
Brown University School of Medicine, Brown, Rhode Island, USA

INTRODUCTION

Beginning in the early 1980s with reports of pneumonia caused by the previously rare organism, *Pneumocystis carinii*[1], opportunistic infections (OI) have been the most common manifestation of infection with the human immunodeficiency virus (HIV). Despite significant improvement in the diagnosis, therapy, and prevention of OIs, they remain the leading cause of death in patients with acquired immunodeficiency syndrome (AIDS). These often life-threatening opportunistic infections are caused by a variety of bacterial, viral, fungal, and protozoan pathogens that are major manifestations of the progressive deterioration of the hosts' immune system. Most opportunistic infections are not commonly seen until significant immunological deterioration has occurred, as reflected by a decreased absolute CD4 lymphocyte count. Infections associated with HIV typically occur at specific levels of immunosuppression and, therefore, knowledge of the patient's CD4 count is important for diagnostic purposes. Specific CD4 thresholds have been developed to guide the institution of various prophylactic interventions.

Many of these opportunistic pathogens are ubiquitous organisms not usually associated with illness in an immunocompetent host, such as *Pneumocystis carinii*, while others are the result of the recurrence of latent infections (e.g., cytomegalovirus (CMV)). In addition, there are differences in the reported rates of infection with various types of opportunistic pathogens in different geographic regions. For example, disseminated coccidioidomycosis is more common in HIV-infected residents or travelers of the south-

AIDS and Malignancies: Current Concepts and Perspectives.
Edited by B.C. Golematis and V.T. DeVita Jr

Table 13.1 Indicator infections included in the 1993 AIDS surveillance case definition

Bacterial pneumonias (recurrent)
Candidiasis of bronchi, trachea, or lungs
Candidiasis, esophageal
Coccidioidomycosis, disseminated or extrapulmonary
Cryptococcus, extrapulmonary
Cryptosporidiosis, chronic intestinal (> 1 month duration)
Cytomegalovirus disease (other than liver, spleen, or nodes)
Herpes simplex: chronic ulcers (> 1 month duration) or bronchitis, pneumonitis, or esophagitis
Histoplasmosis, disseminated or extrapulmonary
HIV-related encephalopathy
Isosporiasis, chronic intestinal (> 1 month duration)
Mycobacterium avium complex or *Mycobacterium kansasi*, disseminated or extrapulmonary
Mycobacterium tuberculosis, any site
Pneumocystis carinii pneumonia
Salmonella septicemia, recurrent
Toxoplasmosis of brain
HIV-related wasting syndrome

Source: Adapted from Centers for Disease Control (1993) revised classification system for HIV infection and expanded surveillance case definition for AIDs among adolescents and adults. *MMWR* 41 (RR-17): 15, 1992.

western USA, while isosporiasis is more prevalent in AIDS patients in Africa. Common pathogens such as *Streptococcus pneumoniae* often cause more severe infection in patients infected with HIV. In addition, many normally non-invasive organisms such as *Candida albicans* may be more virulent and invasive in HIV-infected hosts. Other factors, such as the age at acquisition, various coinfections such as hepatitis C, means of acquisition, and recreational drug abuse likely play a significant role in the infectious manifestations of HIV (Table 13.1).

PNEUMOCYSTIS CARINII

Pneumonia caused by *Pneumocystis carinii* is the most common presenting opportunistic infection in patients infected with HIV in North America. *Pneumocystis carinii* pneumonia (PCP) is associated with a significant level of immunosuppression and is usually seen in patients with a CD4 count of less than 200. The incidence of this infection has stabilized in the past several years due to primary and secondary prophylaxis, though it remains the most common cause of death in patients with AIDS. It is estimated that 80% of patients with AIDS will develop at least one episode of PCP in their lifetime without adequate prophylaxis[2].

Pneumocystis carinii is a ubiquitous organism that was a rare cause of disease in humans prior to the HIV epidemic. Before 1980, infection secondary to this organism was primarily described in malnourished children and severely immunosuppressed patients such as leukaemic children and organ transplant recipients. In this population, PCP was typically an abrupt infection limited to the lungs[3]. In patients with HIV, *Pneumocystis carinii* has been isolated in extrapulmonary sites as well as the respiratory tract. Most Americans have antibodies against *Pneumocystis carinii* by the age of four and thus serological screening is of no benefit[4].

The life cycle of *Pneumocystis* is poorly understood and its classification has been a subject of much conjecture. Molecular and genetic evaluation of the organism suggests it is more closely related to fungi than protozoa; however, its antimicrobial sensitivity pattern is more consistent with the latter. In a recent editorial, it was suggested that '*Pneumocystis* appears to be a phylogenetically old parasite without close relatives'[5]. In nature, *Pneumocystis* undergoes both sexual and asexual reproduction and its exact life cycle and site of maturation are still being elucidated.

The clinical presentation of primary pneumonia caused by *Pneumocystis carinii* is commonly insidious in onset. Patients typically report a syndrome of non-productive cough accompanied by progressive dyspnea with exertion, worsening over several weeks, in association with weakness, fever, and malaise. While the abrupt onset of PCP in patients with HIV has been described, this presentation is more common in HIV-negative patients. Spontaneous pneumothorax presenting in a patient with HIV infection should be evaluated for PCP and is more common in patients receiving aerosolized pentamidine prophylaxis.

Radiographic manifestations of PCP vary with primary versus recurrent infection and whether the patient was previously taking prophylactic therapy. In primary PCP, the chest radiograph typically demonstrates bilateral interstitial infiltrates in a diffuse pattern. This pattern is similar to the radiographic pattern described with atypical respiratory pathogens such as *Mycoplasma pneumoniae* and *Legionella pneumophila*. In patients receiving aerosolized pentamidine, the radiographic pattern is less predictable but often reveals significant upper lobe involvement since aerosolized therapy results in lesser concentrations of the agent in the upper airways.

The diagnosis of PCP can be confirmed by direct visualization of the organism using appropriate stains or by immunofluorescence[6]. In many institutions, because it is inexpensive and non-invasive, induced sputum is the initial specimen tested[7]. If the induced specimen is negative, then a bronchoscopy with bronchoalveolar lavage or biopsy is usually the next choice[8]. Various staining procedures are available for identifying *Pneumocystis carinii*, with the Giemsa and the Gomori methenamine silver stain being the most common utilized. Recent advances in immunofluorescent techniques have led to increased utilization of this procedure; it has a sensitivity of 99% and is less labor intensive than older staining procedures[9].

The primary therapy for PCP is trimethoprim–sulfamethoxazole; however, more than 30% of patients are unable to tolerate this agent because of allergic reactions, the most common of which is a maculopapular rash[10]. There are now several other regimens with documented efficacy such as pentamidine and clindamycin–primaquin, all of which inhibit folic acid biosynthesis[11]. The recently released agent, atavaquone, is approved for use in mild to moderate PCP and a liquid suspension formulation recently released appears to improve this agent's absorption, a significant problem with the initial preparation[12]. Several studies have shown benefit utilizing trimetrexate with leucovorin for salvage therapy in patients failing more standard therapy[13].

The benefit of adjuvant corticosteroids in the treatment of moderate to severe PCP has been well documented[14]. Patients with an ateriolar–alveolar gradient of 35 torr or more or a peripheral arterial oxygen saturation of less than 70 torr on room air should be started on steroids. The most effective dose and route of administration have been undergoing intensive study. Based on the results of multiple studies, a consensus report has recently been generated with specific recommendations for adjuvant therapy[15].

The institution of prophylaxis for PCP is perhaps the single most significant intervention to reduce mortality in patients with HIV. Presently, patients with a CD4 count of 200 cells/mm^3 or less, or with a history of previous PCP, should receive prophylactic therapy. Trimethoprim–sulfamethoxazole is effective in 95–99% of patients who are compliant with therapy[16]. Because over one-third of patients on this regimen develop allergic reactions, other agents have been utilized and a variety of trimehoprim–sulfamethoxazole desensitization regimens have been developed. Dapsone has been shown to be effective but breakthrough has been reported, especially at the 50 mg daily dose as compared to 100 mg[17]. Aerosolized pentamidine treatments given once a month are less effective than the regimens noted above and, because of poor upper lobe distribution of the drug, breakthrough disease with spontaneous pneumothorax has been a significant problem[18] (Table 13.2). Monthly intravenous pentamidine prophylaxis is less desirable because of systemic toxicities, such as hypoglycaemia and pancreatitis.

TOXOPLASMOSIS

The protozoan *Toxoplasma gondii* is a frequent cause of encephalitis in patients with HIV. While this organism is most commonly diagnosed in patients who already have an AIDS diagnosis, Centers for Disease Control (CDC) data from 1989 report this as the initial AIDS infection in 5% of all HIV-infected patients[19]. Multiple series have demonstrated a lower incidence of active toxoplasmosis in patients on trimethoprim–sulfamethoxazole, pyri-

Table 13.2 Pulmonary infections in HIV

Pneumocystis carinii
Mycobacterium tuberculosis
Histoplasmosis
Coccidiomycosis
Cryptococcus
Aspergillus
Cytomegalovirus
Herpes simplex virus
Varicella zoster virus
Streptococcus pneumoniae
Haemophilus influenzae
Other bacteria

methamine–dapsone, or sulfadoxine–pyrimethamine for prophylaxis of *Pneumocystis carinii*[20]. This benefit is not present in patients receiving aerosolized pentamidine.

Toxoplasma gondii is an obligate intracellular organism that is ubiquitous in nature. Felines are the natural reservoir for this organism for sporozoite production, and in mammals incidentally infected it exists only in tachyzoites and cysts. Seroprevalence varies between geographic location and in subpopulations within regions; it is more common in European and African AIDS patients than those in North America[21]. AIDS-associated toxoplasmosis in the USA is more common in immigrants from the Caribbean. Immunocompetent hosts generally are able to maintain infection in a quiescent stage and encephalitis in patients with HIV is usually from latent reactivation of the organism in a seropositive host, though disease has been reported in seronegative patients.

A wide spectrum of clinical presentations has been reported, including altered behavioral patterns, seizures, motor weakness, cerebellar dysfunction, sensory abnormalities and encephalitis with altered consciousness. The presentation is usually insidious in onset with cognitive defects, confusion, lethargy, and focal neurological manifestations commonly noted. Seizures are the presenting event in approximately 33% of patients with active infection and coma is not uncommon. Hemiparesis is the most common focal neurological presentation but ataxia, visual field deficits, aphasia, tremor and many other findings have been reported[22]. Active disease involving the spinal cord has also been described in addition to the central nervous system,

Toxoplasma gondii has been reported to involve the pulmonary system[23]. This often presents as a protracted febrile illness with cough and dyspnea, and associated extrapulmonary disease is often found. Endocrine disorders involving the pituitary axis have been reported as a late complication of active toxoplasmosis[24]. Ocular disease with necrotizing retinochoroiditis may occur and has been reported to precede encephalitis in some patients[15]. Congenital toxoplasmosis transmitted from a woman with either primary infection during pregnancy or reactivation of latent disease is an important consideration in the neonate of an HIV-infected patient but the relative risk has not been quantified.

Radiographic imaging of the CNS is the most frequent test utilized in the diagnosis of toxoplasmic encephalitis. Computed tomography (CT) scan typically reveals multiple, hypodense bilateral mass lesions that enhance with contrast[26]. Magnetic resonance imaging (MRI) appears to be more sensitive than CT and may reveal lesions otherwise not visualized. On MRI, lesions typically are enhancing, bilateral and are most frequently found in the basal ganglia or the cerebral corticomedullary junction. The finding of a single lesion on MRI should raise the suspicion for other causes of mass lesions such as lymphoma. The CT scan or MRI is commonly used for monitoring therapeutic response to medical treatment and typically shows a reduction by at least 50% after three weeks of appropriate therapy.

The diagnosis of toxoplasmic encephalitis can only be definitive by visualizing the organism in appropriate tissue specimens[27]. Because this would require a brain biopsy, it is not common practice to begin empirical therapy and monitor the radiographic response closely. If patients fail to respond to therapy, a brain biopsy is frequently needed to make a diagnosis. Because toxoplasmic encephalitis usually represents recurrence of latent disease, a single detectable serological level of IgG is not helpful. While IgM to toxoplasmosis is usually elevated in immunocompetent hosts, it is often undetectable in HIV-infected patients with active encephalitis. Rising titers may suggest the diagnosis, and negative serology makes the diagnosis of active toxoplasmosis unlikely.

Primary treatment for active disease is sulfadiazine in combination with pyrimethamine, which inhibits parasitic but not mammalian biosynthesis[18]. Folinic acid is typically administered with pyrimethamine to decrease bone marrow suppression associated with this agent. Corticosteroids are often required to manage intracranial hypertension as a result of mass effect from toxoplasmosis abscesses. Patients often are unable to tolerate sulfadiazine due to allergic reactions. In several studies, clindamycin used with pyrimethamine has been shown to be equally effective to the above combination[29]. In addition, the newer agent atavaquone has been beneficial as salvage therapy in patients either not responding or intolerant to first-line agents[30]. The optimal length of primary therapy is not known and it is common practice to decide duration of primary treatment on clinical and radiographic response. Numerous agents are under investigation for efficacy in treating active encephalitis, including the newer macrolides azithromycin and clarithromycin.

All patients treated for toxoplasmic encephalitis require lifelong maintenance therapy to prevent recurrence. Relapse of active disease is related to persistence of the cyst form of the organism as the first-line agents for primary therapy are not active against the cyst form. Presently, combination therapy with pyrimethamine and sulfadiazine is recommended[31]. Because many patients cannot tolerate this regimen, other regimens have been successfully utilized, including pyrimethamine alone[32] and in combination with either clindamycin, dapsone, atavaquone, clarithromycin or azithromycin. Several studies evaluating regimens utilized for prophylaxis against *Pneumocystis carinii* demonstrated a significant reduction in the incidence of toxoplasmosis[33]. These regimens included pyrimethamine–dapsone, pyrimethamine–sulfadoxine, Fansidar, and trimethoprim–sulfamethoxazole. Further studies to determine optimal therapy need to be done.

CRYPTOSPORIDIOSIS

Cryptosporidiosis is the most common etiology of persistent diarrhea in AIDS patients. *Cryptosporidium parvum* was first recognized as a human pathogen in 1976 and was thought only to produce illness in immunosuppressed patients; however, outbreaks in immunocompetent patients have been reported. One-half of all patients with AIDS get diarrhea and the annual rate of cryptosporidiosis is estimated at 5–10% a year[34]. Cryptosporidiosis in AIDS can occur at all ranges of immunosuppression but chronic persistent diarrhea is associated with CD4 counts of less than 200 cells/mm^3.

The clinical manifestations of cryptosporidial disease are generally limited to the gastrointestinal system. In AIDS patients, it is usually associated with severe voluminous watery diarrhea. Patients also frequently report severe crampy abdominal pain as well as weight loss, anorexia and low-grade temperature. Biliary involvement, as well as extracolonic disease, have also been noted in AIDS patients.

There is presently no satisfactory treatment available for cryptosporidial diarrhea. Paromomycin has been reported to improve symptoms in several small series but relapse is common. Oral bovine transfer factor has also been used in AIDS patients and produced symptomatic improvement in five of eight patients in one small series, with one patient achieving complete resolution of disease and no further evidence of *Cryptosporidium* for two years[36]. The newer macrolides are also under study for the treatment of this infection.

Prevention of cryptosporidiosis in AIDS patients is the most effective way to control this pathogen. In 1993, a well-publicized outbreak of infectious diarrhea was reported secondary to contamination of the Milwaukee public water supply with *Cryptosporidium*[37]. There have been six well-documented outbreaks of *Cryptosporidium* related to public water supply systems in the USA and it is likely that others have gone undocumented. Recommendations for decreasing exposure to this pathogen have recently been published[38] (Table 13.3).

Table 13.3 Common infections, causes of diarrhea in AIDS

Bacterial	Viral	Parasitic
Salmonella species	Cytomegalovirus	Microsporidia
Shigella	HIV	*Cryptosporidium*
Campylobacter jejuni	Herpes simplex virus	*Isospora belli*
Clostridium difficile		*Entamoeba histolytica*
Mycobacterium tuberculosis		*Giardia lamblia*

MICROSPORIDIOSIS

Microsporidia are obligate intracellular spore-forming protozoans that cause a myriad of clinical disease in AIDS patients. There are four genera of *Microsporidium* and prior to the AIDS epidemic there were only 10 cases of well-documented human microsporidiosis. The incidence and prevalence of this pathogen are not yet defined and likely will increase with heightened awareness and improved diagnostic tests. The majority of cases have been reported in males with AIDS and usually occur in patients with less than 100 CD4 cells/mm^3 [39].

The clinical manifestations of microsporidiosis are variable, with organ system involvement with the gastrointestinal tract being most frequently affected. Weight loss, chronic diarrhea and anorexia frequently occur with abdominal pain and fever in microsporidiosis[40]. Sclerosing cholangitis and cholecystitis have also been documented in AIDS patients[41]. Dry eyes, blurred vision, ocular pain, increased tearing, and photophobia may be present when the eyes are involved[42]. Microsporidiosis has also been reported to involve the kidneys, bronchial tree, sinuses, bladder, liver, prostate, and peritoneum.

The diagnosis of microsporidiosis is difficult and often not easy to confirm. Stool analyses using special stains may reveal the agent, but electron microscopy is frequently needed. Giemsa or hematoxylin and eosin (H&E) stained biopsies examined by experienced personnel can be used to make the diagnosis. There is little information available for treatment of microsporidiosis, but albendazole appears to be the most effective agent available thus far.

CRYPTOCOCCAL NEOFORMANS

Infection with *Cryptococcus neoformans* is the most common systemic fungal disease in patients with AIDS[43]. Histoplasmosis and coccidioidomycosis are also recognized as a cause of significant illness in their endemic regions. In general, these fungi are associated with severely compromised cell-mediated immunity and are usually not active until the CD4 count is less than

$200/mm^3$. Clinical disease with these pathogens depends on the specific fungus and organ system involved.

Cryptococcus neoformans is an encapsulated round or oval yeast that is often a cause of meningitis in AIDS patients. Prior to the HIV epidemic, this organism was mainly a pathogen in patients with lymphoreticular malignancies or these on high doses of corticosteroids. *Cryptococcus* is distributed throughout the USA and it is uncertain if there are regional variations in the incidence rate. Active disease is generally associated with acute infection, the portal of entry is the respiratory tract, and the most significant reservoir is pigeon feces and soil contaminated with this excreta. Five to ten per cent of patients with AIDS will develop active cryptococcal infection.

The clinical manifestations of *Cryptococcus neoformans* varies by organ system involved. The CNS is the most commonly involved site and, in general, the onset of disease is insidious and symptoms often wax and wane. Patients typically report a prolonged febrile illness with headache and malaise[44]. Meningitis caused by this organism is often subtle in presentation, which is markedly different from bacterial meningitis, and timely diagnosis requires a high index of suspicion[45]. In clinical practice, all patients with an undiagnosed febrile illness and headache should undergo a lumbar puncture to exclude this disease. The respiratory tract—the typical portal of entry—is involved in active disease in 20–30% of patients. Other reported sites of involvement include the pericardium, myocardium, skin, joints, oral cavity and genitourinary system.

The diagnosis of cryptococcal meningitis is confirmed by evaluation of the cerebrospinal fluid (CSF). In clinical practice, patients with AIDS, fever and a headache usually have an imaging study such as a computed axial tomography (CAT) scan or MRI prior to a lumbar puncture to exclude space-occupying lesions such as toxoplasmosis or lymphoma. These occur with increased frequency in AIDS patients and may be a contraindication to performing a spinal tap because of elevated intracranial pressure. The CSF in patients with cryptococcal meningitis reveals few white blood cells and normal chemistries in up to 50% of cases, and a normal-appearing CSF does not exclude the diagnosis. An India ink evaluation, which demonstrates *Cryptococcus neoformans* in 70–80% of cases, should be done by technicians experienced with this study and cultures for fungus should be obtained[46]. Cryptococcal antigen testing should also be routinely performed as this test has a greater than 90% sensitivity rate in culture-proven disease. While the specific titer is not clinically useful to follow as it does not reliably predict response or treatment failure, a negative serum cryptococcal antigen makes the diagnosis of active disease extremely unlikely and is often used as a screening test in AIDS patients with a fever and headache[47].

The treatment of cryptococcal meningitis requires therapy for the acute infection and chronic lifelong suppressive treatment. The optimal regimen for acute cryptococcal meningitis is controversial and still being investigated.

Amphotericin B alone or in combination with flucytosine has been shown to be effective in 40–75% of cases[48]. The toxicity of these agents has been problematic as over 50% of patients must discontinue flucytosine because of significant bone marrow suppression, and amphotericin B causes significant nephrotoxicity. Fluconazole, an azole available in both oral and intravenous form, has been well studied in the treatment of acute cryptococcal meningitis. Early studies demonstrated high failure rates, leading to the suggestion that amphotericin B-based regimens be the first-line therapy. In 1992 the NIAID Mycosis Study Group (MSG) and AIDS Clinical Trials Group (ACTG) published the results of the largest comparison trial, which revealed similar efficacy rates between the two regimens tested[49]. Patients receiving amphotericin B sterilized their CSF cultures earlier than those treated with fluconazole and there was a higher mortality rate in the first two weeks of treatment in the fluconazole arm of the study but overall survival was similar for the two groups (82% of fluconazole versus 84% for amphotericin B). The use of amphotericin B for the first two weeks followed by fluconazole, as well as the role of the new azole, itraconazole, are under investigation.

All AIDS patients treated for acute cryptococcal disease should be treated with lifelong maintenance therapy. Relapse rates range between 50% and 75% within one year in patients not receiving therapy after treatment for acute disease[44]. Fluconazole dosed at 200 mg per day is presently the recommended therapy for long-term suppression[50]. Amphotericin B given weekly is an alternative regimen. Itraconazole is still under investigation as an alternative prophylactic agent; however, initial reports have not been favorable.

Primary prophylaxis against systemic fungal infections is not yet routinely recommended[51]. In several series oral fluconazole has been shown to decrease the rate of disseminated cryptococcal infection. A recent study comparing fluconazole to clotrimazole troches demonstrated a significant benefit in the fluconazole arm. The development of fluconazole resistance to *Candida* and *Cryptococcus* and breakthrough infection has been reported and may limit the benefit of prophylaxis.

CANDIDIASIS

Candida is a genus of yeast that normally colonize the gastrointestinal and genitourinary tracts of humans. In patients infected with HIV, *Candida* species frequently cause superficial mucocutaneous infections though, rarely, invasive life-threatening disease has been reported. The incidence of *Candida* infection varies by clinical syndrome and 54–93% of AIDS patients will develop oropharyngeal cutaneous candidiasis at some point in their clinical course[52]. Vaginal candidiasis, estimated to involve one in two immunocompetent women during life, occurs with more frequency and often recurs in HIV-infected women[53]. Esophageal candidiasis accounts for 15% of AIDS-defining disease in the USA.

Oropharyngeal candidiasis, typically referred to as thrush, has several different manifestations. The most common presentation is pseudomembranous, which appears as removable white or yellow plaques that frequently bleed when scraped, and may be seen on any mucosal surface. The erythematous form is frequently missed on initial examination and appears as confluent red patches on the buccal mucosa, the dorsal surface of the tongue and the hard or soft palate. *Candida* may also present as a hyperplastic lesion or may cause angular cheilitis, erythematous cracks and fissures seen at the corners of the mouth.

The diagnosis of oropharyngeal candidiasis is made by scraping the lesions, performing a potassium hydroxide smear, Gram stain, or calcofluor stain, and observing the *Candida*. Cultures of scrapings will provide information on the involved species and sensitivity testing can be performed on cultured isolates if resistance to commonly used therapy is suspected.

Primary therapy for oropharyngeal candidiasis utilizes topical antifungal agents such as nystatin and clotrimazole. If these are inadequate, oral ketoconazole or fluconazole may be initiated and these are highly effective. *Candida* strains resistant to the above treatments have been reported and in these cases amphotericin B may be used.

Dysphagia, odynophagia, and retrosternal chest pain are the most frequent symptoms of esophageal candidiasis. Patients frequently report progressive difficulty with swallowing and the sensation of food getting stuck. Concomitant thrush is frequently noted and it is common in clinical practice to treat empirically. The differential diagnosis includes esophageal herpes, CMV, lymphoma, Kaposi's sarcoma, histoplasmosis and squamous cell carcinoma.

The diagnosis of esophageal candidiasis is made by clinical response to empirical therapy in many cases but occasionally patients require further testing. Barium swallow may suggest the diagnosis but cannot confirm it. Patients not responding to therapy should undergo endoscopy, which usually reveals large yellow-white friable plaques. Biopsies and stains or cultures of brushings will demonstrate the organism in active cases.

The treatment of esophageal candidiasis is oral ketoconazole or fluconazole and patients should generally be treated for 10–14 days. In cases where the initial therapy was empirical, if response to therapy is not adequate a diagnostic endoscopy should be performed and histopathological studies done to document infection rather than colonization and to rule out concomitant infection with other mucocutaneous pathogens (e.g. CMV, herpes simplex virus (HSV)). Amphotericin B is reserved for patients not responding to, or intolerant of, oral azoles.

HISTOPLASMOSIS

Histoplasmosis is a significant cause of morbidity and mortality in patients with AIDS in endemic regions. In the USA, histoplasmosis is endemic in the central portion of the country extending from Canada in the areas adjacent to the major river basins to Texas and Mexico in the south. In these regions, infection and disseminated disease must be considered high in the differential diagnosis for systemic febrile illnesses in patients with AIDS. Histoplasmosis is an opportunistic infection in 5–25% of AIDS patients in high-risk geographic regions[54].

Primary infection with histoplasmosis is more common than latent disease, usually by inhalation of organisms into the lung. Patients with normal T-cell function are able to control the initial infection, but with significant T-cell dysfunction as seen in AIDs the organism is able to disseminate. In patients with previous exposure to histoplasmosis, the progressive loss of T-cell-mediated immunity with progression of HIV may lead to late recurrences with dissemination.

The clinical manifestations of disseminated histoplasmosis in AIDS are usually non-specific. Fever, weight loss and malaise are common and respiratory complaints are present in 50% of patients[55]. The CD4 count is generally less than 100 cells/mm^3 at the time of diagnosis. Hepatosplenomegaly as well as lymphadenopathy are frequently noted and neurological disease such as meningitis or cerebritis is reported in 15–20% of cases. The chest radiograph is frequently abnormal, with a diffuse interstitial pneumonitis most commonly noted; alveolar or reticulonodular patterns may also be seen.

The diagnosis of histoplasmosis can be confirmed in several different ways but requires a high index of suspicion, especially in non-endemic regions. Blood cultures are positive in over 85% of patients with disseminated disease utilizing lysis–centrifugation systems but frequently take several weeks[54]. Culture of the organism from tissue specimens as well as identification using histopathological examination also may reveal the diagnosis. Standard serological testing does not differentiate between active disease and previous infection and is of limited value. Wheat *et al.* reported a new histoplasma antigen test that may be performed on serum or urine and he reported a 97.3% sensitivity in 72 patients with HIV coinfection. The histoplasma antigen test may also be of value in following response to therapy[56].

Treatment of histoplasmosis requires therapy for the acute disease as well as lifelong suppression in AIDS patients. In patients with mild to moderate disease, itraconazole has been shown to be equally effective to amphotericin B in several clinical trials[57]. In patients with moderate to severe disease including CNS involvement, amphotericin B should be utilized first and intraconazole utilized for maintenance therapy. Fluconazole is less effective than the above therapies and should not be utilized unless no other options are feasible. Ketoconazole, an effective therapy in immunocompetent hosts, has also had poor results in AIDS patients.

COCCIDIOIDOMYCOSIS

Coccidioides immitis, an organism endemic in the southwestern USA and areas of Mexico, Central and South America, is the organism responsible for coccidioidomycosis. In endemic regions, coccidioidomycosis is a frequent clinical disease, with as many as 24% of patients infected with HIV developing this illness in one study from Arizona[58]. The organism enters through the respiratory system, multiplies within the alveolar space, and forms a spherule. When T-cell-mediated immunity is inadequate, the organism may disseminate and lead to multisystem infection. Coccidioidomycosis is most common in AIDS patients when the CD4 count is below 250/cells/mm^3, and it is uncertain whether this is related to primary infection or recurrence of latent disease. Outside of endemic areas, coccidioidomycosis probably represents reactivation of latent disease.

The clinical manifestations of disseminated coccidioidomycosis are varied in both severity and organ system involved[59]. The most common presentation is respiratory disease with diffuse pneumonitis. Patients typically report a progressive syndrome of fever, malaise, and non-productive cough similar to PCP as well as disseminated histoplasmosis. The chest radiograph may reveal cavitary disease, focal infiltrates and, uncommonly, pleural effusions or hilar adenopathy are noted. Involvement of the CNS—coccidioidal meningitis—is associated with elevated CSF white blood cell counts and protein as well as suppressed CSF glucose. Cutaneous manifestations can be seen as well as lymph node involvement and liver disease.

The diagnosis of coccidioidomycosis is generally made by demonstration of the organism utilizing histopathological stains of involved tissue. The organism can be cultured from appropriate clinical specimens but is extremely infectious and represents a hazard to laboratory workers unless precautions to prevent the spread of the organism are in place. The complement fixation test and the tube precipitin test will demonstrate positive serological results for most patients with active disease.

Amphotericin B is presently the treatment of choice for acute disseminated coccidioidomycosis. As with other systemic mycoses, chronic lifelong maintenance therapy is necessary after treatment of the acute illness[60]. Itraconazole and fluconazole appear to be effective for maintenance therapy but their role as first-line therapy of acute disease is unclear. Ketoconazole does not appear to be effective in coccidioidomycosis in AIDS patients.

HERPES SIMPLEX

Herpes simplex virus types one and two (HSV-1, HSV-2) are a significant cause of morbidity in HIV-infected patients. The majority of AIDS patients are infected with these viruses prior to acquiring HIV and active disease is a result of reactivation of the latent virus. In immunosuppressed patients, reactivation may lead to severe disease and a prolonged course of illness with viral shedding. Homosexual AIDS patients have a higher prevalence rate of infection than the general population and thus are at high risk for reactivation of HSV-1 and HSV-2. In addition, herpes simplex infections in HIV-infected patients are often atypical compared to the immunocompetent host.

Orolabial ulcerative disease is a frequent manifestation of recurrent disease. Patients may describe a prodrome of pain, tingling, or numbness at the site of impending disease one to two days prior to the onset of active lesions. Painful vesicular eruptions occurring on the lip, tongue, pharynx, and buccal mucosa are common and these frequently coalesce into a large ulcer covered by a necrotic film. Fever, malaise, cervical lymphadenopathy, and pharyngitis often accompany active lesions.

Genital herpes typically present as multiple papules that rapidly form painful vesicles with an erythematous base. Systemic signs such as fever, malaise, headache, meningismus, myalgias and tender inguinal adenopathy are frequently reported with primary infection. In HIV-infected patients, severe recurrences with a prolonged duration can occur compared to the normal host. Persistent viral shedding, even in asymptomatic patients, has been documented.

Perianal herpes, manifested by anorectal pain, tenesmus, constipation, and ulcerations is the most common cause of non-gonococcal proctitis in homosexual men. HSV-2 is the more frequently identified virus but HSV-1 has been identified. Sacral radiculopathy and neurogenic bladder secondary to herpes virus involvement of the sacral plexus can occur. In addition to proctitis, shallow perianal ulcerations which are painful, pruritic, non-healing, and associated with painful defecation are frequently seen with active genital herpes. Perianal herpetic lesions are often atypical in appearance in HIV-infected hosts and the diagnosis should be confirmed by culture or direct antigen determination.

Dysphagia, odynophagia and retrosternal pain are common symptoms of herpes esophagitis. *Candida*, CMV, and other causes of esophagitis can cause a similar picture and endoscopic evaluation with culture and histopathological evidence of viral disease is needed to confirm the diagnosis.

Herpes encephalitis is a potentially life-threatening complication of herpes infection, but is not more common in AIDS patients than in the general population. The clinical manifestations vary from an insidious onset with subtle personality changes and headache to an abrupt illness with fever, meningismus, altered mental status, coma, and death. The diagnosis is difficult as the CSF is non-specific and cultures are frequently negative. Recent advances utilizing polymerase chain reaction (PCR) technology for diagnosing herpetic encephalopathy appear promising.

Acyclovir is the drug of choice for most herpes infections and is available as an oral[61], intravenous[62], and topical agent[63]. The dose and route of delivery depend on the site of infection and the severity of disease. Acyclovir is well distributed throughout the body, including the brain and CSF. Strains of herpes virus resistant to acyclovir have been reported and should be treated with foscarnet[64] or topical fluorothymidine. In addition, patients with frequent recurrences of herpes often benefit from chronic oral suppressive therapy, but may relapse with resistant infections.

VARICELLA ZOSTER VIRUS

Primary infection with varicella zoster virus (VZV) is a common childhood disease, with 90% of cases occurring in children under 15 years of age, and most adults are not susceptible to primary disease[65]. In immunocompetent children, VZV infection is usually a self-limiting illness manifested by a generalized pruritic vesicular rash and is highly contagious, with attack rates approaching 90% in susceptible household contacts. Complications of primary VZV infection, such as pneumonia or CNS involvement, are uncommon. In HIV-infected patients, active disease commonly represents reactivation of latent VZV due to progressive immunosuppression. While VZV may recur at any level of immunosuppression, complications are more frequent with low CD4 counts.

The clinical manifestations of VZV ranges from a self-limited case of zoster to life-threatening pneumonia or encephalitis. In AIDS patients, shingles is seen at higher prevalence rates than in age-matched immunocompetent cohorts and is concerning not only because of pain with the initial outbreak but because of a significant risk of developing post-herpetic neuralgia. Complications of VZV infection in AIDS patients include ocular involvement, hepatic involvement, chronic atypical skin lesions, pneumonia, dissemination, and varied neurological disease.

The diagnosis of VZV disease is commonly made with the appropriate clinical setting; however, in atypical cases, culture of the virus from lesions or antigen testing may be necessary. Treatment of active VZV with oral acyclovir requires higher doses than used for herpes simplex. Patients frequently require hospitalization and intravenous therapy to control symptoms and all patients with disseminated disease, cutaneous or visceral, should be treated with intravenous therapy. In patients with acyclovir-resistant VZV, foscarnet is beneficial. A vaccine has recently been licensed by the US Food and Drug

Administration but its clinical utility in HIV-infected patients has not been determined.

CYTOMEGALOVIRUS

CMV is the most significant cause of viral-induced illness in patients with AIDS. Most infections with this pathogen are due to recurrence of latent infection. CMV is a ubiquitous organism with a high seroprevalence rate in the general population. Prior to the AIDS epidemic, serious illness related to CMV infection was most commonly reported in immunosuppressed patients such as transplant recipients and patients receiving chronic immunosuppressive therapy.

CMV causes several distinct clinical syndromes in patients infected with HIV[66]. While these different clinical patterns reflect various types of organ system involvement, serious illness is rarely reported until a severe level of immunosuppression exists, usually with an absolute CD4 count below 50 cells/mm^3. Several studies report that up to 90% of patients with AIDS develop active CMV infection, with chorioretinitis being the most common serious infection. Complicating the diagnosis of active CMV disease is the knowledge that blood, tissue, and urine cultures which reveal this organism often do not correlate with active disease.

Ophthalmic disease caused by CMV is the leading cause of blindness in patients with HIV. This illness is generally not present until the absolute CD4 count is less than 50 and is often associated with systemic CMV disease. Patients typically report decreased visual acuity and often note 'floaters' which increase in number as the disease progresses. While CMV retinitis often presents with unilateral involvement, progression to bilateral disease is common, even on therapy. The diagnosis of CMV retinitis is generally made with the appropriate clinical history and ophthalmological examination. The typical appearance of CMV retinitis includes yellow to creamy-white large granular lesions with perivascular hemorrhages and exudates. This had been described as a 'cottage cheese and catsup' appearance.

Gastrointestinal involvement of CMV may present as either involvement of the upper and/or lower gastrointestinal tract. CMV colitis occurs in 5–10% of patients with AIDS and is often difficult to distinguish from other infections of the lower gastrointestinal tract. Diarrhea and associated weight loss are common and patients frequently report crampy abdominal pain, fever and anorexia. Endoscopic examination frequently reveals diffuse submucosal hemorrhages and ulcerations, though abnormal appearing mucosa has been noted in active disease. The diagnosis requires visualization of CMV inclusion bodies in biopsy specimens.

CNS involvement of CMV is a well-recognized complication in patients with AIDS. A subacute encephalitis manifested by headaches, confusion, decreased level of consciousness, and changes in personality has been reported. Isolation of CMV from CSF is suggestive but not diagnostic of active infection. The diagnosis can only be confirmed by brain biopsy revealing perivascular hemorrhages, intracellular inclusion bodies and identification of the virus. A polyradiculopathy manifested by spasticity, lower extremity weakness, urinary retention and sensory deficits is a more recently recognized complication of CMV. CSF evaluation reveals a polymorphonuclear pleocytosis and a moderately depressed glucose, which is unusual for a viral infection.

Pulmonary manifestations of CMV in AIDS have not been clearly defined. Isolation of CMV by culture in sputum or bronchoalveolar lavage fluid is common but the clinical significance of this finding is unclear. Other causes of pulmonary infection are frequently found and resolution of disease usually occurs without anti-CMV therapy. Presently it is common to treat CMV pneumonitis when there is progression of disease with no other identifiable etiology detected.

Treatment of active CMV disease requires an initial induction period followed by lifelong maintenance to attempt to prevent progression. Gancyclovir, a nucleoside analog with 50 times more activity than acyclovir against CMV, is usually the first agent employed[67]. Patients are typically treated with a 14-day induction period and then re-evaluated. If they achieve stabilization or improvement, they are then placed on a lifelong maintenance regimen that is half the induction dose. Gancyclovir results in clinical stabilization or improvement in more than 80% of patients treated, but one-third have the medication discontinued because of toxicity[68]. The primary toxicity of gancyclovir is neutropenia, which often results in the total neutrophil count falling below 1000 cells/mm^3. While newer cytokines such as granulocyte CSF (GCSF) and granulocyte–macrophage CSF (GM-CSF) have been used with varying degrees of success to counter this toxicity, it remains a significant clinical problem. Studies have shown that the combination of zidovudine (AZT) and gancyclovir induces more toxicity than either agent used alone, and this combination should be avoided when possible in clinical practice. Thrombocytopenia, CNS abnormalities such as confusion, and nausea with vomiting are other common toxicities.

Foscarnet, a pyrophosphate that inhibits CMV DNA polymerase, has been used in patients with active CMV disease unable to tolerate gancyclovir or in whom disease progresses despite therapy, usually because of gancyclovir resistance[69]. Studies have demonstrated essentially equal efficacy between foscarnet and gancyclovir but patients receiving foscarnet had on the average a four-month improvement in overall survival[70]. The cause of this difference in survival is not entirely clear. Severe nephrotoxicity, possibly leading to chronic renal failure requiring dialysis, is the most significant toxicity related to prolonged foscarnet use. A newer agent, HPMPC—a nucleotide analog—is also being studied for the treatment of resistant CMV disease, but its nephrotoxicity has limited its wider use.

BACTERIAL INFECTIONS

Bacterial infections are a significant cause of morbidity and mortality in patients infected with HIV. Several immunological factors lead to the increase in incidence of significant bacterial infections when compared to immunocompetent hosts[71]. Impaired complement activation, diminished B-cell function, impaired neutrophil function, and decreased IgA mucosal production all contribute to this increased incidence and severity.

The most frequent cause of invasive bacterial infections in AIDS is *Streptococcus pneumoniae*[72]. HIV-infected patients have up to a 100-fold increase in pneumococcal bacteremia compared to normal hosts. The role of pneumococcal vaccine in HIV-infected patients is under investigation; however, failures have been reported, particularly in severely immunodeficient AIDS patients. Hence, if any vaccination is to be given, it should be administered at the time that a new HIV diagnosis is made.

The incidence of *Salmonella* bacteremia, a significant cause of morbidity early in the HIV epidemic[73], has been decreasing and is now uncommon. This change in incidence appears to be related to the use of trimethoprim–sulfamethoxazole for PCP prophylaxis as well as a possible antibacterial effect of AZT[74].

Bloodstream infections with *Staphylococcus aureus* occur more frequently in AIDS patients and are frequently associated with the use of long-term intravascular access devices. *Pseudomonas aeruginosa*[75] as well as *Haemophilus influenzae* are more frequently associated with invasive and recurrent disease in AIDS patients than in normal hosts. The *Haemophilus influenzae* type B vaccine is recommended in HIV-infected patients but there is presently no data to support its efficacy.

MYCOBACTERIUM AVIUM COMPLEX

Mycobacterium avium complex (MAC) is a significant cause of morbidity in patients with AIDS. Prior to the HIV era, infection with this ubiquitous soil and water contaminant was a rare cause of serious illness. With the progressive decrease in macrophage function seen in AIDS, this atypical mycobacteria has become an emerging pathogen, with disseminated disease being diagnosed in up to 39% of patients in a recent series[76]. In CD4-matched cohorts, patients with disseminated MAC have significantly shorter overall survival than those who are MAC bacteremia free. MAC has been isolated from blood, sputum, stool, urine, spleen, liver, lung, kidney, lymph nodes, adrenals, colon, and bone marrow of infected patients. Involved organs in disseminated MAC often show no granuloma formation or poorly formed lesions.

Patients with a CD4 count of less than 50 cells/mm^3 are at the highest risk for disseminated MAC, though the risk for disease increases at CD4 counts of 75 cells/mm^3 or less[77]. The most common clinical presentation is fever, malaise, weight loss and anemia[78]. MAC has been associated with a wasting syndrome including chronic diarrhea with abdominal pain and malabsorption, as well as extrahepatic biliary obstruction secondary to lymphadenopathy or hepatic infiltration. The most common laboratory abnormalities noted are anemia, neutropenia, and an elevated alkaline phosphatase.

The diagnosis of disseminated MAC is usually made by recovery of the organism from appropriate clinical specimens. Newer blood culture systems such as the Bactec system, which may require up to two weeks for adequate growth, allow more rapid identification of MAC than older diagnostic systems[79]. Isolation from blood as well as organ systems with clinical evidence of disease warrants the institution of appropriate therapy; however, sputum, stool, and urine cultures with MAC need to be evaluated clinically as these may often be positive without invasive or disseminated active disease being present. In the appropriate clinical setting of a patient with a CD4 count of less than 50 cells/mm^3 with persistent fevers and a negative fever work-up, it is common clinical practice to initiate empirical therapy while waiting for cultures to become positive for MAC. A clinical dilemma in advanced AIDS patients is deciding between MAC and *Mycobacterium tuberculosis* infection when acid-fast bacilli are identified and cultures are not yet positive.

Disseminated MAC is generally resistant to agents used to treat tuberculosis, with the exception of ethambutol. In early therapeutic regimens, intravenous amikacin was a mainstay of treatment but recent advances have allowed less toxic and more easily administered therapies to be utilized[80]. Rifabutin, a drug thought to be ineffective when tested at 100–300 mg initially, appears to be better tolerated and effective at higher doses (300–600 mg)[81], but may cause hepatitis and uveitis, the latter occurring when blood levels increase because of concomitant fluconazole or macrolide use. The new macrolides azithromycin and clarithromycin have excellent bactericidal activity against most clinical MAC isolates. Clofazamine as well as many of the quinilones also demonstrate some limited activity against MAC isolates. Rapid resistance to monotherapy has led to the use of multiple drug regimens which usually include a macrolide in combination with at least two other agents with anti-MAC activity[80], preferably including ethambutol.

The significant morbidity associated with disseminated MAC as well as the high prevalence of this disease had led to the study of prophylactic regimens for patients at high risk. Randomized, placebo-controlled trials have demonstrated a significant reduction in disseminated MAC in patients receiving Rifabutin for primary prophylaxis[77]. Based on these trials, it is presently recommended to treat all AIDS patients with a CD4 count of less than 100 prophylactically with this agent[82]. The use of the newer macrolides and quinilones for primary prophylaxis continues to be under investigation but several series using clarithromycin have demonstrated excellent clinical efficacy. Clofazamine has been found to be ineffective for prophylaxis.

BACILLARY ANGIOMATOSIS

Bacillary angiomatosis (BA) is an emerging disease attributed to infection with organisms from the genus *Bartonella*. In 1983, Stoler *et al*. first described this illness in a patient presenting with multiple subcutaneous nodules[83]. Utilizing Warthin–Starry staining, Gram-negative bacilli were seen and successfully treated with erythromycin. The organism was initially classified in the genus *Rochalimaea* but recently was reclassified as a *Bartonella*. BA is associated with severe immunosuppression and CD4 cell counts of less than 100 cells/mm^3 are usually noted[84]. It is now known that BA can affect many organs, including skin, bone, bone marrow, lymph nodes, the gastrointestinal tract, and the CNS. In addition, bacteremia with or without endocarditis has been noted, as well as involvement of the bronchial tree[85].

Cutaneous BA is the most common manifestation of infection with *Bartonella* in AIDS patients[84]. The lesions are frequently described as a vascular proliferative lesion with a red to purple smooth or eroded surface. In addition, papules that form large friable exophytic lesions are commonly described. These lesions are difficult to differentiate from Kaposi's sarcoma and a biopsy with histopathological studies is needed to distinguish between BA and Kaposi's sarcoma.

Bartonella infection of the liver is termed peliosis hepatis and usually is accompanied by abdominal pain and fever[86]. Laboratory evaluation reveals an elevated alkaline phosphatase as well as elevated transaminases[87]. CT of the abdomen reveals multiple hypodense lesions but a biopsy is needed to confirm the diagnosis.

The diagnosis of cutaneous BA requires a biopsy with histopathological evaluation. In liver disease, a biopsy should be performed as other diseases may have a similar presentation in AIDS patients. The CDC has developed an indirect fluorescence antibody test (IFA) that appears promising[88]. Blood cultures of patients with BA may reveal the organism but culture of tissue specimens is difficult.

Erythromycin is the drug of choice for treating BA[83]. In addition, tetracycline, minocycline, and doxycyline have been shown to be effective. There are case reports of clinical response to other agents; however, no controlled trials have been done and no other agents can presently be recommended. The length of therapy as well as dose and route of delivery are under investigation, and relapse to active disease can occur[89]. Because of the high association of BA with cat exposure, especially due to inoculation by scratches, HIV-infected patients should limit such contact, or be sure that any cats that they have as pets remain indoors and are preferably declawed.

REFERENCES

1. Masur H, Michelis MA, Greene JB *et al.* An outbreak of community-acquired *Pneumocystis carinii* pneumonia: initial manifestation of cellular immune dysfunction. *N Engl J Med* 1981; 305: 1431–1438.
2. Glatt AE, Chirgwin K. *Pneumocystis carinii* pneumonia in human immunodeficiency virus-infected patients. *Arch Intern Med* 1990; 150: 271–279.
3. Kovacs JA, Hiemenz JW, Macher AM *et al. Pneumocystis carinii* pneumonia: a comparison between patients with the acquired immunodeficiency syndrome and patients with other immunodeficiencies. *Ann Intern Med* 1984; 100: 663.
4. Kovacs JA, Halpern JL, Swan JC *et al.* Identification of antigens and antibodies specific for *Pneumocystis carinii. J Immunol* 1988; 140: 2023–2031.
5. Frenkel JK, Bartlett MS, Smith JW. RNA homology and the reclassification of pneumocystis. *Diagn Microbiol Infect Dis* 1990; 13: 1–2.
6. Elvin K. Laboratory diagnosis and occurrence of *Pneumocystis carinii. Scand J Infect Dis Suppl* 1994; 94: 1–34.
7. Bigby TD, Margolskee D, Curtis JL *et al.* The usefulness of induced sputum in the diagnosis of *Pneumocystis carinii* pneumonia in patients with the acquired immunodeficiency syndrome. *Am Rev Respir Dis* 1986; 133: 515–518.
8. Blumenfeld W, Wager E, Hadley WK. Use of the transbronchial biopsy for diagnosis of opportunistic pulmonary infections in acquired immunodeficiency syndrome (AIDS). *Am J Clin Pathol* 1984; 81: 1.
9. Ng VL, Virani NA, Chaisson RE *et al. J Clin Microbiol* 1990; 28: 2228–2233.
10. Gordin FM, Simon GL, Wofsy CB, Mills J. Adverse reactions to trimethoprim–sulfamethoxazole in patients with AIDS. *Ann Intern Med* 1984; 100: 495–499.
11. Safrin S. New developments in the management of *Pneumocystis carinii* disease. In Volberding P and Jacobson MA (eds) *AIDS Clinical Review*. New York: Marcel Dekker, 1992; pp. 95–112.
12. Hughes WT, Gray VL, Gutteridge WE *et al.* Efficacy of a hydroxynaphthoquinone, 566C80, in experimental *Pneumocystis carinii* pneumonitis. *Antimicrob Agents Chemother* 1990; 34: 225.
13. Allegra CJ, Chabner BA, Tuazon CU *et al.* Trimetrexate for the treatment of *Pneumocystis carinii* pneumonia in patients with acquired immunodeficiency syndrome. *N Engl J Med* 1987; 317: 978.
14. Bozzette SA, Sattler FR, Chiu J. A controlled trial of early adjunctive treatment with corticosteroids for *Pneumocystis carinii* pneumonia in the acquired immunodeficiency syndrome. *N Engl J Med* 1990; 323: 1451–1457.
15. NIH–University of California Expert Panel for Corticosteroids as Adjunctive Therapy for PCP. Special report: consensus statement on the use of corticosteroids as adjunctive therapy for pneumocystis pneumonia in the acquired immunodeficiency syndrome. *N Engl J Med* 1990; 323: 1500–1504.
16. Fischl MA, Dickinson GM, La Voie L. Safety and efficacy of sulfamethoxazole and trimethoprim chemoprophylaxis for *Pneumocystis carinii* pneumonia in AIDS. *JAMA* 1988; 259: 1185.
17. Kemper CA, Tucker RM, Lang DA *et al.* Low-dose dapsone prophylaxis of *Pneumocystis carinii* pneumonia in AIDS and AIDS related complex. *AIDS* 1990; 4: 1145–1148.
18. Hirschel B, Lazzarin A, Chopard P *et al.* A controlled study of inhaled pentamidine for primary prevention of *Pneumocystis carinii* pneumonia. *N Engl J Med* 1991; 324: 1079.
19. Katz MH, Hessol NA, Buchbinder SP *et al.* Temporal trends of opportunistic

infections and malignancies in homosexual men with AIDS. *J Infect Dis* 1994; 170: 198–201.
20. Hardy WD, Feinber J, Finkelstein DM *et al.* Trimethoprim–sulfamethoxazole versus aerosolized pentamidine for secondary prophylaxis of *Penumocystis carinii* pneumonia in AIDS patients receiving zidovudine: AIDS clinical group protocol 012. *N Engl J Med* 1992; 327: 1842–1848.
21. Clumeck N. Some aspects of the epidemiology of toxoplasmosis and *Pneumocystis* in AIDS in Europe. *Eur J Clin Microbiol Infect Dis* 1991; 10: 177–178.
22. Luft BJ, Brooks RG, Conley FK *et al.* Toxoplasmosis encephalitis in patients with acquired immune deficiency syndrome. *JAMA* 1984; 252: 913.
23. Derouin F, Sarfati C, Beauvais B *et al.* Prevalence of pulmonary toxoplasmosis in HIV-infected patients (Letter). *AIDS* 1990; 4: 1036.
24. Milligan SA, Katz MS, Craven PC. Toxoplasmosis presenting as panhypopituitarism in a patient with AIDS. *Am J Med* 1984; 77: 760–764.
25. Cochereau-Massin I, LeHoang P, Lautier-Frau M. Ocular toxoplasmosis in human immunodeficiency virus-infected patients. *Am J Opthalmol* 1992; 114: 130–135.
26. Elkin CM, Leon E, Grenell SL *et al.* Intracranial lesions in the acquired immunodeficiency syndrome: radiological (CT) features. *JAMA* 1985; 253: 393–396.
27. Cimino C, Lipton R, Williams A *et al.* The evaluation of patients with human immunodeficiency virus-related disorders and brain mass lesions. *Arch Intern Med* 1991; 151: 1381–1384.
28. Eyles DE, Coleman N. An evaluation of the curative effects of pyrimethamine and sulfadiazine alone and in combination on experimental mouse toxoplasmosis. *Antibiot Chemother* 1955; 5: 529–539.
29. Dannemann BR, Israelski DM, Remington JS. Treatment of toxoplasmic encephalitis patients with AIDS: a randomized trial comparing pyrimethamine plus clindamycin to pyrimethamine plus sulfonamides. *Ann Intern Med* 1992; 116: 33–43.
30. Kovacs JA. Efficacy of atovaquone in treatment of toxoplasmosis in patients with AIDS. *Lancet* 1992; 340: 637–638.
31. Leport C, Tournerie C, Raguin G *et al.* Long-term follow-up of patients with AIDS on maintenance therapy for toxoplasmosis. *Eur J Clin Microbiol* 1989; 160: 312–320.
32. de Gans J, Portegies P, Reiss P *et al.* Pyrimethamine alone as maintenance therapy for central nervous system toxoplasmosis in 38 patients with AIDS. *J AIDS* 1992; 5: 137–142.
33. Carr A, Tindall B, Brew BJ *et al.* Low-dose trimethoprim–sulfamethoxazole prophylaxis for toxoplasmic encephalitis in patients with AIDS. *Ann Intern Med* 1992; 177: 106–111.
34. Masur H. Gastrointestinal infections in AIDS. *Ann Intern Med* 1992; 116: 63–67.
35. Flanigan T, Whalen C, Turner J *et al.* *Cryptosporidium* infection and CD4 counts. *Ann Intern Med* 1992; 116: 840–842.
36. Louie E, Borkowsky W, Klesius PH *et al.* Treatment of cryptosporidiosis with oral bovine transfer factor. *Clin Immunopathol* 1987; 44: 329–334.
37. MacKenzie WR, Hoxie JN, Proctor ME *et al.* A massive outbreak in Milwaukee of *Cryptosporidium* infection transmitted through the public water supply. *N Engl J Med* 1994; 331: 161–167.
38. Juranek DD. Cryptosporidiosis: sources of infection and guidelines for prevention. *Clin Infect Dis* 1995; 21: S57–61.
39. Weber R, Bryan RT, Schwartz DA, Owen RI. Human microsporidial infections. *Clin Microbiol Rev* 1994; 7: 426–461.
40. Molina J-M, Sarfati C, Beauvais B *et al.* Intestinal microsporidiosis in human immunodeficiency virus-infected patients with chronic unexplained diarrhea: prevalence and clinical and biologic features. *J Infect Dis* 1993; 167: 217–221.

41. Pol S, Romana CA, Richard S *et al.* Microsporidia infection in patients with human immunodeficiency virus and unexplained cholangitis. *N Engl J Med* 1993; 328: 95–99.
42. Centers for Disease Control. Microsporidian keratoconjunctivitis in patients with AIDS. *MMWR* 1990; 39: 188–189.
43. Centers for Disease Control. HIV/AIDS Surveillance Report, 1991.
44. Chuck SL, Sande MA. Infections with *Cryptococcus neoformans* in the acquired immunodeficiency syndrome. *N Engl J Med* 1989; 321: 794–799.
45. Clark RA, Creer D, Atkinson W *et al.* Spectrum of *Cryptococcus neoformans* infection in 68 patients infected with human immunodeficiency virus. *Rev Infect Dis* 1990; 12: 768–777.
46. Sabetta JR, Andriole VT. Cryptococcal infection of the central nervous system. *Med Clin North Am* 1985; 69: 333–344.
47. Powderly WG, Cloud GA, Dismukes WE *et al.* Value of serum and cerebrospinal fluid cryptococcal antigen measurement in the management of AIDS-associated cryptococcal meningitis. *Clin Infect Dis* 1994; 18: 789–792.
48. Zuger A, Louid E, Holzman RS. Cryptococcal disease in patients with the acquired immunodeficiency syndrome: diagnostic features and outcome of treatment. *Ann Intern Med* 1986; 104: 234–240.
49. Saag MS, Powderly WG, Cloud GA *et al.* Comparison of amphotericin B with fluconazole in the treatment of acute AIDS-associated cryptococcal meningitis. *N Engl J Med* 1992; 326: 83–89.
50. Powderly WG, Saag MS, Cloud GA *et al.* A randomized controlled trial of fluconazole versus amphotericin B as maintenance therapy for prevention of relapse of cryptococcal meningitis in patients with AIDS. *N Engl J Med* 1992; 326: 793–798.
51. Perfect JR. Antifungal prophylaxis: to prevent or not. *Am J Med* 1993; 94: 233–234.
52. Schmidt-Westhausen A, Schiller RA, Pohle HD, Reichart PA. Oral *Candida* and Enterobacteriaceae in HIV-1 infection: correlation with clinical candidiasis and antimycotic therapy. *J Oral Pathol Med* 1991; 20: 469–472.
53. Imam N, Carpenter CCJ, Mayer KH *et al.* Hierarchical pattern of mucosal *Candida* infections in HIV-seropositive women. *Am J Med* 1990; 89: 142–146.
54. Wheat LJ, Connolly-Stringfield P, Baker RL *et al.* Disseminated histoplasmosis in the acquired immune deficiency syndrome: clinical findings, diagnosis and treatment, and review of the literature. *Medicine* 1990; 69: 361–374.
55. Sarosi GA, Johnson PC. Disseminated histoplasmosis in patients with human immunodeficiency virus. *Clin Infect Dis* 1992; 14: S60–67.
56. Wheat LJ, Kohler RB, Tewari RP. Diagnosis of disseminated histoplasmosis by detection of *Histoplasma capsulatum* antigen in serum and urine specimens. *N Engl J Med* 1986; 314: 83–88.
57. Wheat LJ, Hafner RE, Ritchie M *et al.* Itraconazole is effective treatment for histoplasmosis in AIDS: prospective multicenter noncomparative trial. *Program and Abstracts of the 31st Interscience Conference on Antimicrobial Agents and Chemotherapy*, American Society for Microbiology, Anaheim, CA, 1992.
58. Ampel NM, Dols CS, Galgiani JN. Coccidioidomycosis during human immunodeficiency virus infection: results of a prospective study in a coccidioidal endemic area. *Am J Med* 1993; 94: 235–240.
59. Fish DG, Ampel NM, Galgiani JN *et al* Coccidioidomycosis during human immunodeficiency virus infection: a review of 77 patients. *Medicine* 1990; 69: 384–391.
60. Galgiani JN, Ampel NM. Coccidioidomycosis in human immunodeficiency virus-infected patients. *J Infect Dis* 1990; 162: 1165–1169.

61. Straus SE, Seidlin M, Takiff H *et al.* Oral acyclovir to suppress recurring herpes simplex virus infections in immunodeficient patients. *Ann Intern Med* 1984; 100: 522–524.
62. Whitley RJ, Alford CA, Hirsch MS *et al.* Vidarabine versus acyclovir therapy in herpes simplex encephalitis. *N Engl J Med* 1986; 314: 144–149.
63. Whitley RJ, Levin M, Barton N *et al.* Infections caused by herpes simplex virus in the immunocompromised host: natural history and topical acyclovir therapy. *J Infect Dis* 1984; 150: 323–329.
64. Erlich KS, Jacobson MA, Koehler JE *et al.* Foscarnet therapy for severe acyclovir-resistant herpes simplex virus type-2 infections in patients with the acquired immunodeficiency syndrome (AIDS): an uncontrolled trial. *Ann Intern Med* 1989; 110: 710–713.
65. Weller TH. Varicella and herpes zoster: changing concepts of the natural history, control, and importance of a not-so benign virus (parts 1 and 2). *N Engl J Med* 1983; 309: 1362–1368.
66. Mintz L, Drew WL, Miner RC *et al.* Cytomegalovirus infections in homosexual men. *Ann Intern Med* 1983; 99: 326.
67. Masur H, Lane HC, Palestine A *et al.* Effect of 9-(1,3-dihydroxy-2-propoxymethyl) guanine on serious cytomegalovirus disease in eight immunosuppressed homosexual men. *Ann Intern Med* 1986; 104: 41–44.
68. Koretz SH, Buhler WC, Brewin A *et al.* Treatment of serious cytomegalovirus infection with 9-(1,3-dihydroxy-2-propoxymethyl) guanine in patients with AIDS and other immunodeficiencies. *N Engl J Med* 1986; 314: 801–805.
69. Palestine AG, Polils MA, De Smet MD *et al.* A randomized, controlled trial of foscarnet in the treatment of cytomegalovirus retinitis in patients with AIDS. *Ann Intern Med* 1991; 115: 665–673.
70. Jabs D and the Studies of Ocular Complications of AIDS Research Group, in collaboration with the AIDS Clinical Trial Group. Mortality in patients with the acquired immunodeficiency syndrome treated with either foscarnet or ganciclovir for cytomegalovirus retinitis. *N Engl J Med* 1992; 326: 213–220.
71. Janoff EN, Breiman RF, Daley CL, Hopewell PC. Pneumococcal disease during HIV infection: epidemiologic, clinical and immunologic perspectives. *Ann Intern Med* 1992; 117: 313–324.
72. Witt DJ, Craven DE, McCabe WR. Bacterial infections in adult patients with the acquired immune deficiency syndrome (AIDS) and AIDS-related complex. *Am J Med* 1987; 82: 900–906.
73. Angulo FJ, Swerdlow DL. Bacterial enteric infections in persons with human immunodeficiency virus. *Clin Infect Dis* 1995; 21: S84–93.
74. Nightingale ST, Cameron DW, Gordon FM *et al.* Two controlled trials of rifabutin prophylaxis against *Mycobacterium avium* complex infection in AIDS. *N Engl J Med* 1993; 329: 828–833.
75. Franzetti F, Cernuschi M, Esposito R, Moroni M. *Pseudomonas* infections in patients with AIDS and AIDS-related complex. *J Intern Med* 1992; 231: 437–443.
76. Nightingale SD, Byrd LT, Southern PM *et al.* Incidence of *Mycobacterium avium-intracellulare* complex bacteremia in human immunodeficiency virus-positive patients. *J Infect Dis* 1992; 165: 1082–1085.
77. Nightingale SD, Cameron DW, Gordin FM *et al.* Two controlled trials of rifabutin prophylaxis against *Mycobacterium avium* complex infection in AIDS. *N Engl J Med* 1993; 329: 828–833.
78. Bottger EC, Teske A, Kirschner P *et al.* Disseminated *Mycobacterium genavense* infection in patients with AIDS. *Lancet* 1992; 340: 76–80.
79. Young LS. *Mycobacterium avium* complex infection. *J Infect Dis* 1988; 157: 863–867.

80. Kemper CA, Meng TC, Nussbaum J *et al.* Treatment of *Mycobacterium avium* complex bacteremia in AIDS with a four-drug oral regimen. *Ann Intern Med* 1992; 116: 466–472.
81. Sullam P, Gordin F, Wynne B *et al.* Efficacy of rifabutin in the treatment of *Mycobacterium avium* complex (MAC) bacteremia (Abstract PO-B07-1238). *IX International Conference on AIDS*, Berlin, 1993.
82. Masur H, Public Health Service Task Force on Prophylaxis and Therapy for *Mycobacterium avium* Complex. Special report: recommendations on prophylaxis and therapy for disseminated *Mycobacterium avium* complex disease in patients infected with human immunodeficiency virus. *N Engl J Med* 1993; 329: 898–904.
83. Stoler MH, Bonfiglio TA, Steigbigel RT *et al.* An atypical subcutaneous infection associated with acquired immune deficiency syndrome. *Am J Clin Pathol* 1983; 80: 714–718.
84. Koehler JE, Tappero JW. AIDS Commentary: bacillary angiomatosis and bacillary peliosis in patients infected with human immunodeficiency virus. *Clin Infect Dis* 1993; 17: 612–624.
85. Berger TG, Koehler JE. Bacillary angiomatosis. In Volberding P, Jacobson MA (eds) *AIDS Clinical Review 1993/1994*. New York: Marcel Dekker, 1993; pp. 43–60.
86. Perkocha LA, Geaghan SM, Yen Tsb *et al.* Clinical and pathological features of bacillary peliosis hepatis in association with human immunodeficiency virus infection. *N Engl Med* 1990; 323: 1581–1586.
87. Slater LN, Welch DF, Min K-W. *Rochalimaea henselae* causes bacillary angiomatosis and peliosis hepatis. *Arch Intern Med* 1992; 152: 602–606.
88. Regnery RL, Olson JG, Perkins BA *et al.* Serological response to '*Rochalimaea henselae*' antigen in suspected cat-scratch disease. *Lancet* 1992; 339: 1443–1445.
89. Lucey D, Dolan JM, Moss CW *et al.* Relapsing illness due to *Rochalimaea henselae* in immunocompetent hosts: implication for therapy and new epidemiological associations. *Clin Infect Dis* 1992; 14: 683–688.

14

Cutaneous Manifestations of HIV Infection

Clay J. Cockerell* and Alvin E. Friedman-Kien†
*University of Texas Southwestern Medical Center, Dallas, Texas, USA;
†New York University Medical Center, New York, USA

INTRODUCTION

The skin is affected in virtually all patients with human immunodeficiency virus (HIV) infection at some point during the course of their illness. Cutaneous disease may serve as the initial or only problem that these patients may suffer until more serious sequelae develop. Because patients with HIV disease now survive longer, issues related to quality of life are of greater importance.

A variety of cutaneous disorders may serve either as initial clues to the underlying diagnosis of HIV infection itself or to the existence of one or more serious underlying opportunistic infectious diseases. In the immunocompromised host, they are also often the source of severe morbidity, both physical and psychological. Clinicians caring for these patients must be well grounded in how to diagnose and treat these conditions.

VIRAL INFECTIONS

Acute Exanthema of HIV Disease

The earliest manifestation of HIV infection is an acute viral syndrome often associated with an exanthem which is sometimes subclinical and often is unnoticed by patients. A fine morbilliform eruption involving the trunk, chest, back and upper arms develops within two to four weeks following

AIDS and Malignancies: Current Concepts and Perspectives.
Edited by B.C. Golematis and V.T. DeVita Jr

infection and is often accompanied by headache, malaise, fever, diarrhea, myalgias and pharyngitis[2,3]. The acute syndrome generally lasts for five to seven days and usually resolves with complete recovery. Patients are highly infectious during this time. Although the most common manifestation is a pinkish, morbilliform eruption, other manifestations include urticaria, palatal and esophageal ulcers, thrush and perleche[3,4].

Histological evaluation of skin biopsies taken from the morbilliform eruption demonstrates an infiltrate consisting primarily of lymphocytes around blood vessels of the superficial vascular plexus[6]. There is also slight spongiosis and occasional individually necrotic keratinocytes in the epidermis. One study recently reported a dense infiltrate with epidermal necrosis[5]. These findings are similar to those observed in other viral exanthemata as well as in morbilliform drug eruptions.

The differential diagnosis includes other viral exanthemata such as those caused by parvovirus, measles and rubella. Drug eruptions may also cause similar eruptions and must be excluded. Zidovudine and other antiviral agents have been administered to patients with the acute HIV viral exanthem without repeatable success[7,9].

Herpesvirus Infections

Herpesvirus infections may be seen in 20–50% of patients at some point during the course of HIV infection[10]. The prevalence of infection with these viruses ranges from between 20% and 40% with herpes simplex virus (HSV) to virtually 100% with varicella zoster virus (VZV), cytomegalovirus (CMV) and Epstein–Barr virus (EBV)[11].

Recurrent oral, labial and genital herpes simplex infections are commonly seen in both immunocompetent patients as well as in HIV-infected individuals who are relatively immunocompetent. These are manifest as painful grouped vesicles on an erythematous base that rupture and become crusted. Healing is usually complete in less than two weeks. Once significant immune suppression supervenes, however, lesions caused by HSV may become progressive and may be manifest by chronic ulcerative mucocutaneous lesions that may last for months[12].

Up to 13% of patients who develop acquired immunodeficiency syndrome (AIDS) have a prior recent history of having had herpes zoster ('shingles')[13] (Figure 14.2). It may precede the development of oral thrush and oral hairy leukoplakia by more than one year and is predictive of progression from HIV infection to AIDS, having been associated with progression in 23% at two years, 46% at four years and 73% at six years. In addition to zoster, on rare occasions HIV-infected individuals may develop varicella ('chickenpox') that, although most commonly following a benign course, may be associated with pulmonary involvement that may be fatal[14]. If an HIV-infected patient is exposed to VZV for the first time, careful consideration should be given to the

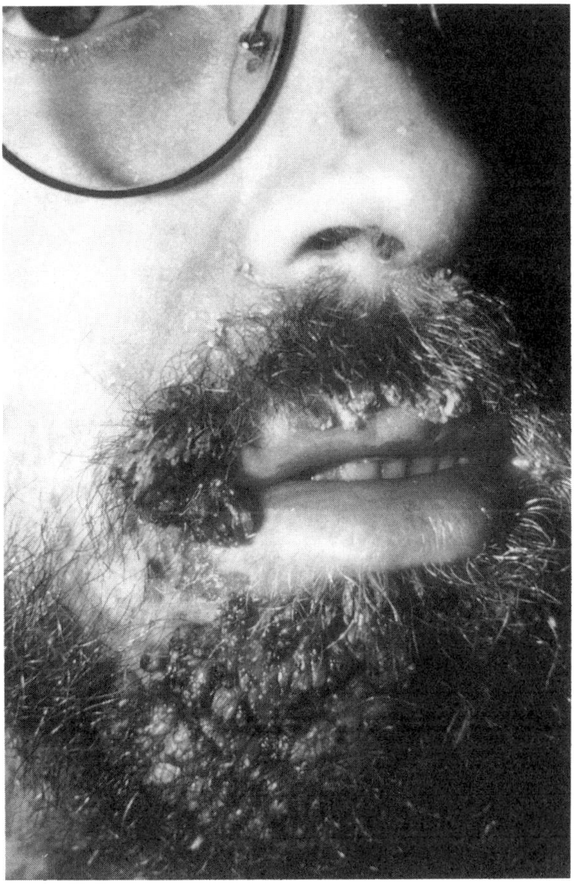

Figure 14.1 *Extensive facial verrucae in a patient with advanced AIDS. Fortunately, this process largely resolved following treatment with* 13-cis-*retinoic acid*

use of varicella zoster immunoglobulin or prophylactic acyclovir or valacyclovir. Administration of the newly released VZV vaccine should be considered for HIV-infected individuals who are still relatively immunocompetent and have not had previous infection with this virus.

Infections with VZV in HIV-infected immunocompromised patients is more serious than in the immunocompetent host (Plate 14.1). Second episodes of varicella, recurrent zoster infections at the same or different sites as well as multidermatomal involvement may occur. Dissemination of virus with development of widespread blisters over large areas of the skin may develop concomitant with the characteristic zosteriform group of vesicles[15,16]. Post-herpetic neuralgia, manifest as persistent, severe pain in an affected dermatome, commonly develops in these patients. This complication is often quite difficult to treat. Painful atrophic scars and persistent ulcerations may also develop following zoster[17,18]. Chronic verrucous lesions that are often resistant to antiviral therapy with acyclovir may also develop[19]. HSV and VZV infections are manifest histologically by intraepidermal acantholytic vesicles associated with characteristic cytopathic effects in epithelial cells. There is margination of the chromatin with ballooning nuclear degeneration and pinkish intracytoplasmic and intranuclear inclusions known as Cowdry bodies. There is an inflammatory infiltrate in the dermis consisting of lymphocytes, histiocytes, eosinophils, neutrophils and plasma cells. Careful inspection of dermal inflammatory infiltrates demonstrates perineural and intraneural inflammation associated with degeneration of nerves[20]. In immunocompromised patients with either HSV or VZV, there is extensive cytonecrosis of the epidermis associated with abundant viral infection of keratinocytes and involvement of hair follicles, sebaceous glands and other cutaneous adnexae[21]. In some lesions, there may be extensive ulceration so that the herpetically infected cells cannot be visualized with routine microscopy. In these cases, immunoperoxidase stains and DNA probes may be useful in detecting viral antigens. Skin lesions caused by both viruses appear identical histologically.

Herpesvirus infections are treated with acyclovir at doses that range from 200 to 1000 mg orally every 4 h while awake. Acyclovir-resistant cases of VZV or HSV require treatment with intravenous foscarnet (180 mg/kg per day in two divided doses for 10–14 days)[22,23]. On occasion, patients with seemingly resistant zoster or herpes simplex infection may be suffering from atrophic gastritis preventing absorption of acyclovir, so that a change to intravenous administration may be effective. Other helpful measures may include local care with cool compresses or sitz baths, topical anaesthetics such as 2–5% lidocaine gel or ointment, and pramoxine ointment or lotion. Sometimes secondary bacterial infections of the ulcerated skin lesions of shingles may require topical or systemic antibiotics especially in the immunocompenent host.

Cytomegalovirus

Up to 90% of patients with AIDS may develop acute active CMV infection at some point during their illness[24]. When the skin is involved, CMV may cause a number of different clinical manifestations including ulcerations, verrucous lesions and palpable purpuric papules[25,26]. Vesicles, bullae, generalized morbilliform eruptions as well as hyperpigmented indurated plaques have been reported[27,28]. Occasionally patients may develop CMV perianal ulcerations secondary to chronic CMV proctocolitis; these ulcers represent contiguous spread of CMV to the skin from the gastrointestinal tract[29]. In spite of the high frequency of CMV viremia in AIDS patients, skin disease caused by CMV is relatively uncommon. Ulcers are often secondarily colonized with the

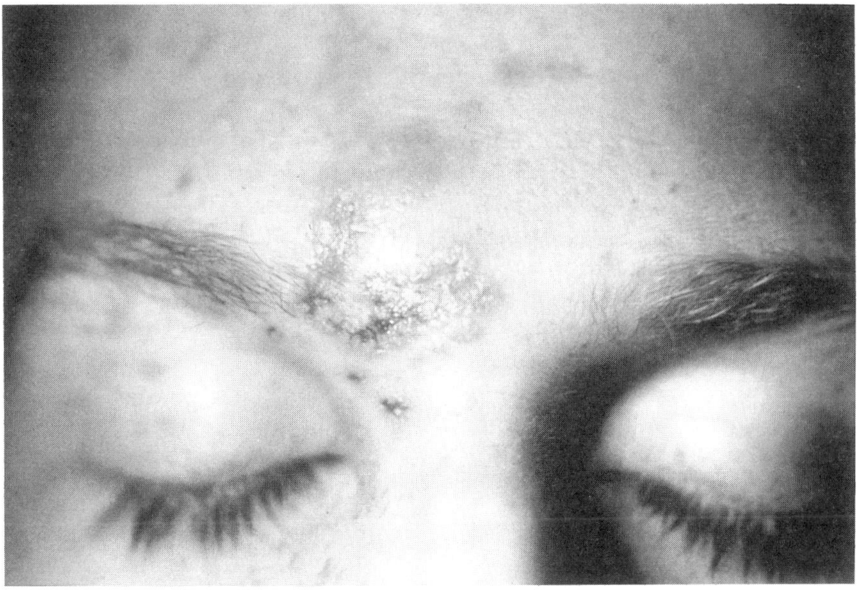

Figure 14.2 *Herpes zoster of the face in a patient with HIV infection. Careful assessment to exclude the possibility of ocular involvement is critical*

virus and many patients have combined herpes simplex and CMV infections[30].

Histopathologically, there is infection of fibroblasts and endothelial cells in the dermis with overlying ulceration. Cutaneous epithelial cells are not infected. Infected cells are enlarged to several times their normal diameter, with purplish intracytoplasmic and intranuclear inclusions having a somewhat crystalline shape. There is a variable degree of inflammation in the dermis. It is important to ensure there is not a 'mixed' infection as it is not uncommon to see both herpes simplex and CMV within the same section.

Oral Hairy Leukoplakia (Epstein–Barr Virus)

With advanced immunodeficiency in HIV-infected patients, latent EBV infection becomes active, leading to either hairy leukoplakia, Burkitt's lymphoma or EBV-associated large cell lymphoma. Oral hairy leukoplakia (OHL) is manifest as one or more whitish plaques usually on the lateral margins of the tongue. The surface is usually corrugated or folded, giving rise to hair-like projections. OHL clinically may simulate other white lesions of the mucous membranes, including true premalignant leukoplakia as well as oral candidiasis (thrush)[31]. Unlike thrush, the lesion of OHL is not easily rubbed off with a tongue depressor, which is a helpful finding in distinguishing it from candidiasis, with which it may be concomitantly infected. The condition is usually asymptomatic but may become verrucous and lead to dysphagia. OHL has been correlated with progression from HIV infection to AIDS as 48% of patients with OHL develop AIDs by 16 months and 83% by 31 months[32].

Histopathologically, OHL is manifest by epithelial hyperplasia with a verrucous appearance[33]. Keratinocytes demonstrate marked ballooning degeneration with pallor. Minimal inflammation is seen in the lamina propria. The differential diagnosis includes other ballooning degenerative lesions of the mouth, including chronic maceration and white sponge nevus. Electron microscopy as well as DNA *in situ* hybridization can be used to demonstrate viral particles in the epithelium[34,35].

OHL often requires no treatment but may respond to treatment with acyclovir at a dosage of 200–400 mg five times a day, topical podophyllin resin 20% in alcohol applied two to three times daily, or application of topical isotretinoin (Retin A) gel. Local destructive measures may also be beneficial[36,37].

Human Papillomavirus Infections

Human papillomavirus (HPV) infections are extremely prevalent in HIV-infected patients. The annual incidence of condylomata acuminata has been reported as high as 106.5 per 100 000 or about 0.1% of the entire population of the USA[38]. Infection with this group of viruses is even more prevalent in HIV-infected individuals. Condyloma acuminata have been demonstrated in 20% of HIV-infected homosexual men[39], and 54% of homosexual men with AIDS were shown to have evidence of HIV infections[41]. HPV types 16 and 18 are the most common viral isolates from anogenital condylomata. The pathogenesis and relationship between HPV and malignancy have been dealt with elsewhere in this text.

Different HPV types tend to be associated with different clinical lesions. Non-genital lesions such as plantar, common or flat warts are most commonly caused by HPV types 1, 2, 3, and 4. Epidermodysplasia verruciformis is induced by HPV types 3, 5, 8 and 10. Mucosal lesions involving either the genital, oral or laryngeal epithelia are caused most commonly by types 6, 11, 16, 18, 31 and 33, some of which are believed to be associated with cervical and rectal malignancies. Bowenoid papulosis—a premalignant condition seen on the genitalia—is almost exclusively associated with HPV types 16 and 18, with 16 being the most frequent[49].

Patients with HIV disease, especially those who are immunocompromised, may present with multiple verrucae vulgares, especially in periungual locations. Multiple plantar warts, including mosaic warts, may develop that may lead to pain on walking. Extensive flat and filiform warts on the bearded area of the face manifest by small verrucous papules are also seen in HIV-infected individuals and may be the first sign of HIV infection.

HPV in men can appear on the penis, urethra, scrotum, perianal, anal and rectal areas. Condyloma acuminata are usually recognized as soft, sessile lesions with surfaces that range from smooth to very rough with finger-like projections. Exuberant cauliflower-like plaques of condylomata acuminata may involve the perianal region as well as flexural areas such as the axillae and angles of the mouth. Extensive perianal condylomata may lead to difficulty with defecation and cause secondary constipation. Subclinical and HPV infection is common in homosexual men and presents as diffuse foci of epithelial hyperplasia that are invisible on routine examination[50]. Subclinical HPV infection as well as intraurethral and vaginal condylomata may serve as a major reservoir for HPV in the population. Treatment failure in women may represent, in some cases, reinfection by a male sexual partner with one of these occult forms of HPV infection.

In women, the spectrum of clinical disease induced by HPV is broad. Classic exophytic lesions of condyloma acuminata of the external genitalia are readily recognized by clinical examination alone. Detection of other intravaginal or cervical forms of HPV infection requires colposcopic and sigmoidoscopic examination. Vulvar condylomata acuminata appear as soft, whitish, sessile tumors with finger-like projections seen most commonly in moist areas such as in the introitus and on the labia[51]. Cervical and intravaginal condylomata acuminata are commonly seen in women with external vulvar condylomata.

Histologically, condylomata acuminata are manifest as dome-shaped papular lesions with acanthosis and koilocytosis. Bowenoid papulosis has architectural features of condyloma but histologically shows changes of squamous cell carcinoma *in situ*. Epidermodysplasia verruciformis appears similar to flat verrucae except there may be atypical keratinocytic changes suggestive of evolving carcinoma *in situ*. Verrucous carcinoma has histological features similar to large condylomata acuminata except such lesions invade into the dermis.

The differential diagnosis of HPV infection includes other benign epithelial neoplasms including seborrheic keratoses, pyogenic granulomata, nevi and various other keratoses and acanthomata. Diagnosis is based on clinical features in the context of histopathological findings. It is important to perform biopsies in any cases that could conceivably represent a malignant HPV-induced condition. In difficult cases, immunoperoxidase stains for HPV antigens, DNA *in situ* hybridization, as well as the polymerase chain reaction (PCR) can be performed to ascertain the types of HPV causing the lesion. Knowledge of the HPV type, however, will not influence the course of the disease or its treatment.

Treatment of HPV infection includes measures which result in diminution of clinical lesions, destruction of premalignant or malignant lesions, reduction of symptoms and minimizing transmission to uninfected individuals. Successful therapy depends upon the ability of the host's immune status to keep the viral infection in check. Frequent recurrences are probably a consequence of reactivation of latent HPV infection. Unfortunately, no treatment has been shown to eradicate HPV entirely. Destructive measures such as application of topical chemicals, i.e. salicylic or trichloroacetic acid, cryotherapy with liquid nitrogen, or ablative surgery are standard measures used for common verrucae. Condylomata acuminata are usually treated by applying topical podophyllin resin 10–50% in tincture of benzoin directly to lesions by a physician or an assistant, to be washed off in 4–6 h. In extensive cases, the entire penile shaft may be 'painted' with the resin. Treatments are administered weekly until resolution or until significant reduction of the number of lesions is noted, at which point secondary destruction with liquid nitrogen cryosurgery or surgical destruction may be performed. While generally safe, complications of severe necrosis and scarring in the anogenital area, 'fistula in ano', dermatitis, balanitis and phimosis may develop, especially if the caustic agent is left on the skin or mucosa for long periods of time[54]. Systemic reactions to podophyllin may rarely occur[55,56]. Podophyllotoxin (Condylox, Oclassen, Ventura, CA), the active ingredient in podophyllin, applied twice a day for three days per week for three to four weeks can be performed by the patient at home[57]. Liquid nitrogen cryotherapy, electrodesiccation and curettage as well as carbon dioxide laser vaporization also may be performed. Care must be taken to avoid adverse consequences of infectious papillomavirus in the laser plume with these latter methods[58,59]. Plantar verrucae are generally treated with topical 40% salicylic acid plaster applied daily with paring of hyperkeratotic areas, although intralesional bleomycin and liquid nitrogen therapy have also been used. Verruca plana and filiform verrucae are treated commonly with topical tretinoin (Retin A) 0.05% cream or 0.01% gel applied daily and increased two to three times per day depending on the amount of irritation that can be tolerated. Topical 5-fluorouracil cream (Efudex) may be applied once or twice per day and may be used in combination with tretinoin. Light electrodesiccation and liquid nitrogen application may be used as an adjunct therapy. Bowenoid papulosis is generally treated by electrodesiccation and curettage, although liquid nitrogen cryodestruction is also usually effective. Verrucous carcinoma requires excisional surgery.

Intralesional interferon also may be used to treat condylomata successfully. The intralesional dosage is approximately 500 000 IU to 1 million units intralesionally three times a week for 8–12 weeks. The frequency of visits and expense are generally prohibitive for this form of therapy except in selected instances[60].

Molluscum Contagiosum

Skin lesions of molluscum contagiosum develop in at least 20% of patients with AIDS[61]. Most patients are severely immunocompromised at the time of infection with $CD4^+$ cell counts of <200 cells/mm^4. The molluscum contagiosum virus is the largest virus known to afflict man and is a member of the pox family of viruses. The virus is spread by direct contact and has a tropism for the epithelial cells where it replicates in the cytoplasm and eventually completely fills it with viral particles known as molluscum or Henderson–Patterson bodies. These compress the nucleus to the periphery of the cell, which subsequently ruptures so that adjacent cells become infected. The epithelia of hair follicles are preferentially infected.

Molluscum contagiosum infection is characterized by dome-shaped umbilicated translucent papules that may develop on any part of the body, especially the genital areas and the face (Figure 14.3). The mucosal surfaces are spared. Lesions may number in excess of 100 and individual ones may become quite large, often greater than 1 cm in diameter[61]. In immunocompetent hosts, lesions generally undergo spontaneous resolution but in HIV-infected patients lesions may persist for months to years.

Histologically, there is a dome-shaped papule with a central crater which arises as a consequence of coalescence of numerous hair follicles and adnexal structures infected by the molluscum virus. Identification of the characteristic molluscum body, a 25 μm structure manifesting as a pinkish, hyaline-like, oval body within the cytoplasm of suprabasilar keratinocytes or floating free within the central crater, is pathognomonic. They are usually present in large numbers near the surface of the center of fully developed lesions.

In patients with HIV infection, waxy lesions of cryptococcosis, cutaneous pneumocystosis and other infectious disorders may appear similar to molluscum contagiosum, so that a biopsy is often necessary to exclude more serious infections. Solitary molluscum lesions may resemble pyogenic granuloma, keratoacanthoma or basal cell carcinoma and may occasionally be difficult to define.

Treatment of molluscum contagiosum is generally by destructive measures. Cryotherapy is the usual method of treatment and may be successful especially if done every one to two weeks until lesions have resolved. Lesions are sprayed with liquid nitrogen for 5–10 s to yield a 15–20 s thaw time. Although the method is generally safe, in dark-skinned individuals dyspigmentation may develop. Unfortunately, discontinuation of therapy is often associated with recurrence. Electrosurgery, application of topical keratolytic preparations and removal by curettage are other effective therapies.

BACTERIAL INFECTIONS

Folliculitis, Abscesses, Furuncles, Impetigo and Related Infections

Most banal bacterial infections such as folliculitis and impetigo are caused by *Staphylococcus* and *Streptococcus*, organisms commonly encountered in immunocompetent hosts. *Staphylococcus aureus* is the most common cutaneous

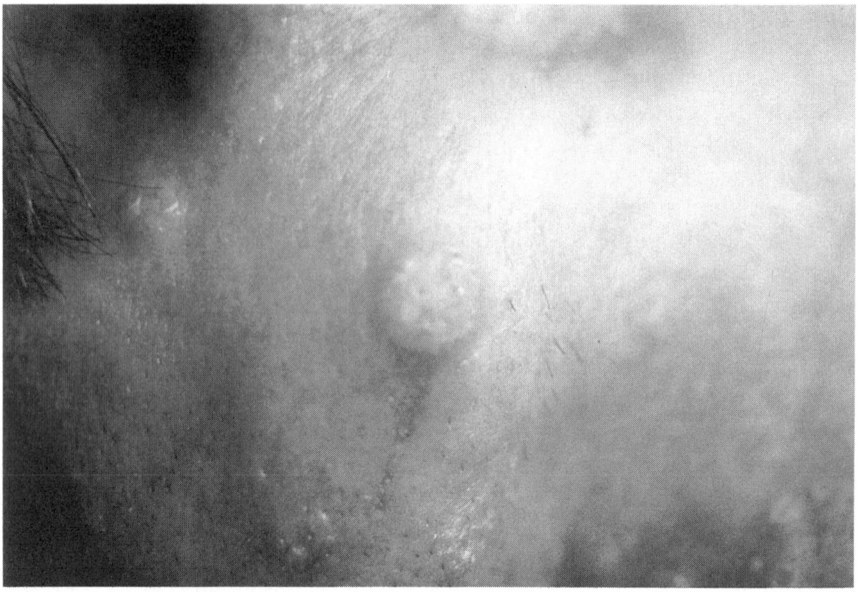

Figure 14.3 *Giant molluscum contagiosum is a common problem in HIV-infected individuals and may be severely cosmetically deforming*

and systemic bacterial pathogen in HIV-infected adults. The initial site of colonization with *S. aureus* is the nares, and the nasal carriage rate in HIV-infected patients is approximately 50%, which is twice that of HIV-seronegative individuals[63]. Up to 83% of patients with AIDS may suffer from some form of *S. aureus* infection at some point during the course of HIV disease[64]. Infection with *Pseudomonas* spp. is also seen with some frequency in patients who are HIV infected and up to 8% of all cases of bacteremia in patients with AIDS are due to these organisms[65]. Aggressive *Haemophilus influenzae* infection of the head and neck has also been observed[66].

Folliculitis is generally manifest as widely distributed acneiform papules and pustules over the skin. Lesions may be pruritic and excoriated. Most cases are confined to the skin superficially but occasionally sepsis may supervene. In some cases the bacterial density may increase significantly as a consequence of immunodepression, leading to more deeply seated skin infections such as botryomycosis or ecthyma[67]. Botryomycosis is most commonly caused by *S. aureus* and represents a manifestation of extension of staphylococcal folliculitis with the formation of bacterial colonies into the dermis[68,69]. Clinically, this is often manifest as a non-descript papule or plaque in the skin that may be surrounded by pustules on the trunk, neck or extremities. Soft tissue and deeply seated bacterial infections such as cellulitis, pyomyositis, deep soft tissue abscesses and necrotizing fasciitis may also develop in HIV-infected hosts[68] and are generally manifest as

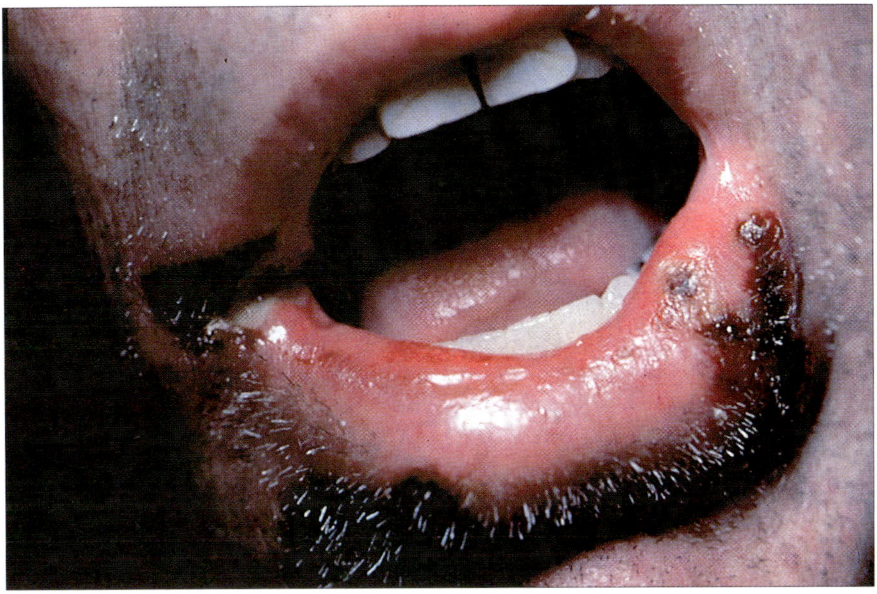

Plate 14.1 Extensive perioral necrotizing herpesvirus infection in a severely immunocompromised patient

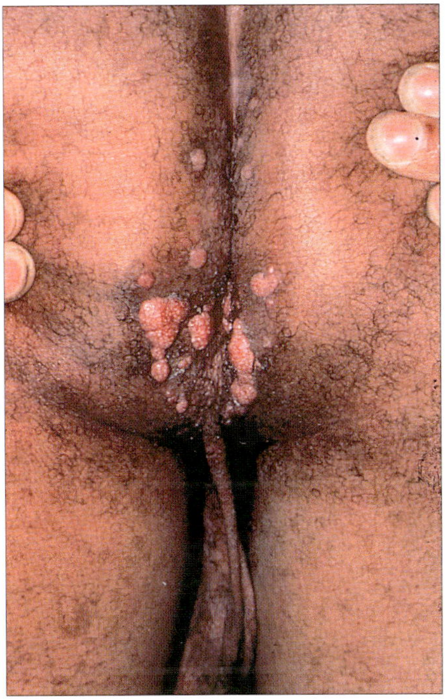

Plate 14.2 Condylomata lata, a manifestation of syphilis, in an AIDS patient. Any individual with syphilis of any form should undergo testing for HIV

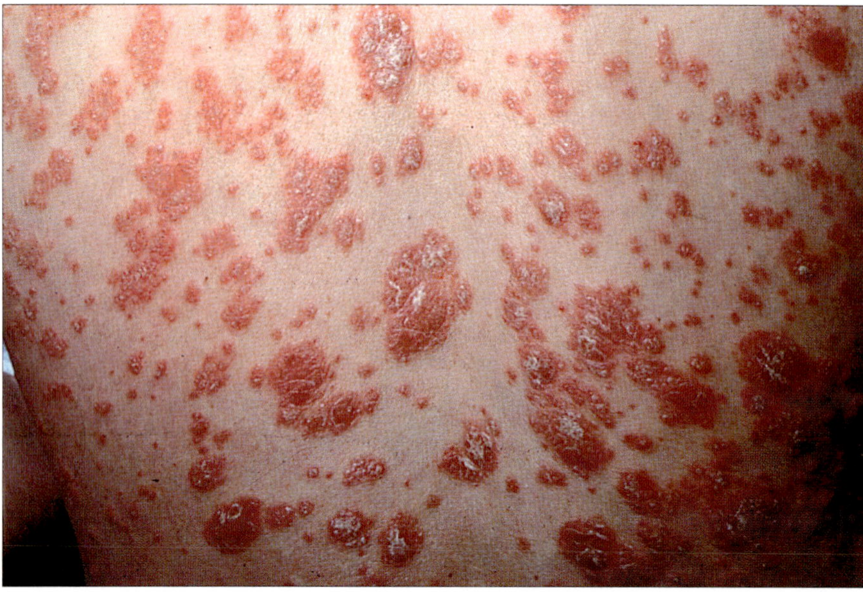

Plate 14.3 Widespread psoriasis which developed eruptively in this patient with AIDS

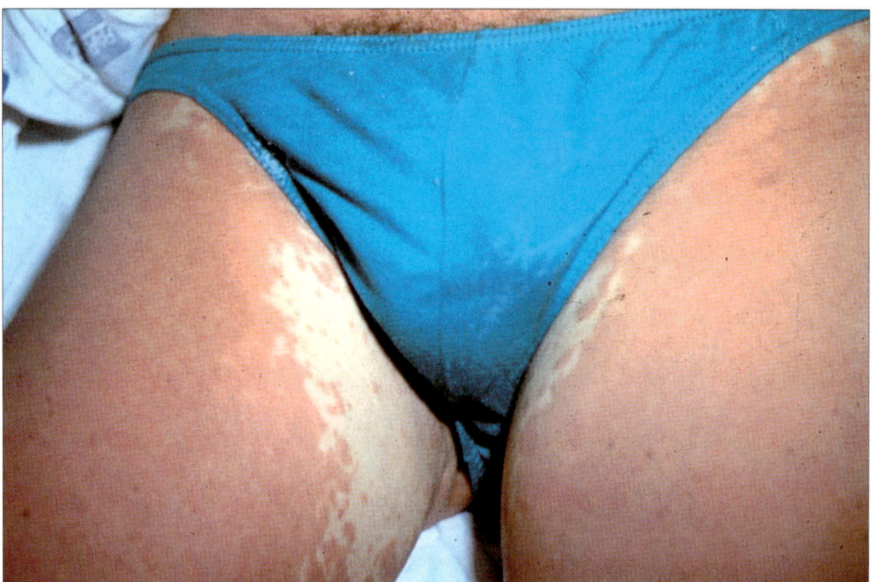

Plate 14.4 An extensive morbilliform drug eruption caused by trimethoprim–sulfamethoxazole in an HIV-infected patient

diffuse, red, warm tender areas in the skin. There is often extreme toxemia, so that early recognition is essential. Streptococcal axillary lymphadenitis presents as diffuse, painful swelling of lymph nodes in the axillae that is usually bilateral[70]. When incised, copious pustular drainage is noted.

Impetigo is manifest as localized or widespread edematous crusted areas of the skin associated with yellowish surface crusts. Although impetigo is seen most commonly on the face in healthy individuals, in patients with HIV disease it is seen more often in the axillary, inguinal and other intertriginous locations. The infection usually begins with painful red macules that may develop superficial vesicles that rupture, oozing serous and purulent fluid that contains potentially infective HIV. A characteristic honey-colored surface crust usually forms and satellite lesions may develop. In some cases, intact bullae and pustules may be observed.

Folliculitis, otitis externa and ecthyma gangrenosum, both primary and secondary to septicemia, may be caused by *Pseudomonas aeruginosa* as well as *P. cepacia* that are frequently acquired from hot tub use[71,72]. The clinical manifestations of these disorders when caused by *Pseudomonas* spp. appear similar to those caused by other pyogenic bacteria, namely firm erythematous papulopustules or nodules, as with localized necrosis. Cultures are essential in making a definitive diagnosis and to insure the administration of appropriate antibiotic therapy[73].

Histologically, there is usually suppurative inflammation in the dermis, often centered within and around hair follicles. There may be rupture in these lesions with secondary granulomatous inflammation. Histologically, impetigo demonstrates a subcorneal pustule with clusters of Gram-positive bacteria seen within the space. Botryomycosis demonstrates diffuse inflammation in the dermis with darkly staining 'grains' which represent colonies of bacteria growing in the skin.

Pyogenic bacterial infections generally respond to treatment with dicloxacillin, cephalexin or ciprofloxacin. Chlorhexidine gluconate washes of the skin and application of topical antibiotics such as polymyxin B sulfate, bacitracin or mupirocin ointment preparations into the nostrils may help to eradicate bacterial colonization. Unfortunately, in immunocompromised hosts recurrence is very common.

Bacillary Angiomatosis

Bacillary angiomatosis is a bacterial infection caused by organisms of the genus *Bartonella* (formerly *Rochalimaea*), specifically *B. quintana* and *B. henselae*. An endocarditis has been associated in one case with *B. elizabethae*[74]. The pathogenesis is not completely known but it has been postulated that either a vasoproliferative factor is produced by the bacterium itself or is induced to be formed by the host as a consequence of bacterial infection.

There are a number of different clinical manifestations of cutaneous disease in bacillary angiomatosis. Cutaneous vascular lesions are the most common and, of these, small pinpoint reddish to purple papules are the earliest lesions. These may assume an appearance similar to pyogenic granulomata and are seen in two-thirds of patients with cutaneous disease[75–77]. They range in number from one to several thousand and range in size from 1 mm to several centimeters. Lesions may ulcerate and be covered by a crust. The second most common skin lesion is the subcutaneous nodule that occurs in approximately 50% of patients with skin lesions. They may be located deep in the subcutis extending to involve soft tissue and bone[79]. Two cases of deeply seated skeletal muscle pyomyositis have been reported[79]. When bone is involved, lesions are generally osteolytic in nature. Non-descript crusted ulcerations, plaques, and cellulitis may also be seen in 5–10% of patients[80]. Viscera may be involved either as disseminated vascular lesions or as bacillary peliosis hepatis of the liver. Although virtually every organ system may be affected, other than the skin, the liver and spleen are the most common sites of involvement. Liver disease is usually manifest by elevated levels of circulating liver enzymes. Patients with bacillary angiomatosis may develop fever, weight loss, and night sweats[81]. These symptoms usually resolve with institution of antibiotic therapy.

Histopathological findings in bacillary angiomatosis are characterized by a lobular proliferation of capillaries associated with enlarged epithelioid-appearing endothelial cells. The background stroma is usually edematous in superficial lesions and more compact in deeper ones. Neutrophils and leukocytoclasis are often seen in the interstitium between vessels. The presence of neutrophils in the body of lesions is a valuable finding that permits distinction from ulcerated pyogenic granulomata that may have similar histological features, although neutrophils are present primarily under areas of ulceration. Granular amphophilic aggregates are characteristically seen adjacent to vessels, often in association with neutrophils which represent masses of *Bartonella* organisms. These appear black after staining with the Warthin–Starry stain. Electron microscopy is confirmatory. Although the diagnosis can usually be made on the basis of microscopic examination of routine hematoxylin and eosin-stained tissue sections, on occasion atypia of endothelial cells may be marked, causing histological confusion with angiosarcoma.

Bacillary angiomatosis must be differentiated from other vascular lesions that develop in patients with HIV infection, especially Kaposi's sarcoma. Generally, the lack of macular and plaque lesions or the presence of lesions oriented along skin lines is helpful in making this distinction. Histopathological findings are also distinct.

Bacillary angiomatosis responds well to systemic treatment with erythromycin ethyl succinate at doses of 500 mg orally four times a day for four weeks to six months depending on the tendency towards relapse. Doxycycline hydrochloride 100 mg orally twice a day is also effective. Other antibiotics that have been shown to have some efficacy include rifampin, ciprofloxacin, trimethoprim–sulfamethoxazole and gentamicin. Azithromycin, rozithromycin and fluoroquinolones such as norfloxacin have also been used with good response. Recent data indicated that trimethoprim–sulfamethoxazole is effective in preventing relapses[82].

Mycobacterial Infections

Any of the mycobacteria including *Mycobacterium avium–intracellulare* and *M. haemophilum* may induce skin lesions in up to 10% of patients with systemic mycobacterial infections[83–85]. This is of importance as the latter organism is more difficult to culture than other mycobacteria, requiring supplementation of media with blood use and other growth factors. Infection with *M. bovis* following BCG vaccination in a patient with HIV infection has also been reported[86].

Mycobacterial skin lesions may assume a number of different appearances. Small papules and pustules that resemble folliculitis, atopic dermatitis-like eruptions, localized cutaneous abscesses, suppurative lymphadenitis, nonspecific ulcerations, palmar and plantar hyperkeratoses and sporotrichoid nodules all have been reported[87–89]. *M. marinum* may cause classic swimming pool granulomata in patients with HIV disease, manifest as verrucous nodules often with a distribution involving ascending lymph nodes on an extremity. Most reported cases behave in a relatively indolent fashion. Lesions may take the form of painful erythematous papules and nodules on the distal extremities and ears[88].

Histologically, cutaneous mycobacterial infections may assume classic patterns of suppurative granulomatous infiltrates in the dermis associated with pseudocarcinomatous hyperplasia, although other patterns may be observed, including dense areas of suppuration with minimal granulomatous infiltrate.

Cutaneous atypical mycobacterial infections demonstrate variable responses to antibiotics, so that it is important to culture the organisms and determine sensitivities.

Syphilis

Syphilis is quite prevalent in patients with HIV infection and of all reported cases of syphilis between the years 1984 and 1993, 25% developed in HIV-infected hosts[90]. Other venereal diseases including lymphogranuloma venereum, chancroid, granuloma inguinale and *Neisseria gonorrhoea* infection all may develop and may be more severe as a consequence of immunocompromise in these patients.

Syphilis may occur in a number of forms in patients with HIV infection, ranging from classic papulosquamous forms with involvement of the palms and soles and mucous membranes to unusual forms that may defy diagnosis. Unusual manifestations of syphilis in these patients include rapid progression from the primary chancre through the secondary stages to advanced late-stage disease in a short period of time, including gummatous tertiary lues, lues maligna (syphilis with vasculitis), sclerodermiform lesions, rupial verrucous plaques, extensive oral ulcerations, keratoderma, deep cutaneous nodules, rubeoliform eruptions and widespread gummata[91–93] (Plate 14.2). Central nervous system (CNS) disease has been noted more frequently and with greater severity in patients with HIV infection[94] and, as in other forms of syphilis, may have an accelerated course, developing over several months as compared to several years in the immunocompetent host.

The histopathology of cutaneous syphilis is usually similar to that seen in immunocompetent hosts, with the characteristic superficial and deep psoriasiform lichenoid pattern of inflammation associated with plasma cells and histiocytes. On the other hand, unusual histological findings have been described, including vasculitis as well as very sparse inflammatory infiltrates with minimal numbers of plasma cells and abundant spirochetes.

Syphilis may have protean manifestations in patients with HIV infection just as it may in immunocompetent hosts. The list of diseases that may be simulated includes many other bacterial and fungal infections as well as connective tissue diseases, Kaposi's sarcoma and lymphoma. It responds to penicillin at higher doses that must be continued for longer courses than in immunocompetent hosts.

PARASITIC INFECTIONS AND ECTOPARASITIC INFESTATIONS

Scabies

Scabies is one of the most frequent skin conditions to develop in patients with HIV infection and is the most common ectoparasitic infestation in these individuals. The causative agent is the mite *Sarcoptes scabiei*, var. *humanus*. Although the data regarding the overall incidence of scabies and HIV infection is not well determined, in one study it was reported in 20% of patients[95].

Scabies may have a number of different clinical manifestations in patients with HIV infection. Hyperkeratosis on the palms, soles, trunk or extremities may develop, having an appearance similar to crusted scabies in other settings. In other patients, only scattered pruritic papules accompanied by slight scale of the trunk and extremities may be seen. A widespread papulosquamous eruption that may resemble atopic dermatitis as well as scalp and facial scaling that may mimic seborrheic dermatitis have also been reported[99,102–104]. Characteristic burrows may be difficult to identify, so that virtually any patient with a scaly persistent pruritic eruption should have skin lesions scraped and examined histologically in search of mites of scabies. Severe forms of scabies may be associated with secondary infection, bactermia and fatal septicemia, especially in severely compromised hosts[105]. Patients complain of intractable pruritus that is worse at night. Usually contacts are infested, especially in the context of the number of mites present on the skin of these individuals. In crusted scabies there is usually a superficial and mid-to-deep perivascular and interstitial infiltrate of lymphocytes with numerous eosinophils. The epidermis is hyperplastic with prominent crusting and many scabetic mites visible in the cornified layer. In patients with post-scabetic 'id' reactions, a spongiotic dermatitis may be noted, and in nodular scabies a dense mixed inflammatory infiltrate with numerous eosinophils in a nodular configuration resembling a pseudolymphoma may be seen. In nodular scabies, the number of mites is few and it may be difficult to find them. Scabies in patients with HIV infection must be distinguished from a wide variety of disorders. Norwegian (crusted) scabies may appear similar to palmoplantar hyperkeratotic disorders such as psoriasis. Diffuse scabies may mimic atopic dermatitis as well as other spongiotic dermatitides such as nummular dermatitis. Occasionally, scabies may involve the scalp with scaling and may simulate seborrheic dermatitis. Nodular scabies may mimic lymphomatoid papulosis as well as other insect bite reactions.

Scabies generally responds to treatment with lindane cream or lotion or 5% permethrin cream applied from head to toe, left in place for 8–12 h and then washed off. The treatment is repeated in one week. In some patients, recurrences develop as a consequence of failure to treat under the fingernails and the intertriginous zones although resistance to scabicidal medications may develop. Some have recommended alternating treatment with lindane and permethrin. Multiple treatments may be required. A recent report of the use of oral ivermectin for this disorder is highly encouraging. Post-scabetic id reactions must be treated with antihistamines such as doxepin 10–25 mg orally three to four times a day with topical application of corticosteroid preparations to diminish inflammation. In cases of nodules, injection of triamcinolone acetonide may be required. Careful laundering of linen and clothing is necessary and household and other contacts should be treated. In cases of crusted scabies, entire wards of patients may require therapy[106]. Adjunctive therapies are also important as pruritus is often severe. Topical application of corticosteroid preparations as well as antipruritic agents containing menthol and phenol, pramoxine and antihistamines may be required. Four per cent doxepin cream (Zonalon) is a valuable antipruritic agent that may be used in patients with refractory pruritus. Exposure to ultraviolet B irradiation and PUVA is also helpful.

Pneumocystosis

Approximately five cases of cutaneous *Pneumocystis carinii* infection have been reported in patients with HIV infection. *P. carinii* may involve the skin preferentially in patients who use aerosolized pentamidine for prophylaxis of *P. carinii* pneumonia. By creating a more unfavorable environment in the lung, organisms spread more widely to involve visceral organs as well as the skin. The disorder may have several different cutaneous manifestations, the most common of which is friable reddish papules or nodules seen in the ear canal or the nares. Small translucent molluscum contagiosum-like papules, bluish cellulitic plaques and deeply seated abscesses have also been observed. Histologically, *P. carinii* in the skin has an appearance similar to that in the lung, with a diffuse infiltrate of foamy appearing cells which, when stained with Gomori's methenamine silver or Steiner stains, highlight the microorganisms resulting in the 'teacup and saucer' appearance.

Pneumocystosis responds to the usual treatment for *P. carinii* pneumonia, namely intravenous pentamidine. Strongyloidiasis requires treatment with thiabendazole 25 mg/kg twice a day for four to five days to several weeks depending in the immune status of the host. Amebiasis responds to metronidazole at a dosage of 750 mg p.o. twice a day for 10 days but, as these patients are often quite immunocompromised, response to therapy may be poor.

Other Parasitic Infestations

Cutaneous strongyloidiasis, caused by the helminth *Strongyloides stercoralis*, has been reported rarely in patients with HIV infection. Clinically, lesions appear similar to urticaria, figurate erythemata, livedo reticularis and other causes of cutaneous livedo. Histologically, there is a diffuse infiltrate of lymphocytes and eosinophils scattered throughout the dermis. If an organism itself is contained within the biopsy specimen, it is located in the upper papillary dermis.

Acanthamebiasis, caused by *Acanthamoeba castellani*[96–101], a part of the normal oral flora, develops when this organism proliferates abnormally and disseminates to the skin and often the CNS in profoundly immunocompromised patients. Clinically, lesions appear as necrotic nodules or as painful ulcerations of the skin, often involving the extremities. Histologically, there is a diffuse infiltrate of amebic cysts and trophozoites throughout the skin, especially around blood vessels and in the subcutaneous fat. Careful inspection is required as these may appear similar to histiocytes or other normal-appearing structures in the skin. Erythrophagocytosis is often noted.

SYSTEMIC FUNGAL INFECTIONS

The most common systemic opportunistic fungal infections to involve the skin in HIV-seropositive patients are histoplasmosis and cryptococcosis. Nearly 20% of HIV-seropositive individuals with disseminated histoplasmosis and up to 10% of those with disseminated cryptococcosis develop mucocutaneous lesions. Systemic and cutaneous coccidioidomycosis are both recognized periodically in HIV-infected patients. HIV-infected hosts with blastomycosis, paracoccidioidomycosis, or sporotrichosis have also been observed.

Mucocutaneous lesions associated with deep systemic fungal infections may assume a number of different forms. The most common lesions are pustules and ulcers although papules and nodules are also frequently observed. Less often, patches, plaques, and mucosal ulcerations are seen.

Oral 'thrush' involving either the tongue and/or buccal mucosa, with or without esophageal infection, is the most common manifestation of candidiasis in HIV-seropositive patients[107]. Oral candidiasis may be the initial sign of HIV infection in many individuals. Other manifestations that may develop include chronic paronychia and onychodystrophy, chronic refractory vaginal candidiasis, distal urethritis and persistent monilial infection of the axilla, glans penis, groin, and/or inframammary area. Disseminated candidiasis in HIV-infected individuals has been reported in a relatively few number of HIV-infected patients.

Although an increasing number of HIV-infected patients with coccidioidomycosis are being described, only a few of these individuals have been reported with associated skin lesions[108–110]. Some of the manifestations include leukocytoclastic vasculitis, painful erythema of the buttock and papulopustules on the extremities, chest, back, and palm. Other skin manifestations that may be seen in coccidioidomycosis include ulcers, abscesses and nodules.

Cryptococcosis

Cryptococcosis is not uncommon in HIV-infected individuals[111–113]. The incidence of cutaneous involvement was found to be approximately 6–7% when a large series of HIV-infected patients with cryptococcosis were evaluated. Mucocutaneous lesions of cryptococcosis are polymorphous and may appear as erythematous papules, nodules, pustules, and/or ulcers of the skin and mucosa[114]. Cutaneous cryptococcosis, like other opportunistic infections that develop in these patients, may mimic the cutaneous morphology of other disorders such as herpes simplex virus, cellulitis or molluscum contagiosum infection, as well as soft tissue hypertrophic lesions such as rhinophyma and Kaposi's sarcoma[115,116]. In addition to simulating it, *Crypto-*

coccus neoformans has been demonstrated with lesions of cutaneous Kaposi's sarcoma. Cryptococcosis has a characteristic histopathological appearance in most cases. There is diffuse pallor of the dermis that correlates with the mucoid capsular material of the organisms, which are usually present in abundance. Inflammation is usually minimal.

Histoplasmosis

Cutaneous lesions of histoplasmosis may develop in 10–17% of patients with systemic infection with *Histoplasma capsulatum*[117]. Clinically, the lesions have appeared protean, manifest as cutaneous and mucosal ulcers, erythematous macules and patches, fistulae, papules and nodules, pustules, and verrucous plaques[118–121] (Figure 14.4). Patients with AIDS have recently been described in whom *H. capsulatum* and Kaposi's sarcoma were found coexisting in a single skin lesion[121,122]. Histologically, histoplasmosis may exhibit a diffuse dermal infiltrate of histiocytes, neutrophils and leukocytoclasis. Some cases have been histologically confused with leukocytoclastic vasculitis.

Sporotrichosis

Clinical forms of sporotrichosis include lymphocutaneous, fixed cutaneous, disseminated cutaneous and systemic. The latter may present as either localized pulmonary disease or as widespread involvement of numerous organs. In patients with HIV infection, skin lesions may be ulcers, papules, nodules, plaques, and/or pustules[123–125]. These may be widespread, and internal organ involvement may develop that often proves fatal.

With the exception of disseminated candidiasis and sporotrichosis, fungal spores or hyphae are usually present in number either free in the dermis or within histiocytes, multinucleated giant cells, or abscesses. The organisms can often be identified on hematoxylin and eosin-stained sections, although special stains such as the periodic acid–Schiff and Gomori methenamine silver can be used to facilitate their detection. Examination of multiple sections taken from the biopsy specimen may be necessary to find organisms in disseminated candidiasis and sporotrichosis. Nevertheless, both of these organisms grow readily and rapidly when cultured on Sabouraud's medium. In contrast to immunocompetent patients, in some immunocompromised hosts infected with HIV, abundant organisms of sporotrichosis may be present and visualized microscopically[126].

Blastomycosis

Disseminated blastomycosis is also seen in some patients with HIV infection and AIDS. Widespread verrucous papules, nodules and plaques have been seen in a number of patients from endemic areas. One case that was described

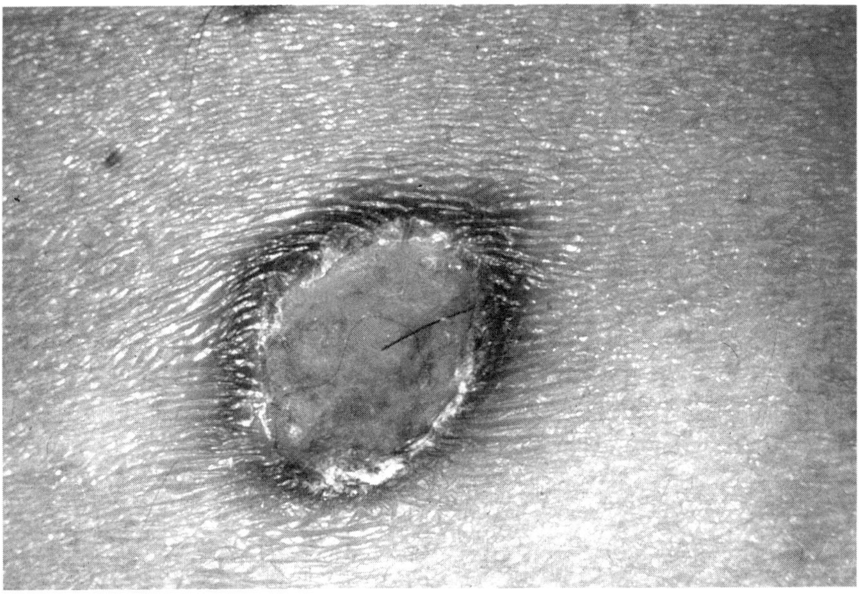

Figure 14.4 *Localized ulceration caused by* Histoplasma capsulatum *in an HIV-infected patient with disseminated histoplasmosis. Serious opportunistic infections in these patients may have very non-descript appearances*

was that of a 30-year-old homosexual HIV-seropositive man who had *Blastomyces dermatitidis*-related pustules, nodules, and cutaneous ulcers. The condition failed to respond well to treatment and eventually proved fatal[196].

Other Fungal Infections

In addition to the fungal infections described above, a number of other fungal infections have been recently reported in patients with HIV disease. Disseminated *Scedosporium inflatum*, *Pseudallescheria boydii* and *Microsporum canis* have been recently observed in these patients, as have infections with other saprophytic fungi[190,191,197]. Disseminated *Aspergillus* infection was the cause of facial palsy in one patient as a consequence of involvement of the mastoid sinus. Zygomycosis infection of the head and neck may develop and may be manifested as local pain, cutaneous necrosis and necrotizing ulcerations[193]. Deep soft tissue muscular aspergillosis has also been noted. These infections are being encountered more frequently as a consequence of better prophylaxis against other opportunistic infections and because of abnormal neutrophil function that has been demonstrated in these patients.

Penicillium marneffei, a fungus that is endemic in Asia, causes an infection that has been reported with increasing frequency in patients with AIDS in

Thailand[194,195]. Seventy-six per cent of affected individuals develop skin disease. Some of the cutaneous manifestations include umbilicated papules that could be confused with molluscum contagiosum, ecthyma-like lesions, folliculitis, subcutaneous nodules and morbilliform eruptions. The diagnosis is established by histological evaluation of skin biopsies and by the performance of cultures.

The treatment of disseminated fungal infections in HIV-infected patients is currently in flux but recent trials with newly released imidazoles such as fluconazole and itraconazole are quite promising[127]. Nevertheless, until these agents have been used to treat significant numbers of HIV-infected individuals, amphotericin B remains the drug of choice for many.

NON-INFECTIOUS SKIN DISORDERS

Seborrheic Dermatitis

Seborrheic dermatitis is the most common skin condition to affect patients with HIV infection, seen in up to 85% of all HIV-infected individuals at some point during the counsel of their disease[128]. Seborrheic dermatitis most commonly is manifested as slightly indurated, diffuse or confluent, pinkish-red scaly plaques involving the face and scalp. These may be large, thickened and heavily crusted and may involve other areas such as the upper anterior chest, back, groin and extremities. Clinically, seborrheic dermatitis must be distinguished from other papulosquamous dermatoses such as psoriasis, dermatophytosis and even scabies.

The histopathological findings of seborrheic dermatitis are similar to those seen in patients with non-HIV-associated disease, namely psoriasiform hyperplasia of the epidermis with mounds of parakeratosis containing neutrophils near ostia of hair follicular infundibula. There is an infiltrate of lymphocytes and scattered plasma cells in the dermis. One finding that is characteristically seen in seborrheic dermatitis in patients with HIV infection and AIDS that is not seen generally in patients with non-HIV-associated seborrheic dermatitis is the presence of scattered individually necrotic keratinocytes[133].

Seborrheic dermatitis is generally treated with topical application of corticosteroid preparations and antifungal creams. Systemic antifungal treatment with imidazoles such as ketoconazole, intraconazole and fluconazole have been reported to be of benefit although patients receiving these medications may develop or present with florid seborrheic dermatitis. Exposure to ultraviolet B phototherapy is also often effective as an adjunct. The disease may be more difficult to control with routine therapy in HIV-infected individuals, a finding which should serve as a clue that a patient might be immunocompromised.

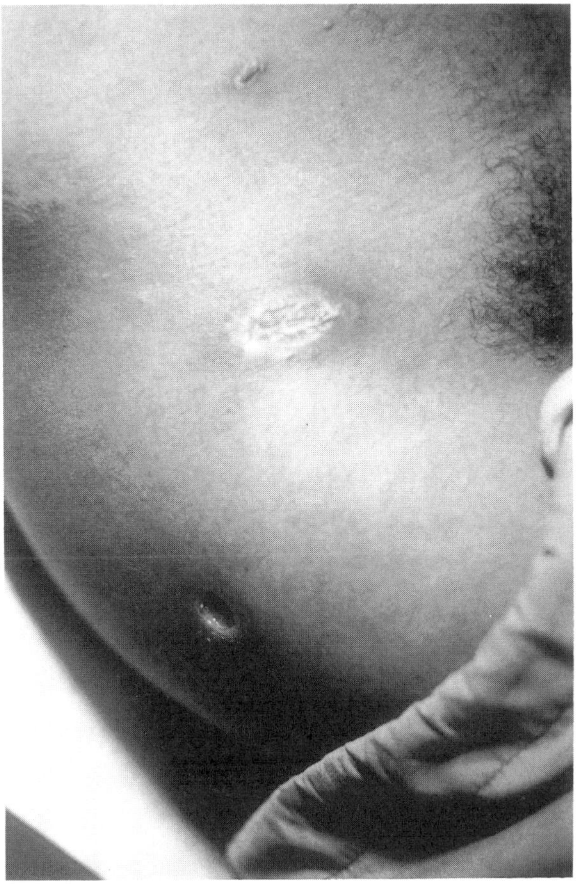

Figure 14.5 *Non-specific ulcers of the buttock in an immunocompromised host caused by infection with atypical mycobacteria*

Psoriasis

Psoriasis develops in 5% of patients with HIV infection[128,129]. Patients with HIV-associated psoriasis may develop arthritis in up to 10%, which is significantly higher than the 1% of immunocompetent patients with psoriasis who develop psoriatic arthritis. Psoriasis may resemble classic psoriasis found in immunocompetent hosts, consisting of reddish plaques with superficial micaceous scale on the extensor surfaces with nail changes of onycholysis, pitting and subungual hyperkeratosis (Plate 14.3). In other patients, severe psoriatic arthritis may be seen. Different forms of psoriasis may be found in the same patient such as guttate psoriasis associated with classic psoriasis vulgaris. Severe exfoliative erythroderma may develop and

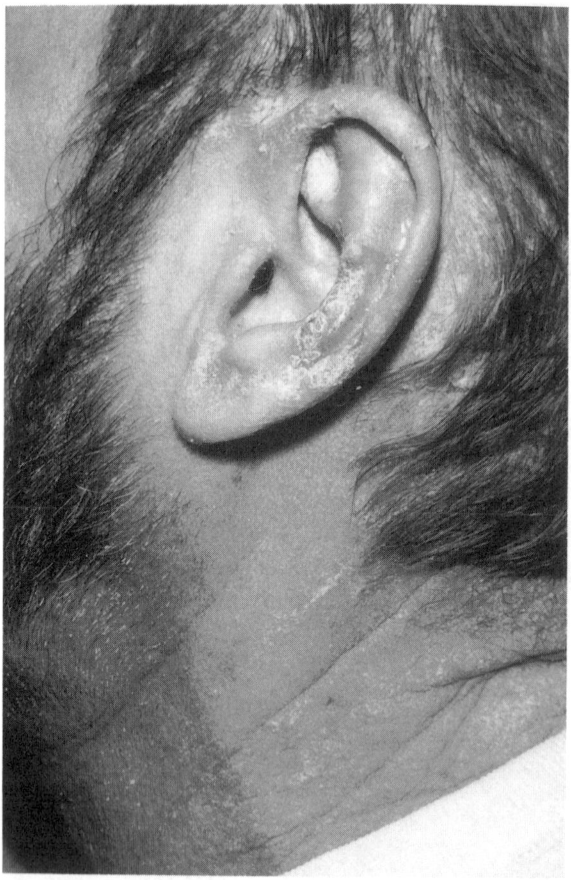

Figure 14.6 *Scaly and crusted plaques of the ear, neck and scalp were due to scabies in this HIV-infected patient. Scabies is notorious for having unusual presentations in these individuals*

acral pustular lesions of keratoderma blenorrhagicum coexisting with psoriasis or sebopsoriasis have been noted. Concomitant seborrheic dermatitis of the scalp is almost always seen. HIV-related psoriasis may develop in patients with mild re-existing psoriasis that suddenly undergoes severe exacerbation in patients once AIDS develops or it may develop spontaneously at some point after HIV seroconversion in an individual who has never before had clinical disease.

Psoriasis has histological features quite similar to those seen in non-HIV-infected patients. The pattern is that of marked acanthosis with regular elongation of epidermal retia associated with dilated tortuous blood vessels in the papillary dermis, thin suprapapillary plates and mounds of parakeratosis containing neutrophils. In pustular cases, spongiform areas in the epidermis containing collections of neutrophils are noted. Psoriasis may have histological features similar to that of other psoriasiform processes, including psoriasiform drug eruptions[121]. Other skin disorders that may progress to widespread erythroderma include cutaneous T-cell lymphoma, drug eruptions and atopic dermatitis and these must also be excluded.

Psoriasis may undergo partial remission in response to zidovudine therapy although recurrence is common[130]. Spontaneous remission as well as complete unresponsiveness to all forms of treatment have both been observed in HIV-infected patients. Emollients such as hydrophilic petrolatum applied several times daily, 3–5% salicylic acid ointment applied once to twice per day for keratolytic effect and application of triamcinolone acetonide ointment 0.025–0.1% or its equivalent for localized short-term therapy are often partially effective. In many cases, systemic drugs such as etretinate at a dosage of 1 mg/kg of body weight daily with or without the addition of dapsone 100–200 mg/day may be required, as may systemic psoralen and ultraviolet A therapy. Methotrexate may be used with extreme caution beginning at a dosage of 5–7.5 mg/week, gradually increasing the dose by 2.5 mg/week as needed. Patients must be monitored very carefully, however, as this drug may cause worsened immunodepression. Concomitant administration of trimethoprim-containing compounds is contraindicated as the folate reductase-inhibiting effect is synergistic with that induced by methotrexate[134].

Reiter's Syndrome

Reiter's syndrome has been reported in 6–10% of HIV-infected patients[131,132]. It is characterized clinically by arthritis (especially sacroiliitis), urethritis, conjunctivitis and pustular scaling lesions of the glabrous skin, glans penis and scalp. Debilitating palmoplantar pustular disease is common and there is generally striking nail dystrophy associated with periungual erythema, inflammation and hyperkeratosis with prominent crusting. Reiter's disease has a histological picture similar to that of pustular psoriasis. Clinically, Reiter's syndrome must be distinguished from other forms of arthritis such as lupus erythematosus and infectious ones such as those due to disseminated gonococcal infection.

Non-infectious Papular Pruritic Disorders ('Itchy Red Bump Disease')

Pruritic conditions in patients with HIV infection are quite common although the precise incidence and prevalence are unknown. Some studies have shown prevalences of up to 20–30%[135,137]. Some of the disorders include eosinophilic folliculitis, atopic dermatitis and xerosis. Xerotic dermatitis is commonly found in patients with advanced HIV disease and AIDS and may be seen to some degree in up to 85% of patients.

The pathogeneses of various pruritic dermatoses seen in patients with HIV infection are not entirely clear. Such patients should be evaluated for the presence of ectoparasites and other pathogens such as scabies and fungi as these may cause itching. Systemic parasites, too, may lead to itching by inducing urticarial reactions or as a consequence of migration through the skin. Other causes of itchy eruptions include hypersensitivity to medications and underlying atopic dermatitis, both of which should be included in differential diagnosis. Patients with HIV infection commonly have elevated circulating IgE antibodies[138]. This may correlate with an increased frequency of IgE-mediated disorders such as worsened atopic dermatitis and other hypersensitivity disorders. Basophils have been shown to be hyperreleasable in patients with HIV disease and it is presumed that the mast cells in some patients may have lowered threshold for release of histamine[139] with attendant inflammatory reactions and pruritus. Patients with HIV disease may also have direct neural infection with HIV leading to neural irritation and enhanced sensations of itching[140]. This may result in chronic excoriation, lichen simplex chronicus and prurigo nodularis. Sometimes, autonomic dysfunction is associated with diminished sweating and sebaceous gland secretion, worsening xerosis and itching. In addition, patients infected with HIV may be under considerable stress which may also lead to urticaria and itching. Finally, patients with HIV infection may develop pruritus secondary to underlying circulating pruritogens associated with different systemic disorders. Chronic liver disease or renal disease and systemic lymphoma may be associated with pruritus. All these factors should be considered when dealing with an itchy HIV-infected patient. In our experience, most patients develop pruritus as a consequence of a primary cutaneous disease rather than secondary to an underlying systemic illness.

Prurigo Nodularis

Prurigo nodularis is a reaction pattern that may be associated with many of the aforementioned underlying causes of itching. Patients chronically rub and scratch lesions, resulting in thickening of the skin. Prurigo nodularis appears as hyperpigmented dome-shaped verrucous and often crusted papules and nodules that are usually associated with lichen simplex chronicus. Lesions are induced by chronic rubbing and scratching.

Eosinophilic Pustular Folliculitis

Eosinophilic pustular folliculitis (EPF) is one of the most common pruritic dermatoses to develop in patients with HIV disease. Patients generally present with widespread excoriated follicular papules that involve the trunk, extremities and head and neck areas[136]. It is important to exclude the diagnosis of scabies, which may look quite similar. Although the condition is called eosinophilic pustular folliculitis, it is rare to find intact pustules as patients are usually so uncomfortable that by the time they present to the dermatologist lesions have been excoriated vigorously. Many patients have clinical appearances manifest mostly as lichen simplex chronicus and prurigo nodularis. The term 'itchy red bumps' has been used to describe the clinical presentation of EPF. Eosinophilic folliculitis has a characteristic histopathological appearance that allows the diagnosis to be made in most cases. Characteristically, within the infundibula of hair follicles there are clusters of eosinophils that may be numerous. There is often a perifollicular inflammatory infiltrate of lymphocytes, neutrophils and some eosinophils, especially in cases in which follicles have ruptured. In some cases, the number of eosinophils may be relatively small, in which case the differentiation from bacterial folliculitis may be difficult. When longstanding lesions are biopsied, the primary finding may be that of lichen simplex chronicus or prurigo nodularis which is manifested by marked acanthosis and hyperkeratosis with coarse thickened collagen bundles in the papillary dermis.

Eosinophilic pustular folliculitis appears similar to a number of other pruritic dermatoses that may be found in both HIV-infected individuals as well as in immunocompetent patients. Bacterial folliculitis may be associated with pruritus and has clinical features similar to EPF. Insect bite reactions, scabies and dermatitis herpetiformis must all be excluded. In the setting of a pruritic dermatosis in an HIV-seropositive patient with skin scrapings that show no evidence of scabies, the diagnosis can generally be assumed to be eosinophilic pustular folliculitis and treated accordingly without a biopsy in most cases.

Therapy of EPF has been the subject of a number of studies because of the frequency of the disorder and the morbidity it induces in HIV-infected individuals. Ultraviolet B exposure has been known to be quite efficacious in relieving the pruritus associated with this condition[136]. Patients are generally treated with gradually increasing exposure to ultraviolet B, usually administered by phototherapy units. Irradiances beginning at one-third of the minimal effective dose with gradual increase by one-third to one-half of the previous dose are instituted and continued until remission is experienced. Because exposure to ultraviolet irradiation may be associated with complications of both photosensitivity as well as theoretically using activation of HIV, indiscriminate use of ultraviolet B or sunlight exposure should be avoided[150]. Nevertheless, several studies have demonstrated that moderate exposure to ultraviolet B is safe in the treatment of HIV-related dermatoses if administered properly[151]. If patients are unable to undergo treatment with ultraviolet B for financial or other reasons, excellent relief may be obtained by exposure to natural sunlight. Use of tanning booths which provide ultraviolet A also may be of benefit. In addition to ultraviolet light, administration of itraconazole in doses of 200 mg orally twice a day has been shown to diminish the pruritus of EPF[152]. The mechanism of action is unknown but it may act by diminishing the concentration of *Pityrosporum* yeasts within follicular infundibula. Recently, oral therapy with isotretinoin has been shown to be efficacious. Administration of antihistamines such as doxepin at doses of 10–20 mg every 6 h by mouth as well as topical application of antipruritic agents such as pramoxine and menthol and phenol-containing lotions may also be beneficial in diminishing sensations of itching.

Atopic Dermatitis

Atopic dermatitis is characteristically manifested by erythematous patches and plaques with fine papulovesicles associated with scaling, crusting and lichen simplex chronicus. Patients often have associated hyperlinear palms, allergic rhinitis and asthma. HIV-infected individuals who develop atopic dermatitis may manifest severe forms of the disorder with erythroderma. Atopic dermatitis has microscopic features of a superficial perivascular infiltrate of lymphocytes and eosinophils with epidermal hyperplasia and foci of spongiosis. Late lesions have a morphology that is primarily that of lichen simplex chronicus. Asteatotic dermatitis or xerotic dermatitis shows very little inflammation in the dermis, with slight epidermal hyperplasia, tiny amounts of spongiosis and small zones of parakeratosis. Atopic dermatitis must be differentiated from other psoriasiform dermatitides such as psoriasis, cutaneous T-cell lymphoma and psoriasiform drug eruptions. In general, the presence of severe pruritus and a history of atopy will aid in this diagnosis.

Atopic dermatitis usually responds to measures used to treat atopic dermatitis in immunocompetent hosts. These consist of avoidance of irritants, application of emollients and topical corticosteroid preparations.

Xerotic Dermatitis

Xerotic dermatitis generally is characterized by diffuse dryness of the skin, with hyperpigmented scales and focal crusting. Many lesions may be fissured and, in some cases, eczema craquelé develops. This latter complication may lead to localized infection as the skin is broken, serving as portals of entry for bacteria and fungi. Clinically, xerotic dermatitis is generally characteristic. Other forms of dry, scaly dermatoses such as the characteristic 'flaky paint' dermatitis seen with kwashiorkor should be excluded. As both conditions occur in individuals with advanced AIDS, evaluation of nutritional status is essential.

Papular Urticaria

Papular urticaria and chronic urticaria are manifested by pinkish red erythematous papules and plaques initially with little surface change. Edema and a *peau d'orange* appearance of the skin are noted. Angioedema may be seen. Although papular urticaria may be excoriated, primary urticaria generally is not.

Chronic Actinic Dermatitis

Chronic actinic dermatitis may be associated with HIV infection and is believed to be related to the exaggerated B-cell immune response that may be present in these individuals. These patients may develop allergies to drugs and other substances and, with alteration of the immune system, underlying allergic phenomena may be recalled. The condition is characteristically manifested by psoriasiform lichenified plaques in the sun-exposed areas of the body which are often hyperpigmented, scaly and pruritic[153,154]. Lesions are generally located on the dorsal surfaces of the hands, forearms, face, upper anterior chest and the posterior neck. Extensive lichenification is often seen and patients may have an appearance similar to what has been described with actinic reticuloid.

Chronic actinic dermatitis is manifested histologically by a superficial and often deep psoriasiform dermatitis with an infiltrate of lymphocytes and abundant eosinophils. Some cases may be associated with a band-like infiltrate and epidermotropism of lymphocytes, many of which may be atypical in appearance, simulating mycosis fungoides. Clinical correlation may be necessary to render a definitive diagnosis. Spongiosis is generally seen and necrotic keratinocytes may be noted. The diagnosis of chronic actinic dermatitis may be corroborated by the performance of phototesting. Thorough questioning is important to elicit a history of recent exposure to potential photoallergens or phototoxins as well as past histories of exposure to such that may have been reactivated.

Treatment of chronic actinic dermatitis consists of avoidance of photoallergens and phototoxins as well as application of topical corticosteroid preparations. Avoidance of ultraviolet light is also important. In some cases, even visible light may precipitate a flare of the condition, so that in these cases complete light avoidance is essential as even light emitted from television monitors may be sufficient to worsen the condition. Paradoxically, the use of psoralen and ultraviolet A therapy may 'harden' the skin and lead to remission. Administration of hydroxychloroquine (Plaquenil) at doses of 200 mg orally every day to twice a day may also be beneficial. Fortunately, the incidence of this often difficult-to-manage condition remains low.

Photoexacerbated drug eruptions often appear lichenoid or erythematous distributed on photoexposed sites.

Porphyria Cutanea Tarda

Porphyria cutanea tarda has been reported in increased incidence in patients with HIV infection. HIV-infected patients are known to produce greater concentrations of porphyrins possibly as a consequence of abnormal liver function secondary to hepatitis such as hepatitis C. The disorder appears virtually identical to that seen in immunocompetent hosts with blisters on the dorsal surfaces of the hands and other sun-exposed areas associated with crusting, milia formation, dyspigmentation and scarring[155–157]. There is also often hyperpigmentation and hypertrichosis of the malar areas of the face. Patients may describe the excretion of dark urine.

Porphyria cutanea tarda has histological findings that are similar to that seen in immunocompetent individuals manifest by a subepidermal blister with minimal inflammation in the dermis. Preservation of dermal papillae, so-called 'festooning', is seen and there are thick hyaline periodic acid–Schiff (PAS)-positive rims surrounding blood vessels in the upper dermis. Elongated aggregations of necrotic keratinocytes are often present in the epidermis overlying the blister that have been referred to as 'caterpillar bodies'[158].

Porphyria is diagnosed on the basis of clinical and histological findings as well as demonstration of elevated urinary uroporphyrins and coproporphyrins.

Porphyria is classically treated by repeated phlebotomy. In patients with HIV infection who are often anemic, this treatment cannot be used. Low doses of hydroxychloroquine beginning at 25 mg weekly and increased to 200 mg weekly may be effective in mobilizing accumulated porphyrin in the liver[159]. Recently, erythropoietin has been shown to be effective in treatment of porphyria cutanea tarda by enhancing heme biosynthesis[160]. This results in mobilization of porphyrins. Thus, although expensive, this might be the most beneficial form of treatment as it will tend to correct the hematological deficit as well as the metabolic one.

Cutaneous Drug Eruptions

Cutaneous drug-induced eruptions are the most common manifestation of drug hypersensitivity. In a recent study, 79% of HIV-infected patients had one or more dermatological diagnoses, many of which included cutaneous reactions to drugs[160]. In some studies, 50–60% of HIV-positive patients have been shown to develop a cutaneous eruption due to this agent[162]. Up to 45% of patients develop morbilliform eruptions with variable numbers of other reactions being reported. Stevens–Johnson syndrome and toxic epidermal necrolysis occur sporadically[163]. Other antibiotics are common offenders as morbilliform eruptions may be seen in 10% of patients taking antituberculous regimens and in 40% of patients treated with amoxicillin–clavulanic acid[164–166].

Trimethoprim–sulfamethoxazole is the best-known and most common allergic drug eruption to develop in patients with HIV infection (Plate 14.4). In some studies, 50–60% of HIV-positive patients have been shown to develop a cutaneous eruption due to this agent[162]. In most cases, a widespread eruption of fine pink to red macules and papules involving the trunk and extremities develops 8–12 days after initiating therapy, reaching maximal intensity one to two days later. In some cases, desquamation may supervene. The eruption may disappear within three to five days even though therapy is continued, although in some cases the eruption may persist for days to weeks following discontinuation of the medication. Cutaneous eruptions due to trimethoprim–sulfamethoxazole do not always recur with drug rechallenge in HIV-infected patients; however, if the agent is to be reinstituted, it should be done under controlled circumstances to monitor for possible anaphylactoid reactions. Stevens–Johnson syndrome and toxic epidermal necrolysis may also develop as a consequence of trimethoprim–sulfamethoxazole administration. Stevens–Johnson syndrome is characterized by fever, widespread blistering of the skin and mucous membranes of the eye, mouth and/or genitals. Toxic epidermal necrolysis (TEN) is a more serious manifestation of the same process which involves widespread areas of the skin with confluent bullae that can lead to loss of skin in massive sheets. Thirty-five cases of TEN have been reported in HIV-infected individuals.

Zidovudine may induce several different cutaneous complications. The most common reaction is hyperpigmentation of the nails. Blue to brown-black nail discoloration has been reported to occur in over 40% of patients[167,168]. It is more common in blacks and usually begins four to eight weeks after initiating treatment or may occur as late as one year. Longitudinal streaks are most common, but diffuse pigmentation and transverse bands may occur. The thumbnails are affected most frequently. Zidovudine may also induce hyperpigmentation of the mucous membranes and the skin that may mimic that seen with adrenal insufficiency[169,170]. In addition to pigmentary abnormalities, severe exanthematous eruptions may develop within one to two weeks following the initiation of zidovudine therapy. Lichenoid papular reactions may appear almost identical to lichen planus with whitish, lacy plaques of the mucous membranes as well as polygonal pink papules on flexural surfaces of glabrous skin[171]. Lichenoid eruptions due to zidovudine must be distinguished from true lichen planus. Zidovudine-induced nail pigmentation must be differentiated from other causes of pigmented bands in the nail plate such as junctional nevi and acrolentiginous melanoma. Other manifestations include acral and periarticular reticulate erythema that may simulate dermatomyositis[172].

The histopathology of the common form of morbilliform drug eruptions typically consists of a superficial perivascular inflammatory infiltrate of lymphocytes with scattered eosinophils associated with vacuolar alteration of the dermoepidermal junction and individually necrotic keratinocytes. The differential diagnosis of morbilliform drug eruptions includes other morbilliform eruptions such as those caused by viruses. In some cases, spongiosis is prominent. Slight parakeratosis may be noted and scattered plasma cells may be seen. Allergic drug eruptions may also clinically appear as erythema multiforme, Stevens–Johnson syndrome or toxic epidermal necrolysis and are all characterized by prominent vacuolar interface changes with extensive keratinocytic necrosis of the epidermis. In toxic epidermal necrolysis, the number of inflammatory cells in the dermis may be minimal although there is confluent epidermal necrosis with no parakeratosis, a consequence of the rapidity of progression of the eruption. Urticarial eruptions are usually characterized by mixed infiltrates of inflammatory cells interstitially in the dermis with minimal epidermal change.

Ulcerations caused by foscarnet used for herpesvirus infections may mimic fixed drug eruptions or ulcers of a number of other causes, including those caused by infectious agents such as HSV, CMV, and in some cases bacteria and fungi. Toxic epidermal necrolysis is generally characteristic but must be distinguished from staphylococcal scalded skin syndrome and toxic strep syndrome. Skin biopsy or frozen section evaluation of the roof of the blister will demonstrate confluent epithelial necrosis in erythema multiforme and sloughing of the stratum corneum in staphylococcal scalded skin syndrome.

The most important aspect of the treatment of a cutaneous drug eruption relates to the avoidance of serious complications that may arise if the diagnosis is not made in timely fashion and the offending agent is not withdrawn. The most serious cutaneous complication is the development of toxic epidermal necrolysis. Other complications include systemic toxicity such as hepatotoxicity or renal damage associated with the sulfone syndrome. Toxic epidermal necrolysis may lead to secondary infection with sepsis, volume depletion and high output cardiac failure as a consequence of widespread denudation of the skin. Patients who develop this must be treated aggressively in intensive care settings. Whether systemic corticosteroids should be used remains controversial.

Hypersensitivity to trimethoprim–sulfamethoxazole has been successfully treated with desensitization. Desensitization to other antibiotics may also be attempted when necessary[172].

Hair and Nail Abnormalities

A number of abnormalities of hair and nails may be encountered in patients with HIV disease. Chronic inflammatory and non-inflammatory alopecia has been observed. The hair may become lusterless and dull and, in patients with curly hair, straightening is often noted[141]. Biopsies of the scalp have shown histological features both of non-inflammatory telogen effluvium-like alopecia as well as dense inflammatory cell infiltrates containing lymphocytes,

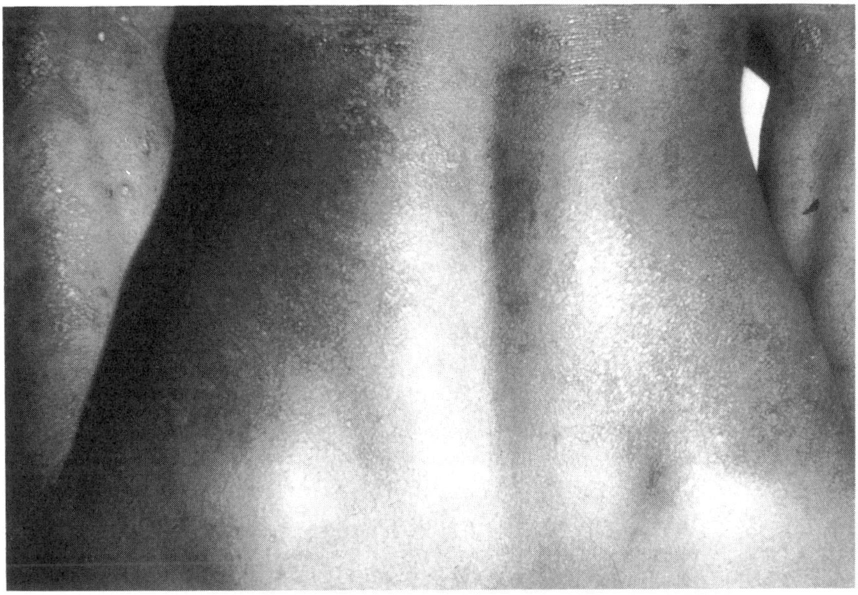

Figure 14.7 *Extensive xerosis associated with scaling, crusting and inflammation*

histiocytes and plasma cells with destruction of follicles[142]. Diffuse fine downy alopecia that may or may not be associated with scaling has also been observed, usually in patients with end-stage AIDS. Finally, patients with HIV infection may develop serious infections with high fevers leading to true telogen effluvium.

In addition to loss of scalp hair, there may be elongation of the eyelashes, a sign of a prolonged anagen phase. This condition has been termed trichomegaly of the eyelashes[143–145]. The cause of this phenomenon is unknown but in some cases it is associated with the administration of drugs such as recombinant interferon A. The frequency with which this problem develops is unclear but it has been reported in as many as 20% of HIV-infected patients in one study[143]. Other changes of the hair seen in HIV-infected patients include premature canities and alopecia areata[143].

Nail disorders commonly develop in patients with HIV infection. Patients receiving zidovudine may develop elongated pigmented grayish streaks of multiple nail plates, as mentioned previously. Nail plate thickening with subungual hyperkeratosis and dystrophy may be associated with fungal infections due to dermatophytes, *Candida* as well as *Scytalidium* spp. and other non-dermatophyte fungi. The yellow nail syndrome secondary to metabolic abnormalities, lymphedema and hypoxia has been reported to develop in HIV-infected patients as has transverse and longitudinal ridging[148,149]. Diminished thickness of the nail plate may also be seen. Increased nail plate opacity as well as both Muehrcke's and Terry's nails have been seen. Ridging and nail thickness changes are most likely a consequence of diminished matrix growth with decreased nail plate turnover. Just as in immunocompetent patients, Beau's lines may be seen two to three months after an episode of a serious infection. Involvement of the periungual tissues by infectious agents, psoriasis and erythema with features similar to Gottron's papules may also be seen.

NEOPLASTIC DISORDERS

Many different neoplasms of the skin are seen in HIV-infected individuals. As patients live for longer periods of time, the opportunity for these patients to develop these disorders will almost certainly increase. Thus, it is likely that this will become a major public health problem over the ensuing years.

As visceral and vascular neoplasms, specifically Kaposi's sarcoma, have been discussed elsewhere in this text, they will not be addressed in detail here.

Primary Cutaneous Neoplasms

The incidence of epithelial neoplasms in patients infected with HIV is markedly increased, most commonly in oral, cervical and anorectal locations. Bowenoid papulosis refers to squamous cell carcinoma *in situ* that develops as a consequence of infections with HPV types 16 and 18 most commonly. Lesions often have morphological features similar to condylomata acuminata and may be clinically confused with them. Generally, lesions are manifest as brownish flat-topped papules on the labia or penile skin. Lesions are often hyperpigmented but in some cases they clinically appear similar to condylomata acuminata. Rarely, brownish macules may be the only manifestation of the disease. Epidermodysplasia verruciformis, a premalignant condition associated with HPV infection, has a clinical appearance of widespread warty papules that are either pink or red. In some cases, diffuse erythematous pruritic areas of the skin may be seen[181]. Ultraviolet irradiation is a major risk factor for the development of carcinomata in patients with this condition. Biopsies are necessary to establish this diagnosis and demonstrate characteristic vacuolated HPV-infected cells in the epidermis. Basal cell carcinomas have been reported in HIV-seropositive patients, often on unexposed sites. Most have had clinical appearances similar to those seen in immunocompetent hosts although multiple primary nodular and/or superficial basal cell carcinomas may develop. In rare cases, metastases of basal cell carcinoma occur, probably as a consequence of immunocompromise[182]. Most metastases have been to draining lymph nodes and the lung.

Melanoma involving HIV-infected patients has also been observed sporadically. While no good data exists about the relative frequency of this neoplasm in these patients, multiple primary and 'early' nodular lesions have been noted. In at least one patient, a highly aggressive, fatal course ensued.

The histopathological findings of these conditions range from subtle atypical intraepithelial proliferations within stratified squamous epithelium that begin at the basal cell layer of full-thickness involvement of the epithelium by atypical neoplastic keratinocytes. Epithelial retia are expanded and replaced by atypical cells, many of which are strikingly pleomorphic and in mitosis. In time, bulbous aggregations of neoplastic cells extend from the epithelium into the underlying lamina propria and reticular dermis. Involvement of deeper soft tissues, nerves and blood vessels may develop in due course. Lesions are often digitated, verrucous and associated with prominent necrosis.

Bowenoid papulosis is manifested histologically by similar cytological features except that lesions have a histological architectural pattern similar to that of condyloma acuminatum. Epidermodysplasia verruciformis is characterized by a diffuse infiltrate of pale-appearing cells in the epidermis that represent koilocytes[52]. There is also dyskeratosis and characteristic 'corps rond-like' structures in the stratum corneum.

Squamous cell carcinoma may have clinical and histological features similar to pseudocarcinomatous hyperplasia including that induced by infectious agents. Giant HPV-induced verrucous carcinoma may have histological features similar to giant condylomata. These lesions are similar clinically to the Buschke–Lowenstein variant of verrucous carcinoma. Epidermodysplasia verruciformis may clinically simulate widespread warts or, in some cases, other forms of erythroderma or widespread erythematous scaly dermatoses. Basal cell carcinoma may mimic molluscum contagiosum as well as non-descript papular lesions of opportunistic infections.

Diagnosis is established primarily on the basis of clinical appearance and skin biopsy. Of interest, recent studies have evaluated the efficacy of exfoliative cytology in determining the presence of intraepithelial neoplasia of both the cervix and anal areas and have found a high rate of false negatives comparing this technique to colposcopically or sigmoidoscopically directed tissue biopsies[183].

Treatment of squamous cell carcinoma usually requires excision or aggressive destructive measures. Cryotherapy, generally used for the management of cervical intraepithelial neoplasia (CIN), has been shown in one study to have an overall efficacy of 25%, significantly below that observed in HIV-seronegative patients[184]. Carbon dioxide laser destruction may be more effective in this setting. Bowenoid papulosis, while generally treated with simple cryosurgical destruction or topical application of 5-fluorouracil, should be treated with either electrodesiccation and curettage or other destructive surgical measures with biopsy confirmation of removal rather than by conservative topical measures. Basal cell carcinoma also should be treated aggressively with destructive measures such as cryosurgery or excision as there is the potential for metastasis in HIV-infected immunocompromised hosts. Epidermodysplasia verruciformis may be refractory to all forms of therapy. Any neoplasms that develop should be destroyed or excised. Systemic administration of retinoids such as etretinate or 13-*cis*-retinoic acid at doses 1–2 mg/kg may be effective in preventing development of carcinomata.

Lymphoreticular Malignancies

Most cases of lymphoma in HIV-infected patients involve visceral sites. When the skin is affected by non-Hodgkin lymphoma, it is usually manifested as pink to purplish papules or nodules. Any site may be involved, including the head and neck, trunk and extremities. Deeply seated soft tissue involvement may expand superficially forming dome-shaped nodules that often ulcerate. Cutaneous Hodgkin's disease appears similar to non-Hodgkin lymphoma either as diffuse nodular lesions or as a 'panniculitis'. HIV-related cutaneous T-cell lymphoma may have a clinical appearance similar to mycosis fungoides manifest as widespread plaques that may progress to erythroderma[186]. HTLV-1-associated lymphoma may also resemble mycosis fungoides, although it may have a clinical picture of an acute viral exanthem with an eruption of morbilliform papules and small fine vesicles[188].

When the skin is involved by lymphoma, histologically there is generally a diffuse infiltrate of atypical lymphoid cells that are monomorphous in appearance. Many of the cells are large, pleomorphic, and in mitosis. The infiltrate tends to be deeply situated involving the lower portions of the dermis and subcutaneous fat and there is often extensive necrosis as well as obliteration of pre-existing adnexal structures. Hodgkin's disease involving the skin may have an appearance similar to an inflammatory infiltrate in the skin although the diffuse nature of the infiltrate as well as the presence of large, atypical cells having a Reed–Sternberg-like morphology generally aid in making the diagnosis. Cutaneous T-cell lymphoma is usually manifest histologically by psoriasiform hyperplasia of the epidermis with a band-like infiltrate of atypical lymphocytes, many having convoluted nuclei with a cerebriform appearance. These cells are also present in the epidermis, where they often form small collections. In some cases, minimal epidermotropism is noted but the atypical nature of the cells allows the diagnosis to be made. In cases of HTLV-1-associated lymphoma, neoplastic lymphocytes are often extremely large and multilobulated, having a 'clover leaf' appearance. There is also usually prominent exocytosis and, in that there is an associated leukemia, atypical lymphoid cells are often seen in blood vessels and lymphatics.

The routine diagnosis of these neoplasms is based on the characteristic clinical appearance taken in the context of histopathological features. In many cases, gene rearrangement studies, flow cytometric immunological analysis and the use of DNA probes are necessary to further characterize and subtype the neoplasm. Immunophenotyping of mycosis fungoides-like cutaneous T-cell lymphoma (CTCL) in HIV patients is usually characterized by an infiltrate of $CD8^+$ lymphocytes but may be comprised of monoclonal $CD4^+$ cells[187]. HTLV-1-associated leukemia/lymphoma is characterized by an infiltrate by $CD4^+$ cells with absent $CD2^+$ and $CD7^+$ antigens[189].

Treatment consists of the usual therapy for systemic lymphoma. Some of the regimens utilized include methotrexate, prednisone, bleomycin, adriamycin, cyclophosphamide and vincristine. Cutaneous T-cell lymphoma may respond to psoralen and ultraviolet A therapy, total body electron beam and topical nitrogen mustard. As expected, however, these lymphomas tend to be more aggressive than in patients who are immunocompetent, with survival generally between 5 and 10 months following diagnosis[190]. As patients are already immunocompromised, administration of many of these agents may cause profound immunocompromise with acceleration of death.

REFERENCES

1. Tindall B, Barker S, Donovan B *et al.* Characterization of the acute clinical illness associated with human immunodeficiency virus infection. *Arch Intern Med* 1988; 148: 945–949.
2. Sinicco A, Palestro G, Caramello P *et al.* Acute HIV-1 infection: clinical and biologic study of twelve patients. *J AIDS* 1990; 3: 260–265.
3. Kinlock S, de Saussure Ph, Vanhems Ph *et al.* Primary HIV infection: a prospective and retrospective study. Poster presentation, *VIIIth International Conference on AIDS*, Amsterdam, 19–24 July 1992.
4. Rabeneck L, Popovic M, Gartner S *et al.* Acute HIV infection presenting with painful swallowing and esophageal ulcers. *JAMA* 1990; 263: 2318–2322.
5. Shapiro P. Histologic findings in the acute exanthem of HIV infection. Poster presentation, *Meeting of the American Society of Dermatopathology*, February 1995, New Orleans, Louisiana.
6. McMillan A, Bishop PE, Aw D, Peutherer JF. Immunohistology of the skin rash associated with acute HIV infection. *AIDS* 1989; 3: 309–312.
7. Henderson DK, Gerberding JL. Prophylatic zidovudine after occupational exposure to the human immunodeficiency virus: an interim analysis. *J Infect Dis* 1989; 160: 321–323.
8. Looke DFM, Grove DI. Failed prophylactic zidovudine after needle-stick injury (Letter). *Lancet* 1990; 335: 1280.
9. Lange J, Boucher CAB, Hollack CEM *et al.* Failure of zidovudine prophylaxis after accidental exposure to HIV-1. *N Engl J Med* 1990; 322: 1375–1377.
10. Safran S, Ashley R, Houlihan C *et al.* Clinical and serologic features of herpes simplex virus infection in patients with AIDS. *AIDS* 1991; 5: 1107–1110.
11. Masur H. Clinical implications of herpes virus infections in patients with AIDS. *Am J Med* 1992; 92(2A): 1S-2S.

12. Siegal FP, Lopez C, Hammer GS *et al*. Severe acquired immunodeficiency in male homosexuals, manifested by chronic perianal ulcerative herpes simplex lesions. *N Engl J Med* 1981; 305: 1439–1444.
13. Friedman-Kien AE, LaFleur FL, Gendler EC *et al*. Herpes zoster: a possible early clinical sign for development of acquired immunodeficiency syndrome in high-risk individuals. *J Am Acad Dermatol* 1986; 14: 1023–1028.
14. Jura E, Chadwick EG, Josephs HS *et al*. Varicella zoster virus infections in children infected with human immunodeficiency virus. *Pediatr Infect Dis J* 1989; 8: 856–590.
15. Williamson BC. Disseminated herpes zoster in a human immunodeficiency virus-positive homosexual man without complications. *Cutis* 1987; 40: 45–46.
16. Gilson IH, Barnett JH, Conans MA *et al*. Disseminated ecthymatous varicella-zoster virus infection in patients with acquired immunodeficiency syndrome. *J Am Acad Dermatol* 1989; 20: 637–642.
17. Janier M, Hilion B, Baccard M *et al*. Chronic varicella zoster infection in acquired immunodeficiency syndrome (Letter). *J Am Acad Dermatol* 1988; 18: 584–585.
18. Cohen PR, Beltranny VP, Grossman ME. Disseminated herpes zoster in patients with immunodeficiency virus infection. *Am J Med* 1988; 84: 1076–1080.
19. Jacobson MA, Berger TG, Fikrig S *et al*. Acyclovir-resistant varicella zoster virus infection after chronic oral acyclovir therapy in patients with the acquired immunodeficiency syndrome (AIDS). *Ann Intern Med* 1990; 112: 187–191.
20. Worrell JT, Cockerell CJ. Histopathologic findings of cutaneous nerves in herpes simplex and varicella zoster virus infection (Abstract). American Society of Dermatopathology, 3 December 1992.
21. Smith KJ, Skelton HG, Angritt P. Histopathologic features of HIV-associated skin disease. *Dermatol Clin* 1991; 9: 551–578.
22. Hardy WD. Foscarnet treatment of acyclovir-resistant herpes simplex virus infection in patients with acquired immunodeficiency syndrome: preliminary results of a controlled, randomized, regimen-comparative trial. *Am J Med* 1992; 92: 30s–35s.
23. Chatis PA, Miller CH, Schrager LE *et al*. Successful treatment with foscarnet of an acyclovir-resistant mucocutaneous infection with herpes simplex virus in a patient with acquired immunodefieincy syndrome. *N Engl J Med* 1989; 320: 297–300.
24. Klatt EC, Shibata D. Cytomegalovirus infection in the acquired immunodeficiency syndrome. *Arch Pathol Lab Med* 1988; 112: 540–544.
25. Lin CS, Pinha PD, Krishnan MN *et al*. Cytomegalic inclusion disease of the skin. *Arch Dermatol* 1981; 117: 282–284.
26. Feldman PS, Walker AN, Baker R. Cutaneous lesions heralding disseminated cytomegalovirus infections. *J Am Acad Dermatol* 1982; 7: 545–548.
27. Muehler-Stamou A, Sen HJ, Emodi G. Epidermolysis in a case of severe cytomegalovirus infection. *Br Med J* 1974; 3: 609–611.
28. Minars N, Silverman JF, Escobar NR *et al*. Fatal cytomegalic inclusion disease: associated skin manifestations in a renal transplant patient. *Arch Dermatol* 1977; 113: 1569–1571.
29. Horn TD, Hood AF. Cytomegalovirus is predictably present in perineal ulcers from immunosuppressed patients. *Arch Dermatol* 1990; 126: 642–644.
30. Lee JY, Peel R. Concurrent cytomegalovirus and herpes simplex virus infections in skin biopsy specimens from two AIDS patients with fatal CMV infection. *Am J Dermatopathol* 1989; 11: 136–143.
31. Greenspan JS, Greenspan D, Lenette ET *et al*. Replication of Epstein–Barr virus within epithelial cells of oral 'hairy' leukoplakia and AIDS associated lesion. *N Engl J Med* 1985; 313: 1564–1571.

32. Greenspan D, Greenspan JS, Overby G *et al.* Risk factors for rapid progression from hairy leukoplakia to AIDS: a nested case–control study. *J AIDS* 1991; 4: 652–658.
33. Cockerell CJ. Mucocutaneous signs of AIDS other than Kaposi's sarcoma. In Friedman-Kien AE (ed.) *Color Atlas of AIDS*. Philadelphia: Saunders, 1989; p. 96.
34. Fowler CD, Reed KD, Brannon RB. Intranuclear inclusions correlate with the ultrastructural detection of herpes-type virions in oral hairy leukoplakia. *Am J Surg Pathol* 1989; 13: 114–119.
35. DeSouza YG, Greenspan D, Feltzen JR *et al.* Localization of Epstein–Barr virus DNA in the epithelial cells of oral hairy leukoplakia via *in situ* hybridization of tissue sac (Letter). *N Engl J Med* 1989; 320: 1559.
36. Kessler HA, Benson CA, Urbanksi P. Regression of oral hairy leukoplakia during treatment with azidothymidine. *Ann Intern Med* 1988; 148: 2496–2497.
37. Schofer H, Ochsendorf FR, Elm EB *et al.* Treatment of oral hairy leukoplakia in AIDS patients with vitamin A acid (topically) or acyclovir (systemically) (Letter). *Dermatologica* 1987; 174: 150–151.
38. Beutner KR, Becker TM, Stone KM. Epidemiology of HPV infections. *Dermatol Clin* 1991; 9: 211–218.
39. Mattes WL, Triana A, Shapiro R *et al.* Dermatologic findings associated with human immunodeficiency virus infection. *J Am Acad Dermatol* 1987; 17: 746–751.
40. Palefsky JM, Gonzales J, Greenblatt RM *et al.* Anal intraepithelial neoplasia and anal papillomavirus infection among homosexual males with group IV HIV disease. *JAMA* 1990; 263: 2911–2916.
41. Oreal JD. Natural history of genital warts. *Br J Vener Dis* 1971; 47: 1–13.
42. Dyson N, Hoelwy PM, Munger K, Harlow E. The human papillomavirus-16-E7 Oncoprotein is able to bind to the retina blastoma gene products. *Science* 1989; 243: 934–937.
43. Chardonnet Y, Viac J, Staqnet MJ. Cell mediated immunity to human papillomavirus. *Clin Dermatol* 1985; 3: 156–161.
44. Sillman FH, Sedliss A. Anogenital papillomavirus infection and neoplasia in immunodeficient women. *Obstet Gynecol Clin North Am* 1987; 14: 537–558.
45. Byrne MA, Taylor-Robinson D, Munday PE, Harris JR. The common occurrence of human papillomavirus in intraepithelial neoplasia in women infected by HIV. *AIDS* 1989; 3: 379–382.
46. Frazer JH, Medley G, Cratper RM. Association between anorectal dysplasia, human papillomavirus and immunodeficiency virus infection in homosexual men. *Lancet* 1986; ii: 657–660.
47. Doherty R, Tanskanen E, Churchill MJ, Deacon NJ. Interactions between human immunodeficiency virus and human papillomavirus. Poster presentation, *VIIIth International Conference on AIDS*, Amsterdam 19–24 July 1992.
48. Tornesello ML, Buonaguro FM, Galloway DA *et al.* HIV and HPV Interaction: transactivation of HPV long control region by HIV-*tat* protein. Poster presentation, *VIIIth International Conference on AIDS*, Amsterdam, 19–24 July, 1992.
49. Rütlinger R, Buchmann P. HPV 16-positive Bowenoid papulosis and squamous cell carcinoma in an HIV-positive man. *Dis Colon Rectum* 1989; 32: 1042–1045.
50. Rosemberg SK. Subclinical papilloviral infection of male genitalia. *Urology* 1985; 26: 552–557.
51. Campion MJ. Clinical manifestations and natural history of genital human papillomavirus infection. *Obstet Gynecol Clin North Am* 1987; 14: 363–388.
52. Berger TG, Sawchuk WS, Leonardi C *et al.* Epidermodysplasia verruciformis-associated papillomavirus infection complicating human immunodeficiency virus disease. *Br J Dermatol* 1991; 126: 79–83.
53. Grusendorf-Conen EI. Papillomavirus-induced tumors of the skin: cutaneous

warts in epidermodysplasia verruciformis. In Syrjanen K, Gisman L, Kist LG (eds) *Papillomaviruses in Human Disease*. Berlin: Springer-Verlag, 1987; pp. 158–181.
54. Melchers W, Van Den Brule A, Walboomers J *et al*. Increased detection rate of human papillomavirus in cervical scrapes by the polymerase chain reaction as compared to modified FISH and Southern blot analysis. *J Med Virol* 1989; 27: 329–335.
55. Stoeh GP, Peterson AL, Taylor WJ. Systemic complications of local podphyllin therapy. *Ann Intern Med* 1978; 89: 362–363.
56. Slater GE, Rumack BH, Peterson RG. Podopyllin poisoning: systemic toxicity following cutaneous application. *Obstet Gynecol* 1987; 52: 94–96.
57. Beutner KR, Conant M, Friedman-Kien AE *et al*. Patient-applied Podofilox for treatment of genital warts. *Lancet* 1989; i: 831–838.
58. Baggish MS. Improved laser techniques for the elimination of genital and extragenital warts. *Am J Obstet Gynecol* 1985; 153: 545–550.
59. Sawchuck WS, Weber RJ, Lowry DR *et al*. Infectious papillomavirus in the vapor of warts treated with carbon dioxide laser or electrocoagulation: detection and protection. *J Am Acad Dermatol* 1989; 21: 41–49.
60. Friedman-Kien AE, Eron LJ, Conant M *et al*. Natural interferon alfa for treatment of condylomata acuminata. *JAMA* 1988; 259: 533–538.
61. Katzman M, Carey JT, Elmets CA *et al*. Molluscum contagiosum and AIDS: clinical and immunologic details of two cases. *Br J Dermatol* 1987; 116: 131–138.
62. Fivenson DP, Weltman RE, Gibson SH. Giant molluscum contagiosum presenting as basal cell carcinoma in an AIDS patient (Letter). *J Am Acad Dermatol* 1988; 19: 912–914.
63. Ganesh R, Castle D, Gibbon D *et al*. Staphylococcal carriage in HIV infection. *Lancet* 1989; ii: 558.
64. Nichols SL, Balog K, Silverman M. Bacterial infection and AIDS: clinical pathologic correlations in a series of autopsy cases. *Am J Clin Pathol* 1989; 92: 787–790.
65. Pitrack DL, Pall AK, Back PA. Serious *Pseudomonas aeruginosa* infection complicating AIDS. Poster presentation, *IXth International Conference on AIDS*, Berlin, 6–12 June 1993.
66. Steinhart R, Reingold AL, Taylor F *et al*. Invasive *Haemophilus* influenza infections in men with HIV infection. *JAMA* 1992; 268: 3350–3352.
67. Patterson JW, Kitces EN, Neafie RC. Cutaneous botryomycosis in a patient with acquired immunodeficiency syndrome. *J Am Acad Dermatol* 1987; 16: 238–242.
68. Weitzner JM, Dhawan SS, Rosen LB, Reznick L. Successful treatment of botryomycosis in a patient with acquired immune deficiency syndrome. *J Am Acad Dermatol* 1989; 21: 1312–1314.
69. Patterson JW, Kitces EN, Neafie RC. Cutaneous botryomycosis in a patient with acquired immune deficiency syndrome. *J Am Acad Dermatol* 1987; 16: 238–242.
70. Janssen F, Zelinsky-Gurung A, Caumes E, Decazed JM. Group A streptococcal cellulitis–adenitis in a patient with the acquired immunodeficiency syndrome. *J Am Acad Dermatol* 1991; 24: 363–365.
71. el Baze P, Thyss A, Vinti H *et al*. A study of nineteen immunocompromised patients with extensive skin lesions caused by *Pseudomonas aeruginosa* with and without bacteremia. *Acta Derm Venereol* 1991; 71: 411–415.
72. Kielhofner M, Atmar RL, Hamill RF, Musher DM. Life-threatening *Pseudomonas aeruginosa* infections in patients with human immunodeficiency virus infection. *Clin Infect Dis* 1992; 14: 403–411.
73. Sangeorzan JA, Bradley SF, Kaufman CA. Cutaneous manifestation of *Pseudomonas* infection in the acquired immune deficiency syndrome. *Arch Dermatol* 1990; 126: 832–833.

74. Adal K, Cockerell CJ, Petrie WP. Bacillary angiomatosis: ten years later. *N Engl J Med* (In Press).
75. Cockerell CJ, LeBoit PE. Bacillary angiomatosis: a novel pseudoneoplastic, infectious vascular disorder. *J Am Acad Dermatol* 1990; 22: 501–519.
76. Cockerell CJ, Whitlow MA, Webster GF, Friedman-Kien AE. Epithelioid angiomatosis: a distinct vascular disorder in patients with acquired immunodeficiency syndrome or AIDS-related complex. *Lancet* 1987; 329: 654–656.
77. LeBoit PE, Berger TG, Egbert BM *et al*. Bacillary angiomatosis: the histopathology and differential diagnosis of a pseudoneoplastic infection in patients with human immunodeficiency virus disease. *Am J Surg Pathol* 1989; 13: 909–920.
78. Behren AL, Steinbach LS, LeBoit PE *et al*. Osteolytic lesions in bacillary angiomatosis in AIDS patients: a basis for radiologic differentiation from Kaposi's sarcoma. *Radiology* 1990; 177: 77–81.
79 Berger TG, Taparo JW, Kayman A *et al*. Bacillary (epithelioid) angiomatosis and concurrent Kaposi's sarcoma in acquired immunodeficiency syndrome. *Arch Dermatol* 1989; 125: 1543–1547.
80. Schwartzman WA, Marchevski A, Meyer RD. Epithelioid angiomatosis or cat-scratch disease with splenic and hepatic abnormalities in AIDS: case report or review of the literature. *Scand J Infect Dis* 1990; 22: 121–133.
81. Knobler EH, Silvers DN, Fein KC *et al*. Unique vascular skin lesions associated with human immunodeficiency virus. *JAMA* 1988; 260: 524–527.
82. Tim Berger. Personal Communication, 1995.
83. Barbaro DJ, Orcutt VL, Colder BM. *Mycobacterium avium–intracellulare* infection limited to the skin and lymph nodes in patients with AIDS. *Rev Infect Dis* 1989; 11: 625–628.
84. Rogers PL, Walker RE, Wayne HC *et al*. Disseminated *Mycobacterium haemophilum* infection in two patients with AIDS. *Am J Med* 1988; 84: 640–642.
85. Rohatgi PK, Palazzolo JV, Saini NB. Acute miliary tuberculosis of the skin in acquired immunodeficiency syndrome. *J Am Acad Dermatol* 1992; 26: 285–287.
86. Boudes P, Sobel A, Deforges L *et al*. Disseminated *Mycobacterium bovis* infection from BCG vaccination and HIV infection (Letter). *JAMA* 1989; 262: 2386.
87. Roth C, Theodore C, Aitkin C *et al*. Presumed disseminated *Mycobacterium tuberculosis* infection presenting with cutaneous lesions in a patient with AIDS. Abstract, *VIIIth International Conference on AIDS*, Amsterdam, 19–24 July 1992.
88. Rogers PL, Walker RE, Lane HC *et al*. Disseminated *Mycobacterium haemophilum* infection in two patients with AIDS. *Am J Med* 1988; 84: 640–642.
89. Piketty C, Lons Danic D, Weiss L *et al*. Atypical sporotrichosis-like infection caused by *Mycobacterium avium* in AIDS. Abstract, *VIIth International Conference on AIDS*, Amsterdam, 19–24 July 1992.
90. Quinn TC, Cannon RO, Glasser D *et al*. The association of syphilis with risk of human immunodeficiency virus infection in patients attending sexually transmitted disease clinics. *Arch Intern Med* 1990; 159: 1297–1302.
91. Gregory N, Sanchez M, Buchness MR. The spectrum of syphilis in patients with human immunodeficiency virus infection. *J Am Acad Dermatol* 1990; 22: 1061–1067.
92. Glover RA, Piaquadio DJ, Kern S, Cockerell CJ. An unusual presentation of secondary syphilis in a patient with human immunodeficiency virus infection: a case report and review of the literature. *Arch Dermatol* 1992; 128: 530–534.
93. Ficarra G, Zaragoza AM, Stendardi L *et al*. Early oral presentation of lues maligna in a patient with HIV infection: a case report. *Oral Surg Oral Med Oral Pathol* 1993; 75: 728–732.
94. Johns DR, Tierney M, Felsenstein D. Alteration of the natural history of neuro-

syphilis by concurrent infection with the human immunodeficiency virus. *N Engl J Med* 1987; 316: 1569–1572.

95. Gherman CR, Ward RR, Bassis ML. *Pneumocystis carinii* otitis media and mastoiditis as the initial manifestation of the acquired immunodeficiency syndrome. *Am J Med* 1991; 127: 250–252.
96. Hennessey NP, Parro EL, Cockerell CJ. Cutaneous *Pneumocystis carinii* infection in patients with acquired immunodeficiency syndrome. *Arch Dermatol* 1991; 127: 1699–1701.
97. Litwin MA, Williams CM. Cutaneous *Pneumocystis carinii* infection mimicking Kaposi's sarcoma. *Ann Intern Med* 1992; 117: 48–49.
98. Hirschmann JV, Chu AC. Skin lesions with disseminated toxoplasmosis in a patient with the acquired immunodeficiency syndrome. *Arch Dermatol* 1988; 124: 1446–1447.
99. Portnoy BL, Micheletti GA. Acanthamoeba infection of skin and sinuses in an AIDS patient: diagnosis and treatment. (Abstract), *VIIIth International Conference on AIDS*, Amsterdam, 19–24 July 1992.
100. Glezerov V, Masci JR. Disseminated strongyloidiasis and other selected unusual infections in patients with acquired immunodeficiency syndrome. *Prog AIDS Pathol* 1990; 2: 137–142.
101. Insera DW, Bickley LK. Crusted scabies in acquired immunodeficiency syndrome. *Int J Dermatol* 1990; 29: 287–289.
102. Raur C, Baird IM. Crusted scabies in a patient with acquired immunodeficiency syndrome (Letter). *J Am Acad Dermatol* 1986; 15: 1058–1059.
103. Jucowics P, Ramon ME, Donn PC *et al.* Norwegian scabies in an infant with acquired immunodeficiency syndrome. *Arch Dermatol* 1989; 125: 1670–1671.
104. Skinner SM, DeVillez RL. Sepsis associated with Norwegian scabies in patients with acquired immunodeficiency syndrome. *Arch Dermatol* 1992; 50: 213–216.
105. O'Donnell BF, O'Loughlin S, Powell FC. Management of crusted scabies. *Int J Dermatol* 1990; 29: 258–266.
106. Klein RS, Harris CA, Small CB *et al.* Oral candidiasis in high-risk patients as the initial manifestation of the acquired immunodeficiency syndrome. *N Eng J Med* 1984; 311: 354–358.
107. Wolf JE, Little JR, Pappagianis D, Kobayashi GS. Disseminated coccidioidomycosis in a patient with the acquired immune deficiency syndrome. *Diag Microbiol Infect Dis* 1986; 5: 331–336.
108. Prichard JG, Sorotzkin RA, James RE III. Cutaneous manifestations of disseminated coccidioidomycosis in the acquired immunodeficiency syndrome. *Cutis* 1987; 39: 203–205.
109. Fish DG, Ampel NM, Galgiani JN *et al.* Coccidioidomycosis during human immunodeficiency virus infection: a review of 77 patients. *Medicine* 1990; 69: 384–391.
110. Manrique P, Mayo J, Alvarez JA *et al.* Polymorphous cutaneous cryptococcosis: nodular, herpes-like, and molluscum-like lesions in a patient with the acquired immunodeficiency syndrome. *J Am Acad Dermatol* 1992; 26: 122–124.
111. Cusini M, Cagliani P, Grimalt R *et al.* Primary cutaneous cryptococcosis in a patient with the acquired immunodeficiency syndrome (Letter). *Arch Dermatol* 1991; 127: 1848–1849.
112. Jones C, Orengo I, Rosen T, Ellner K. Cutaneous cryptococcosis simulating Kaposi's sarcoma in the acquired immunodeficiency syndrome. *Cutis* 1990; 45: 163–167.
113. Lynch DP, Naftolin LZ. Oral *Cryptococcus neoformans* infection in AIDS. *Oral Surg Oral Med Oral Pathol* 1987; 64: 449–453.

114. Rico NJ, Penneys NS. Cutaneous cryptococcosis resembling molluscum contagiosum in a patient with AIDS. *Arch Dermatol* 1985; 121: 901–902.
115. Mares M, Sartori MT, Carretta M *et al.* Rhinophyma-like cryptococcal infection as an early manifestation of AIDS in a hemophilia B patient. *Acta Haematol* 1990; 84: 101–103.
116. Cohen PR, Grossman ME, Silvers DN. Disseminated histoplasmosis and human immunodeficiency virus infection. *Int J Dermatol* 1991; 30: 614–622.
117. Hazelhurst JA, Vismer JF. Histoplasmosis presenting with unusual skin lesions in acquired immunodeficiency syndrome (AIDS). *Br J Dermatol* 1985; 113: 345–348.
118. Kalter DC, Tschen JA, Klima M. Maculopapular rash in a patient with acquired immunodeficiency syndrome. *Arch Dermatol* 1985; 121: 1455–1456.
119. Lindgren AM, Fallon JD, Horan RF. Psoriasiform papules in the acquired immunodeficiency syndrome: disseminated histoplasmosis in AIDS. *Arch Dermatol* 1991; 127: 722–723, 725–726.
120. Chaker MB, Cockerell CJ. Concomitant psoriasis, seborrheic dermatitis and disseminated cutaneous histoplasmosis in a patient infected with human immunodeficiency virus. *J Am Acad Dermatol* 1993; 29: 311–313.
121. Cole MC, Cohen PR, Satra KH, Grossman ME. The concurrent presence of systemic disease pathogens and cutaneous Kaposi's sarcoma in the same lesion: *Histoplasma capsulatum* and Kaposi's sarcoma coexisting in a single skin lesion in a patient with AIDS. *J Am Acad Dermatol* 1992; 26: 285–287.
122. Lipstein-Kresch E, Isenberg HD, Singer C *et al.* Disseminated *Sporothrix schenckii* infection with arthritis in a patient with acquired immunodeficiency syndrome. *J Rheum* 1985; 12: 805–808.
123. Shaw JC, Levinson W, Montanara A. Sporotrichosis in the acquired immunodeficiency syndrome. *J Am Acad Dermatol* 1989; 21: 1145–1147.
124. Fitzpatrick JE, Eubanks S. Acquired immunodeficiency syndrome presenting as disseminated cutaneous sporotrichosis. *Int J Dermatol* 1988; 27: 406–407.
125. Bibler MR, Luber HJ, Glueck HI, Estes SA. Disseminated sporotrichosis in a patient with HIV infection after treatment for acquired factor VIII inhibitor. *JAMA* 1986; 256: 3125–3126.
126. Terrell CL, Hughes CE. Antifungal agents used for deep-seated mycotic infections. *Mayo Clin Proc* 1992; 67: 69–91.
127. Mathes BM, Douglass MC. Seborrheic dermatitis in patients with acquired immunodeficiency syndrome. *J Am Acad Dermatol* 1985; 13: 947–951.
128. Duvic M, Johnson TM, Rapini RP *et al.* Acquired immunodeficiency syndrome-associated psoriasis and Reiter's syndrome. *Arch Dermatol* 1987; 123: 1622–1623.
129. Kaplan MH, Sadik NS, Weider J *et al.* Antiposoriatic effects of zidovudine in human immunodeficiency virus associated psoriasis. *J Am Acad Dermatol* 1989; 20: 76–82.
130. Kaye BR. Rheumatologic manifestations of infection with human immunodeficiency virus (HIV). *Am Intern Med* 1989; 111: 158–167.
131. Herman LE, Curbin AK. Erythroderma as a manifestation of the AIDS-related complex. *J Am Acad Dermatol* 1987; 17: 507–508.
132. Rao BK, Cockerell CJ. Histologic findings in inflammatory dermatoses in a patient with HIV infection. Poster presentation, *VIIth International Conference on AIDS*, Florence, Italy, 1991.
133. Auerbach R. Personal communication, 1993.
134. Soeprono FF, Schinella RA. Eosinophilic pustular folliculitis in patients with acquired immunodeficiency syndrome. *J Am Acad Dermatol* 1986; 14: 1020–1022.

135. Rosenthal D, LeBoit PE, Klumpp L, Berger TG. Human immunodeficiency virus-associated eosinophilic folliculitis: a unique dermatitis associated with advanced human immunodeficiency infection. *Arch Dermatol* 1991; 127: 206–209.
136. Buchness MR, Lim HW, Hatcher VA *et al.* Eosinophilic pustular folliculitis in the acquired immunodeficiency syndrome. *N Engl J Med* 1988; 318: 1183–1186.
137. Sadik NS, McNutt NS. Cutaneous hypersensitivity reactions in patients with AIDS. *Int J Dermatol* 1993; 32: 621–627.
138. Miadonna A, Zeger E, Tedeschi A *et al.* Enhanced basophil releasability in subjects infected with human immunodeficiency virus. *Clin Immunol Immunopathol* 1990; 54: 237–246.
139. Tateno M, Gonzales-Scarano F, Levy JA. Human immunodeficiency virus type 1 can infect CD-4 negative human fibroblastoid cells. *Proc Natl Acad Sci* 1989; 11: 4287–4290.
140. Leonidas JR. Hair alteration in black patients with acquired immunodeficiency syndrome. *Cutis* 1987; 39: 537–538.
141. Cockerell CJ. Personal observation, 1993.
142. Casanova JM, Puig T, Rubio M. Hypertrichosis of the eyelashes in acquired immunodeficiency syndrome. *Arch Dermatol* 1987; 123: 1599–1601.
143. Foon KA, Dougher G. Increased growth of eyelashes in a patient given leukocyte A interferon (Letter). *N Engl J Med* 1984; 311: 1259.
144. Kaplan MH, Sadik NS, Talmor M. Acquired trichomegaly of the eyelashes: a cutaneous marker of acquired immunodeficiency syndrome. *J Am Acad Dermatol* 1991; 25: 801–804.
145. Schonwetter RS, Nelson EB. Alopecia areata and the acquired immunodeficiency syndrome related complex (Letter). *Ann Intern Med* 1986; 104: 287.
146. Sadick NS. Clinical and laboratory evaluation of AIDS trichopathy. *Int J Dermatol* 1993; 32: 33–38.
147. Chernosky ME, Findley VK. Yellow-nail syndrome in patients with AIDS. *J Am Acad Dermatol* 1985; 13: 731–737.
148. Scher RK. Acquired immunodeficiency syndrome and yellow nails. *J Am Acad Dermatol* 1988; 18: 758–759.
149. Valerie K, Delers A, Bruck C *et al.* Activation of human immunodeficiency virus type 1 by DNA damage in human cells. *Nature* 1988; 333: 78–81.
150. Meola T, Soter NA, Ostrecher R *et al.* The safety of UVB phototherapy in patients with HIV infection. *J Am Acad Dermatol* 1993; 29: 216–220.
151. King DA, Ion D, Berger TG, Conant M. Itraconazole for treatment in HIV-associated eosinophilic folliculitis. Poster presentation, *IXth International Conference on AIDS*, Berlin, Germany, 6–12 June, 1993.
152. Toback AC, Longley J, Cardello AC *et al.* Severe chronic photosensitivy in association with acquired immunodeficiency syndrome. *Arch Dermatol* 1986; 15: 2056–2057.
153. Tojo N, Yoshimura N, Yoshizawa M *et al.* Vitiligo and chronic photosensitivity in human immunodeficiency virus infection. *Jpn J Med* 1991; 30: 255–259.
154. Lobato MN, Berger TG. Porphyria cutanea tarda associated with the acquired immunodeficiency syndrome. *Arch Dermatol* 1988; 124: 1009–1010.
155. Herranz MT, el Amrani A, Aranegui P *et al.* Porphyria cutanea tarda and acquired immunodeficiency syndrome: pathogenetic mechanisms. *Arch Dermatol* 1991; 12: 1585–1586.
156. Picard C, Crickx B, Fegueuz S *et al.* Porphyria cutanea tarda in HIV infection. Poster presentation, *VIIth International Conference on AIDS*, Florence, Italy, 16–21 June, 1991.

157. Egbert BM, LeBoit PE, McCalmont T *et al.* Caterpillar bodies: distinctive basement membrane-containing structures in blisters of porphyria. *Am J Dermatopathol* 1993; 15: 199–202.
158. Cockerell CJ. Successful treatment of HIV-related porphyria cutanea tarda with low-dose oral hydroxychloroquine. Submitted for publication.
159. Anderson KE, Goeger DE, Carson RW *et al.* Erythropoietin for the treatment of porphyria cutanea tarda in a patient on long-term haemodialysis. *N Engl J Med* 1990; 322: 315–317.
160. Coopman SA, Johnson RA, Platt R, Stern RS. Cutaneous disease and drug reactions in HIV infection. *N Engl J Med* 1993; 328: 1670–1674.
161. Gordin FM, Simon GL, Wofsy CD, Mills J. Adverse reactions to trimethoprim sulfamethoxazole in patients with the acquired immunodeficiency syndrome. *Ann Intern Med* 1984; 100: 495–499.
162. Raviglione MC, Dinan WA, Pablo-Mendez A *et al.* Fatal toxic epidermal necrolysis during prophylaxis with pyrimethamine and sulfadoxine in a human immunodeficiency virus-infected person. *Arch Intern Med* 1988; 148: 2683–2685.
163. Nunn P, Wasunna K, Kwanyah G *et al.* Cutaneous hypersensitivity reactions to thiacetazone among HIV-1 seropositive tuberculosis patients in Nairobi. Poster presentation, *VIIth International Conference on AIDS*, Florence, Italy, 16–21 June 1992.
164. Snyder DE, Graczyk J, Beck E *et al.* Supervised six-month treatment of newly diagnosed pulmonary tuberculosis using isoniazid, rifampin and pyrazinamide with and without streptomycin. *Am Rev Respir Dis* 1984; 130: 190–194.
165. Battegay M, Opravil M, Wuthrich B *et al.* Rash with amoxicillin–clavulanate therapy in HIV-infected patients (Letter), *Lancet* 1989; ii: 1100.
166. Donn PC, Fusco F, Fried P *et al.* Nail dyschromia associated with zidovudine. *Ann Intern Med* 1990; 112: 145–146.
167. Furth PA, Kazakis AM. Nail pigmentation changes associated with azidothymidine (zidovudine). *Ann Intern Med* 1987; 107: 350.
168. Greenberg RG, Berger TG. Nail and mucocutaneous hyperpigmentation with azidothymidine therapy. *J Am Acad Dermatol* 1990; 327: 330.
169. Merenich JA, Hannen RN, Gentry RH *et al.* Azidothymidine-induced hyperpigmentation mimicking primary adrenal insufficiency. *Am J Med* 1989; 86: 469–470.
170. Gaglioti D, Ficarra G, Adler-Storthz K *et al.* Zidovudine-related oral lichenoid reactions. Poster presentation, *VIIth International Conference on AIDS*, Florence, Italy, 16–21 June 1991.
171. Bessen LJ, Greene JB, Louis E *et al.* Severe polymyositis-like syndrome associated with zidovudine or AIDS or ARC (Letter). *N Engl J Med* 1988; 311: 708.
172. Feingold I. Oral desensitization of trimethoprim-sulfamethoxasole in a patient with acquired immunodeficiency syndrome (Letter). *J Allergy Clin Immunol* 1986; 78: 905.
173. Nelson AM, Mvula M, St Louis M *et al.* Increased rates of cervical dysplasia associated with clinical and immunological evidence of immunodeficiency. Poster presentation, *VIIIth International Conference on AIDS*, Amsterdam, 19–24 July 1992.
174. Galfetti M, Irion O, Beguin F. Vulvar and cervical pathologies in HIV-seropositive (HIV+) women followed in a colposcopy outpatient clinic (Abstract, Vol. II), *VIth International Conference on AIDS*, San Francisco, California, 20–24 June 1990; p. 337.
175. Palefsky JM, Gonzales J, Greenblatt RM *et al.* Anal intraepithelial neoplasia and anal papillomavirus infection among homosexual males with group IV HIV disease. *JAMA* 1990; 263: 2911–2916.

176. Beck DE, Jaso RF, Zajac RA. Surgical management of anal condylomata in the HIV-positive patient. *Dis Colon Rectum* 1990; 33: 180–183.
177. Marte C, Cohen M, Fruchter R *et al.* Pap test and STD findings in HIV positive women at ambulatory care sites (Abstract Vol. I), *VIth International Conference on AIDS*, San Francisco, California, 20–24 June 1990; p. 211.
178. Goedert JJ, Caussy D, Palefsky J *et al.* Interaction of HIV and papillomaviruses: association with anal intraepithelial abnormality in homosexual men (Abstract, Vol. I), *VIth International Conference on AIDS*, San Francisco, California, 20–24 June 1990; p. 201.
179. Yabe Y, Tanimura Y, Sakai A. Molecular characteristics and physical state of human papillomavirus DNA change with progressing malignancy: studies in a patient with epidermodysplasia verruciformis. *Int J Cancer* 1989; 43: 1022–1028.
180. Pandya AG and Cockerell CJ. Personal observation, 1993.
181. Sitz KV, Keppen M. Metastatic basal cell carcinoma in acquired immunodeficiency syndrome-related complex. *JAMA* 1987; 257: 340–343.
182. Fink MJ, Fretcher R, Mamand M *et al.* Cytology, colposcopy and histology in HIV-positive women. Poster presentation, *IXth International Conference on AIDS*, Berlin, Germany, 6–12 June 1993.
183. Guinness K, LaGuardia K. Cryotherapy in the management of cervical dysplasia in HIV-infected women. Poster presentation, *IXth International Conference on AIDS*, Berlin, Germany, 6–12 June 1993.
184. Chadbourne A, Metroka C, Nmuradian J. Progressive lymph node histology and its prognostic value in patients with acquired immunodeficiency syndrome and AIDS-related complex. *Hum Pathol* 1989; 20: 579–587.
185. Bernheim A, Berger R. Cytogenic studies of Burkitt's lymphoma/leukemia in patients with acquired immunodeficiency syndrome. *Cancer Genet Cytogenet* 1988; 32: 67–74.
186. Parker SC, Fenton DA, McGibbon DH. L'homme rouge and the acquired immunodeficiency syndrome. *N Engl J Med* 1989; 321: 906–907.
187. Kobayashi M, Yoshimoto S, Fujishita M *et al.* HTLV-positive T-cell lymphoma/leukemia in an AIDS patient. *Lancet* 1984; i: 1361–1362.
188. Nagatani T, Miyazawa T, Matsuzaki T *et al.* Adult T-cell leukemia/lymphoma (ATL): clinical, histopathological, immunological and immunohistochemical characteristics. *Exp Dermatol* 1992; 1: 248–252.
189. Knowles DM, Chamulak G, Subar M *et al.* Clinical pathologic immunophenotypic and molecular genetic analysis of AIDS-associated lymphoid neoplasia: clinical and biologic implications. *Pathol Ann* 1988; 23: 33–67.
190. Scherr GR, Evans SG, Kiyabu MT, Klatt EC. *Pseudallescheria boydii* in the acquired immunodeficiency syndrome. *Arch Pathol Lab Med* 1992; 116: 535–536.
191. Hevia O, Kligman D, Penneys NS. Non-scalp hair infection caused by *Microsporum canis* in a patient with acquired immunodeficiency syndrome. *J Am Acad Dermatol* 1991; 24: 789–790.
192. Sachot LJ, Hadderingh RJ, Devriese PP. Facial palsy and HIV infection (Abstract), *VIIIth International Conference on AIDS*, Amsterdam, 19–24 July 1992.
193. Sanchez MR, Ponge-Wilson I, Moy JA. Zygomycosis and HIV infection. *J Am Acad Dermatol* 1994; 30: 904–908.
194. Liu MT, Wong CK, Fung CP. Disseminated *Penicillium marneffei* infection with cutaneous lesions in an HIV-positive patient. *Br J Dermatol* 1994; 131: 280–283.
195. Borradori L, Schmit JC, Stetzkowski M *et al.* *Penicilliosis marneffei* infection in AIDS. *J Am Acad Dermatol* 1994; 31: 843–846.
196. Fraser VJ, Keath EJ, Powderly WG. Two cases of blastomycosis from a common

source: use of DNA restriction analysis to identify strains. *J Infect Dis* 1991; 163: 1378–1381.
197. Wood GM, McCormack JG, Muir DB *et al*. Clinical features of human infection with *Scedosporium inflatum*. *Clin Infect Dis* 1992; 14: 1027–1033.

15

Critical Care of AIDS Patients: Clinical and Ethical Problems

Robert M. Wachter and John M. Luce

San Francisco General Hospital, Medical Center and University of California, San Francisco, California, USA

INTRODUCTION

Despite the availability and effectiveness of prophylactic regimens to prevent *Pneumocystis carinii* pneumonia (PCP), this infection remains the most common index diagnosis and cause of mortality among patients with the acquired immunodeficiency syndrome (AIDS). Since most patients who die of PCP generally succumb to severe respiratory failure, questions related to the use of intensive care for PCP have been debated since the start of the AIDS epidemic.

In this chapter, we will review the outcome of critical care for patients with AIDS, PCP, and respiratory failure, the predictors of mortality in such patients, and some of the ethical issues that arise in decision-making about life-sustaining treatments in AIDS.

It should be stated that AIDS patients may require intensive care for a wide variety of indications beyond PCP[1]. However, there is little recent data concerning the outcome of such patients, and thus we will concentrate on PCP and respiratory failure, the most common indication for the use of the intensive care unit (ICU) in patients with AIDS.

AIDS and Malignancies: Current Concepts and Perspectives.
Edited by B.C. Golematis and V.T. DeVita Jr

OUTCOMES OF INTENSIVE CARE

We have defined three eras in describing the outcomes of ICU care for patients with AIDS, PCP, and severe respiratory failure. In era I (1981–1985), a number of studies[2–8] demonstrated a survival rate to hospital discharge of approximately 10%. Not surprisingly, once patients and physicians learned of this data, the use of the intensive care unit fell precipitously[7].

Over the following few years, more than a dozen studies were published which demonstrated a marked improvement in survival rates for patients with AIDS, PCP, and respiratory failure[9–22]. The reasons for the improved survival rate of approximately 40% in era II (1986–1988) were not completely defined by these studies, but the adjuvant use of corticosteroids seemed to play an important role. As patients and physicians learned of the improved outcomes, ICU utilization rose in the USA[13].

Recently, there have been indications that we have entered a third era, in which the outcome of ICU care for patients with PCP and respiratory failure has once again deteriorated. At San Francisco General Hospital, for example, the survival rate for such patients fell from 39% in 1986–1988 to 24% in 1989–1991. Similarly poor outcomes were seen in recent studies from Paris[23] and Vancouver[24]. We have been unable to fully define the reasons for the declining survival rate in era III, since patients appeared to be no more ill at the time of ICU admission in recent years than in the previous era. We suspect that the reason has to do with the availability of effective prophylaxis for PCP, as well as effective adjuvant therapy for severe PCP in the form of corticosteroids. Today, the need for mechanical ventilation generally implies that an HIV-infected person failed (or failed to receive) PCP prophylaxis, and then failed (or failed to receive) corticosteroids in addition to anti-*Pneumocystis* antibiotics. The declining survival rate in era III may be due to the fact that patients who slip through these multiple pharmacological safety nets are members of a cohort destined to do poorly.

PREDICTORS OF ICU MORTALITY

A number of studies have looked for factors that might predict which patients would or would not survive their stay in the ICU for severe PCP. In our most recent study from San Francisco General Hospital (R.M. Wachter, unpublished data), we found that having a low CD4 cell count was the strongest predictor of hospital mortality. Specifically, only one of the 18 patients with a CD4 count of less than 50 left the hospital alive, while seven of nine patients with CD4 counts greater than 50 survived their hospitalization. The other strong predictor of mortality at our hospital in recent years has been the development of a pneumothorax while on mechanical ventilation. In our experience between 1986 and 1991, none of the 16 patients who suffered this complication survived to hospital discharge.

A number of other studies have analyzed predictors of ICU mortality for patients with AIDS, PCP, and severe respiratory failure requiring mechanical ventilation. Based on our analysis of these studies, we presently cite an average hospital survival rate of about 10–25% for such patients. We would be inclined to be even more pessimistic when counseling a patient with a CD4 count below 50 (as noted above), a serum albumin below 2.0[13], a lactate dehydrogenase above 1000[20], a pH below 7.35[21], multisystem organ failure[20], or failure of at least five days of anti-*Pneumocystis* therapy and corticosteroids[23]. Once a patient is in the ICU, we believe that the development of pneumothorax (as noted above) or a stay of more than two weeks in the ICU on mechanical ventilation bespeak a poor prognosis.

ETHICAL ISSUES IN CRITICAL CARE FOR AIDS PATIENTS

We believe that the decisions of informed, competent patients or their designated proxies regarding the use of life-sustaining treatments should be respected. In our experience, many such patients or proxies, when informed of the poor outcomes expected with the use of the ICU for PCP and respiratory failure, choose to forego critical care. This is especially true when one or more of the negative prognostic variables are present and when compassionate comfort care is readily available.

There is general agreement that patients need not be offered care that is futile. However, given the small numbers of AIDS patients receiving critical care at any one site, it has been difficult to define a subgroup of patients for whom the prognosis is truly futile[25]. For example, even though none of our 16 patients who developed a pneumothorax in the ICU between 1986–1991 survived, the upper bound of the 95% confidence interval for the true survival rate after this complication is 19%. As if to highlight this uncertainty, we recently saw a patient who did survive such a complication after an ICU stay of more than a month.

We recently examined the cost-effectiveness of intensive care for patients with PCP and respiratory failure. At our hospital, the cost per year of life saved rose from $95 000 (US) in 1986–1988 to $215 000 in 1989–1991 (R.M. Wachter, unpublished data). Whether and how this sort of information should be integrated into clinical decision-making represents one of the most vexing challenges in medicine and health policy. At the present time, our practice is to encourage HIV-infected patients to complete advance directives, designating someone to make decisions for them should they lose competence and indicating their preferences regarding the use of life-sustaining treatment. We then offer intensive care to virtually all of our patients with PCP and respiratory failure, provide patients or their proxies with sufficient prognostic information to make informed choices, and respect these choices. However, with the cost of American health care now topping one trillion dollars each year, it is possible—perhaps likely—that society will ultimately choose to limit the availability of expensive, low-yield technology such as the use of the ICU for patients with severe PCP.

REFERENCES

1. Wachter RM, Luce JM, Hopewell PC. Critical care of patients with AIDS. *JAMA* 1992; 267: 541–547.
2. Murray JF, Felton CP, Garay SM *et al.* Pulmonary complications of the acquired immunodeficiency syndrome. *N Engl J Med* 1984; 310: 1682–1688.
3. Stover DE, White DA, Romano PA *et al.* Spectrum of pulmonary diseases associated with the acquired immune deficiency syndrome. *Am J Med* 1985; 78: 429–437.
4. Schein RM, Fischl MA, Pitchenik AE, Sprung CL. ICU survival of patients with the acquired immunodeficiency syndrome. *Crit Care Med* 1986; 14: 1026–1027.
5. Rosen MJ, Cucco RA, Teirstein AS. Outcome of intensive care in patients with the acquired immunodeficiency syndrome. *J Intensive Care Med* 1986; 1: 55–60.
6. Garay S. Respiratory failure in AIDS. *Am Rev Respir Dis* 1986; 133: A344.
7. Wachter RM, Luce JM, Turner J *et al.* Intensive care of patients with the acquired immunodeficiency syndrome: outcome and changing patterns of utilization. *Am Rev Respir Dis* 1986; 134: 891–896.
8. Baggott LA, Baggott BB. *Pneumocystis carinii* pneumonia in AIDS patients in intensive care. *Chest* 1987; 92: 132S.
9. Bennett RL, Gilman SC, George L *et al.* Improved outcomes in intensive care units in AIDS-related *Penumocystis carinii* pneumonia: 1987–1991. *J AIDS* 1993; 6: 1319–1321.
10. Curtis JR, Greenberg DL, Fisher LD *et al.* Trends in survival rates and intubation rates for HIV-infected patients with pneumocystis pneumonia. *Am Rev Respir Dis* 1993; 147: A1002.
11. Friedman Y, Franklin C, Freels S, Weil MH. Long-term survival of patients with AIDS, *Pneumocystis carinii* pneumonia, and respiratory failure. *JAMA* 1991; 226: 89–92.
12. Rogers PL, Lane HC, Henderson DK *et al.* Admission of AIDs patients to a medical intensive care unit: causes and outcome. *Crit Care Med* 1989; 17: 113–117.
13. Wachter RM, Russi MB, Hopewell PC, Luce JM. *Pneumocystis carinii* pneumonia and respiratory failure in AIDS: improved outcomes and increased use of intensive care units. *Am Rev Respir Dis* 1991; 143: 251–256.
14. El-Sadr W, Simberkoff MS. Survival and prognostic factors in severe *Pneumocystis carinii* pneumonia requiring mechanical ventilation. *Am Rev Respir Dis* 1988; 137: 1264–1267.
15. Montaner JS, Russell JA, Lawson L, Ruedy J. Acute respiratory failure secondary to *Pneumocystis carinii* pneumonia in the acquired immunodeficiency syndrome: a potential role for systemic corticosteroids. *Chest* 1989; 95: 881–884.
16. Friedman Y, Franklin C, Rackow EC, Weil MH. Improved survival in patients with acquired immunodeficiency syndrome, *Pneumocystis carinii* pneumonia, and severe respiratory failure. *Chest* 1989; 96: 862–866.
17. Efferen LS, Nadarajah D, Palat DS. Survival following mechanical ventilation for

Pneumocystis carinii pneumonia in patients with the acquired immunodeficiency syndrome: a different perspective. *Am J Med* 1989; 87: 401–404.
18. Bozzette SA, Feigal D, Chiu J *et al.* Length of stay and survival after intensive care for severe *Pneumocystis carinii* pneumonia: a prospective study. California Collaborative Treatment Group. *Chest* 1992; 101: 1404–1406.
19. Gachot B, Clair B, Wolff M *et al.* Continuous positive airway pressure by face mask or mechanical ventilation in patients with human immunodeficiency virus infection and severe *Pneumocystis carinii* pneumonia. *Intensive Care Med* 1992; 18: 155–159.
20. Montaner JS, Hawley PH, Ronco JJ *et al.* Multisystem organ failure predicts mortality of ICU patients with acute respiratory failure secondary to AIDS-related PCP. *Chest* 1992; 102: 1823–1828.
21. Peruzzi WT, Skoutelis A, Shapiro BA *et al.* Intensive care unit patients with acquired immunodeficiency syndrome and *Pneumocystis carinii* pneumonia: suggested predictors of hospital outcome. *Crit Care Med* 1991; 19: 892–900.
22. Tucker KJ, Anton B, Tucker HJ. The effect of human immunodeficiency virus infection on the distribution and outcome of pneumonia in intensive care units. *West J Med* 1992; 157: 637–640.
23. Staikowsky F, Lafon B, Guidet B *et al.* Mechanical ventilation for *Pneumocystis carinii* pneumonia in patients with the acquired immunodeficiency syndrome: is the prognosis really improved? *Chest* 1993; 104: 756–762.
24. Hawley PH, Ronco JJ, Guillemi SA *et al.* Decreasing frequency but worsening mortality of acute respiratory failure (ARF) secondary to AIDS-related *Pneumocystis carinii* pneumonia. *Chest* 1994; 106: 1456–1459.
25. Schneiderman LJ, Jecker NS, Jonsen AR. Medical futility: its meaning and ethical implications. *Ann Intern Med* 1990; 112: 949–954.

16

Vaccine Strategies for HIV Infection

Barton F. Haynes

Duke University Arthritis Center and the Duke University Center for AIDS Research, Duke University Medical Center, Durham, North Carolina, USA

INTRODUCTION

Human immunodeficiency virus (HIV) vaccine development is at a crossroads due to new insights into the complex nature of HIV-host interactions[1]. New data have demonstrated that HIV mutates into variant quasispecies at an alarming rate[2], and that the correlates of immunity of HIV are not simple, but rather are a complex interaction of viral, immune and genetic factors[3]. Moreover, it has become apparent that envelope neutralizing determinants on monomeric recombinant (r) gp120 as well as on HIV grown in laboratory T-cell lines do not reflect neutralizing determinants found on HIV primary isolates grown in peripheral blood mononuclear cells[4]. Thus, large-scale National Institutes of Health (NIH)-sponsored efficacy trials of rgp120 of envelope of two prototype laboratory strains, HIVMN and HIVSF2, were not pursued because anti-HIV antibodies induced in phase I and phase II trials of these immunogens did not induce antibodies that neutralized HIV primary isolates grown in peripheral blood mononuclear cells (PBMC), and did not induce anti-HIV cytotoxic T-lymphocyte (CTL) responses[4,5].

Prospective analysis of cohorts of subjects at risk for HIV infection have demonstrated that there is spectrum of clinical courses of HIV infection, ranging from rapid loss of $CD4^+$ cells and progression to AIDS within the first three years of infection (rapid progressors), to stable $CD4^+$ cell levels as long as 10–12 years after infection (non-progressors)[6,7]. Since initial approaches to

AIDS and Malignancies: Current Concepts and Perspectives.

HIV vaccine development have not resulted in vaccine candidates that would be predicted to be efficacious[2], HIV vaccine developers are spending considerable efforts on the study of rapid progressors to acquired immunodeficiency syndrome (AIDS) (RP) as well as non-progressors to AIDS (NP) in order to understand the correlates of protective immunity to HIV. If it can be understood how the immune system controls HIV, then the rational design of an effective preventive HIV immunogen would be possible. This chapter summarizes some of the complexities of HIV–host interactions, and briefly discusses select aspects of future HIV vaccine development research goals and strategies.

HIV QUASISPECIES VARIATION IS A MAJOR PROBLEM FOR HIV VACCINE DEVELOPMENT

Recent estimates of HIV diversity have suggested that original estimates of HIV quasispecies present in infected individuals were underestimated. Taking the entire HIV genome into consideration, Wain-Hobson has estimated that in any infected patient there may be from 10^5 to 10^6 HIV variants present[2]. In a recent analysis of the HIV third variable (V3) loop of gp120 (a key target for anti-HIV neutralizing antibodies on laboratory-adapted HIV strains grown in PBMC), there were 147 variants when only the eight amino acids in the V3 loop were taken into account[8]. A vaccine strategy targeted at variable regions of HIV proteins, regardless of whether the strategy is targeted at inducing anti-HIV neutralizing antibodies, anti-HIV T-helper cell responses, or anti-HIV CTL responses, must take into account the extraordinary level of HIV sequence variability, the speed at which HIV mutates, and the potential problem of HIV epitope primer-induced suppression of immune responses.

Kilbourne *et al.* have described a form of primer-induced antibody suppression termed 'original antigenic sin', whereby boosting humans with a second influenza immunogen after priming with a first led to boosting the antibody response to the priming immunogen while interfering with production of antibody to the boosting immunogen[9–11]. A second type of primer-induced antibody suppression of HIV antibody has been described whereby priming with gp120 immunogens of certain HIV isolates suppressed subsequent antibody responses to other HIV isolates [12,13]. Primer-induced antibody suppression phenomena have been shown to occur in humans sequentially immunized with multiple forms of gp120[14], and been postulated in HIV infection to limit the long-term effectiveness of neutralizing antibody responses over time[15]. A recent study of comparison of sequential administration of HIV immunogens versus simultaneous administration of a multivalent immunogen demonstrated that both forms of primer-induced immune suppression could be abrogated by administration of the multivalent immunogen together as a mixture[12].

Not only is HIV variation extensive, but analysis of HIV variants in adjacent areas of spleen[16] and skin[17] showed that HIV quasispecies vary in the same individual in different locations in these tissues. Therefore, the variants seen in the blood may or may not reflect HIV variants in tissues, and variants in one tissue, and even one location in one tissue, may not reflect variants in other tissues, or in other locations in the same tissue. Thus, vaccine developers are beginning to study ways to present near-infinite variants of neutralizing determinants and CTL epitopes as an HIV immunogen, and at the same time to search for widely conserved HIV epitopes for use in immunogens.

TARGETING THE TRANSMITTED HIV VARIANT IS KEY FOR HIV VACCINE DEVELOPMENT

Some HIV variants preferentially infect monocytes and PB mononuclear cells *in vitro* and are termed *monocytotropic*, while other variants preferentially infect T-cell lines, and are termed *T-cell tropic*[18] (Table 16.1). Monocytotropic (MT) and T-cell tropic HIV variants vary in replication rate, and vary in ability to induce syncytia in certain cell types[18]. Recent data have demonstrated that the virus types transmitted by sexual contact and from HIV-infected mothers to newborns are usually monocytotropic (MT), non-syncytium inducing (NSI), slowly replicating HIV variants[19,20]. There appears to be a selection mechanism for MT, NSI variants at genital mucosal surfaces and at the mother–fetus interface[19,21]. These data, together with data that most HIV spread of infection *in vivo* is via infected cells, have suggested to HIV vaccine developers that the appropriate target of immune responses induced by HIV vaccines is the transmitted virus, i.e. MT, NSI HIV in infected monocyte/macrophages and PB T-cells[3].

THE HIV gp120 ENVELOPE V3 LOOP AND THE gp120 CD4 BINDING SITE ARE WEAKLY EXPRESSED ON HIV PRIMARY ISOLATES

The HIV gp120 V3 loop and the gp120-CD4 binding site have been the two major targets of prototypic vaccine candidates for induction of neutralizing antibodies until recently, when it was found that neither of these antibody specificities neutralized HIV primary isolates grown *in vitro* in PBMC[4]. Most neutralization assays have been performed using HIV grown in laboratory T-cell lines, and these cell types have small amounts of monomeric gp120 that

Table 16.1 Characterization of monocytotropic versus T-cell tropic HIV isolates

Monocytotropic	T-cell tropic
Replicate slowly	Replicate rapidly
Non-syncytium inducing	Syncytium inducing
Usually transmitted in infection	Rarely transmitted in infection
Frequently isolated in primary HIV infection	Frequently isolated in late stages of HIV infection
Frequently isolated from CNS	Rarely isolated from CNS

Data from references reviewed in references 1 and 3.

are easily bound by anti-V3 and anti-CD4 binding site neutralizing antibodies[22,23]. In contrast, gp120 on HIV primary isolates grown in PBMC is oligomeric, and both the V3 loop and CD4 binding site are in such a conformation as to be largely inaccessible to antibodies induced by monomeric gp120 or other gp120 subunit immunogens[22,23]. Thus, conformational and other neutralizing determinants on the surface of HIV primary isolates grown in PB mononuclear cells are now being avidly sought in order to determine appropriate targets for neutralizing antibodies that will prevent the infectivity of a wide spectrum of HIV MT and T-cell tropic HIV primary isolates (Table 16.2).

GENETIC, IMMUNE AND VIRAL FACTORS THAT DETERMINE THE CLINICAL COURSE OF HIV INFECTION

A major stumbling block in the development of a successful HIV vaccine has been the lack of knowledge of the correlates of protective immunity to HIV[1]. Indeed, there is debate regarding whether there are *any* correlates of protective immunity to HIV, with the concern that all HIV-infected patients will eventually develop AIDS[6].

Table 16.3 shows some of the immunological virological and genetic factors that have been associated with either rapid progression (RP) to AIDS or non-progression (NP) to AIDS[3]. While the full answer is not yet known, the picture is emerging that there is no single or simple correlates of protective immunity to HIV. Rather, salutary anti-HIV immune responses that limit HIV replication after primary HIV infection in *usual progressors* to AIDS (those that progress to AIDS within 7–10 years of infection) likely eventually also participate in immune-mediated damage to immune generative microenvironments and synergize with several HIV-mediated pathological processes (apoptosis, T-cell anergy, direct $CD4^+$ killing) that lead to $CD4^+$ immune cell loss and profound immune deficiency[3]. In general, RP to AIDS have low levels of neutralizing antibody responses, have homogenous HIV quasi-

Table 16.2 Targets of neutralizing antibodies on HIV envelope proteins

Epitope	T-cell lines	Accessible on HIV grown in PB mononuclear cells	References
gp120 V3 loop	Yes	Weakly	22,23
gp120-CD4 binding site	Yes	Weakly	22,23
V2 neutralizing epitope	Yes	Unknown	27
gp41	Yes	Yes	28
Mab A32-defined conformational determinant on gp120	Yes	Yes	23

Table 16.3 Immunological, virological, and genetic characteristics of rapid progressors and non-progressors to AIDS

Characteristic	Rapid progressors	non-progressors
Immunological	Rapid loss of CD4+ cells	Stable CD4+ cells
	High level of polyclonal immune activation	Low level of polyclonal immune activation
	Anti-HIV CTL low levels	Anti-HIV CTL high levels
	Low levels of anti-HIV neutralizing antibodies	High levels of anti-HIV neutralizing antibodies
	High levels of enhancing antibodies	Low levels of enhancing antibodies
	Progressive destruction of LN germinal centers	No destruction of LN germinal centers
Virological	High viral load	Low viral load
	Few HIV variants	Many HIV variants
	T cell tropic, SI rapidly replicating variants	MT, NSI, slowly replicating HIV variants
Genetic	Usually have MHC genes that predispose to RP	Usually do not have MHC genes that predispose to RP
	Usually do not have protective MHC genes	Usually have protective MHC genes

Data summarized from reference 18 and from references cited in reference 3.

species, and frequently have major histocompatibility complex (MHC)-encoded genes that predispose to RP to AIDS coupled with lack of protective MHC alleles[3,24,25]. RP to AIDS may also have lower levels of CTL against HIV-infected cells. In contrast, NP to AIDS have higher levels of anti-HIV immune responses than RP, slower replicating HIV variants, heterogeneous

HIV variants, do not have MHC-encoded genes that predispose to AIDS, and do have protective MHC alleles[3,24,25]. Taken together, data are emerging that a complex interaction of immune, genetic and viral factors converge in each patient to determine the precise clinical manifestations and clinical course of HIV infection. The MHC background of the host likely determines the quantity of the immune responses made (the intensity of antibody and CTL responses and the epitopes recognized) as well as the quality of immune responses (i.e. whether *salutary* or *pathogenic* or both types of immune responses are made)[3,24–26]. Thus, the concept is emerging that to make a successful HIV vaccine the nature of the interactions of host genetic, immune, and viral factors in HIV infection need to be understood, in order to design an immunogen that has the capacity to induce only salutary long-lived anti-HIV immune responses.

SUMMARY AND FUTURE RESEARCH DIRECTIONS

While there are many scientific problems ahead in the quest for a successful HIV preventive vaccine, basic and clinical investigative work is underway that will lead to insights into the pathogenesis of HIV infection, and hopefully will lead to insights into design of strategies to both prevent and treat HIV infection. Specifically, it is critical to continue to study the genetic, virological and immunological determinants of HIV-positive RP and NP. In addition, understanding the nature of gp120–gp41 interactions on HIV primary isolates, determining the host cells that are involved in HIV transmission in blood and at genital surfaces, determining the role that CTL versus neutralizing antibodies play in salutary and pathological anti-HIV immune responses, and determining the structures of conserved conformational determinants of HIV envelope on primary isolates that can serve as targets for broadly neutralizing antibodies are all current HIV vaccine development research goals.

ACKNOWLEDGEMENT

This work was supported by NIH grants AI28662, 2PO1-CA43447, U01-AI35351 and DAMD17-94-J-4467.

REFERENCES

1. Haynes BF. The scientific and social issues of HIV vaccine development. *Science* 1993; 260: 1279–1286.
2. Wain-Hobson S. Is antigenic variation of HIV important for AIDS and what might

be expected in the future? In Morse SSB (ed.) *The Evolutionary Biology of Retroviruses*. New York: Raven Press, 1994; pp. 185–209.
3. Haynes BF, Fauci AS. Towards an understanding of the correlates of protection immunity to HIV. *Science* 1996; 271: 324–328.
4. Matthews TJ. Tenth anniversary perspectives on AIDS: Dilemma of neutralization resistance of HIV-1 field isolates and vaccine development. *AIDS Res Hum Retroviruses* 1994; 10: 631.
5. Graham BS, Matthews TJ, Belshe RB *et al.* and NIAID AIDS Vaccine Clinical Trials Network. Augmentation of human immunodeficiency virus type 1 neutralizing antibody by priming with gp160 recombinant vaccinia and boosting with rgp160 in vaccinia-naive adults. *J Infect Dis* 1993; 167: 533–537.
6. Sheppard HW, Ascher MS, McRae B *et al.* The initial immune response to HIV and immune system activation determine the outcome of HIV disease. *J AIDS* 1991; 4: 704.
7. Phair JP. Variations in the natural history of HIV infection. *AIDS* 1994; 10: 883–885.
8. Korber B, Wolinsky S, Haynes B *et al.* HIV-1 intrapatient sequence diversity in the immunogenic V3 region. *AIDS Res Hum Retroviruses* 1992; 8: 1461–1465.
9. Kilbourne ED. Comparative efficacy of neuraminidase-specific and conventional influenza virus vaccines in induction of antibody to neuraminidase in human. *J Infect Dis* 1976; 134: 384–394.
10. Kilbourne ED, Cereni CP, Khan MW *et al.* Immunologic response to the influenza virus neuraminidase is influenced by prior experience with the associated viral hemagglutinin. I. Studies in human vaccine. *J Immunol* 1987; 138: 3010–3013.
11. Johanssan BE, Moran TM, Bona CA *et al.* Immunologic response to influenza virus neuraminidase is influenced by prior experience with the associated viral hemagglutinin. II. Sequential infection of mice stimulates human experience. *J Immunol* 1987; 139: 2010–2014.
12. Haynes BF, Moody MA, Heinley CS *et al.* HIV type 1 V3 region primer-induced antibody suppression is overcome by administration of C4-V3 peptides as a polyvalent immunogen. *AIDS Res Hum Retroviruses* 1995; 11: 211–221.
13. Klinman DM, Higgins KW, Conover J. Sequential immunization with rgp120s from independent isolates of human immunodeficiency virus type 1 induce the preferential expansion of broadly cross-reactive B cells. *J Exp Med* 1991; 173: 881–887.
14. Schwartz D, Clements ML, Belshe R *et al.* and NIAID AIDS Vaccine Evaluation Group. Antibody responses to neutralizing domains of gp120 in HIV(–) vaccines boosted with homologous or heterologous rgp120. *IXth International Conference on AIDS*, Berlin (PO-A29-0690), 1993.
15. Kohler H, Goudsmit J, Nara P. Clonal dominance cause: for a limited and failing immune response to HIV-1 infection and vaccination. *J AIDS* 1992; 5: 1158–1168.
16. Cheynier R, Henrichwark S, Hadida F *et al.* HIV and T-cell expansion in splenic white pulps is accompanied by infiltration of HIV-specific cytotoxic T lymphocytes. *Cell* 1994; 78: 373–387.
17. Sala M, Zambruno G, Vartanian JP *et al.* Spatial discontinuities in human immunodeficiency virus type 1 quasispecies derived from epidermal Langerhans cells of a patient with AIDS and evidence for double infection. *J Virol* 1994; 68: 5280–5283.
18. Schuitmaker H. Macrophage-tropic HIV-1 variants: initiators of infection and AIDS pathogenesis. *J Leuko Biol* 1994; 56: 218.
19. Wolinsky SM, Wike CM, Korber BT *et al.* Selective transmission of human immunodeficiency type-1 variants from mothers to infants. *Science* 1992; 255: 1134.

20. Zhu T, Mo T, Wing N *et al.* Genotypic and phenotypic characterization of HIV-1 in patients with primary infection. *Science* 1993; 261: 1179.
21. Pauza D, Trivedi P, Meyer KK *et al.* Selection of SIV during transmission across the mucosal barrier. *AIDS Res Hum Retroviruses* 1994; 10: 585.
22. O'Brien WA, Mao S-H, Cao Y, Moore JP. Macrophage-tropic and T cell line adapted chimeric strains of human immunodeficiency virus type-1 differ in their susceptibilities to neutralization by soluble CD4 at different temperatures. *J. Virol* 1994; 68: 5264.
23. Liao H-X, Jones DM, Robinson JE *et al.* Passage of HIVIIIB/LAI in activated peripheral blood mononuclear cells leads to decreased expression of multiple HIV neutralizing determinants on HIV-infected cells (Abstract). *NCVDG Meeting*, 4–7 November 1994.
24. Kaslow R. Presented at NIAID Workshop on HIV/SIV Pathogenesis and Mucosal Transmission, Washington, DC, 14–17 March 1994; Kaslow R, Mann D. *J Infect Dis* 1994; 169: 1332.
25. Saah A. Presented at the National Academy of Science, Institutes of Medicine Roundtable For the Development of Drugs and Vaccines Against AIDS, 10 December 1993.
26. Haynes BF. Immune responses to HIV. In DeVita VT, Hellman S, Rosenberg SA (eds) *AIDS, Etiology, Diagnosis, Treatment, and Prevention.* Philadelphia: Lippincott, 1992; pp. 77–86.
27. Pincus S, Messer KG, Nara PL *et al.* Temporal analysis of the antibody response to HIV envelope protein in HIV-infected laboratory workers. *J Clin Invest* 1994; 93: 2505.
28. Conley AJ, Kessler JA, Boots LJ *et al.* Neutralization of divergent human immunodeficiency virus type-1 variants and primary isolates by IAM-41-2F5, an anti-gp41 human monoclonal antibody. *Proc Natl Acad Sci USA* 1994; 91: 3348.

Index

Index compiled by A.C. Purton